MICHAEL'S WOMEN

Love Stories of a Dreamer

A Novel by

PETER LYNN

ISBN: 1-4107-1474-8 (e-book)
ISBN: 1-4107-1475-6 (Paperback)

This book is printed on acid free paper.

Published by 1stBooks Library, 2003

Originally published by Rampant Horse Ltd.

Typeset and Designed by Harold Martin & Redman Ltd

1stBooks - rev. 08/26/03

For Hildegard and Roxane

"Woman, in the picture language of mythology, represents the totality of what can be known. The hero is the one who comes to know… She lures, she guides, she bids him burst his fetters. And if he can match her import, the two, the knower and the known, will be released from every limitation. Woman is the guide to the sublime acme of sensuous adventure. By deficient eyes she is reduced to inferior states; by the evil eye of ignorance she is spellbound to banality and ugliness. But she is redeemed by the eyes of understanding. The hero who can take her as she is, without undue commotion but with the kindness and assurance she requires, is potentially the king, the incarnate god, of her created world."

Joseph Campbell, *The Hero with a Thousand Faces*.

PREFACE

My name is Michael. It is the third of the four names my father thought I should have, all recorded on my birth certificate. Untouched for decades, the original parchment is brittle, awaiting crumbling decay, archival sleep, in the dreamless sacristy of a church in Vienna. A piece of paper, really, merely registering a new life, mine to live.

I do not know if there was a previous Michael in my family, but my father, a Jewish convert to Catholicism, wanted to cover all bases; since he had affection for all things Irish, Michael had to be one of his son's names. My mother could not be consulted in this matter: she had died while giving me the dubious opportunity to make my way onto this planet.

I am long past middle age. My life has been colorful, adventurous, and modestly fulfilling. True, I would have preferred to be given the vocal cords of a great tenor, or be renowned as a physician who discovered the secret of malignant cells, eliminating all cancers. As it was, I became a healer of souls, and several hundred people are grateful that I enriched their lives. But my richness is in my dreams, which my training as a healer has taught me to interpret, adding understanding to what I know about myself consciously. They are powerful dreams, and always of women: women as lovers; as friends; as casual affairs;

as Goddesses who have captured my heart, broken it through betrayal, or cherished it; and through them I have been reborn many times over.

Sometimes the line between my dreams and reality is blurred. When that happens, I go out and seek my dream on the street, in the park, on an aeroplane, or in the personal ads of a magazine. The latter is always a delicious challenge: will my dream be found in the copy written by a woman who is seeking me, or must I provide the copy to which my dream will reply? The namesake of my city, New York, is the magazine of choice where dreams intersect, match or collide; unpredictable effects of a mysterious cause.

Some time ago, my dreams presented me with the stories of eight women to whom my love has flowed, at different times and in diverse ways; from the first love of my teens, to the grand transformations of my ageing self. In the dreams, my life with these women is not merely a recapturing, a memoir of actual events: in the nocturnal world of unconscious sleep, there are corrections for past mistakes; compensations for attitudes too narrow or too broad; or dangerous cliffs on which my love has foundered, but can still be redeemed as the treasure hard to attain.

The first dream which had me in its grip is the one which reopened the story of Christina. I was to learn then about the power of the unconscious; that bottomless shadowy part of the mind; a lesson I was never to forget again. I remember the dream lingered for days, pulling at my consciousness, making me feel both blissfully transported and terrified. Though the dark portents of political events about to happen were on display everywhere, I could not grasp their personal relevance. I was blind to the pair of opposites the dream had presented – the joy and the fear.

CHRISTINA

The gurgling of water is loud and insistent. The image before my eyes is of a large bluish pool. Sculpted nymphs of many fountains spout sulphurous liquid, refilling the pool with healing thermal water, its smell strong but not unpleasant. I recognize Baden, a spa famous since Roman times, nestled in a valley close to the Vienna woods. I stand at the pool's edge, and swimming towards me is the first, moon-embracing love of my life, Christina. Tall, with blond curls cascading to her shoulders, she is the archetype of Schnitzler's sweet Viennese girl. A blue bathing suit shows off her full figure, high breasts, never-ending legs. Sleek and wet, she steps out of the pool. We kiss with the tremulous passion only first love can awaken: shy, with a fearful intimacy, fragile and seemingly unbreakable at the same time. I cannot let go of her, we tumble into the sand, and create an indecent spectacle for the elderly nannies who are fully dressed on this summer day as they care for their charges, knitting furiously.

Suddenly, our tumble in the sand becomes a nightmare. We roll over and over; the sky is dark, the pool gone, the sand a sticky mess, yet our rolling momentum is not slowed. There is a macabre rhythm to it, curiously in ¾ time. On and on we roll; I hear the Emperor waltz pushing us forward, and now I see a burning castle, Valhalla is burning, and still we roll; a cliff is ahead and we tumble over it, falling, helplessly clamped down by a huge Swastika flag which is being tightened, choking us.

The year was 1937, and I had been in love with Christina for an entire year. Courting her without letup after we'd met in Mlle. Bourdeau's private French class, I used to send a ceaseless flow of letters, poems and flowers to the spa town where she lived, half an hour south of Vienna. Two or three times a week she came to the city, visiting friends and taking French lessons. We were both eighteen.

I was not Christina's only admirer. An entire movie company was after her. Not for her acting experience, but merely for her incredible looks, a budding Austrian film outfit had signed her for a walk-on part in a comedy called, *Music for You,* and she reported daily to the studio. George, my chief rival for her affection, and I kept hanging around the set. California had its leggy surfgirls, Budapest its dark gypsy types, but only Vienna could boast of Christina's blond sweetness. I would proclaim this to my father – who was impressed with my good taste-, to my friends, and anyone else willing to listen to the praise that emanated from someone who was sick with love.

But Christina was a virgin, and though I had long ago been granted the greatest favor she was willing to bestow, kissing, she had firmly drawn the line at being touched anywhere below the neck. So sleeping with Christina was relegated to the far horizon of my shimmering fantasies. Still, I was content that along with hated George I was evidently at the top of the crowd that was pursuing her.

My happiness reached dizzying heights when Christina implied at Christmas, a holiday kissing feast, that I was the one who truly mattered to her. However, I was soon to learn a very different meaning of "dizzying heights."

There was one area in Christina's life from which I was barred. She was a superb ballroom dancer and had been chosen, along with other Viennese beauties, to partake in the great entrance waltz which opened Vienna's famous opera ball. By woeful contrast, I was a total zero on the dance floor. But being in love with Christina had caused me to enroll in Frau Hollreiser's dance school, where I took private lessons from Fraeulein Cissy. An attractive brunette, she succeeded in teaching me the fox-trot and the slow-fox. But when it came to moving in ¾ time, I developed a frightening dizziness, especially when the tempo speeded up, as it does in the famous "Linkswalzer"; left turns only, and absolutely *de rigeur* in Vienna. Only an instant cessation of all movement would prevent a dead faint. Cissy was baffled by this phenomenon, but try as she might, her efforts were in vain.

In desperation, I sought medical help from my father's friend, Professor Hirschhorn, who held the prestigious chair of neurology at the university. The famous man promised discretion, but concluded after a lengthy examination that I had some inner ear trouble for which there was no remedy. He predicted that if I stood at a high place like the aerie of St. Stephen's cathedral, I would be unable to look down to street level without experiencing the same symptom. He was right.

I was crushed. After wrestling with my anxiety, I decided to confide in Christina, hoping that in matters of true love, not being able to dance the waltz could be seen as a minor inconvenience. Christina made light of my despair. She said I should just practice some more, and if I wanted, she herself would teach me. This was a delicious proposal but fraught with even greater anxiety. After all, my young ego would be exposed to the potential humiliation of fainting in the arms of the woman I hoped to conquer. Eventually I gave in.

The tutoring was a total failure. I did not faint, but neither could I keep up the circling motions without getting dizzy. Still, the sensation of holding Christina in my arms, or more accurately, being held by her, was so enchanting that I hit upon a trick which turned my embarrassment to advantage. Once we started the damned turns and my dizziness increased along with the tempo of the accursed Emperor waltz, I would pull Christina down onto the nearby couch, showering her with kisses and admitting defeat on the waltz thing. I vowed that my love for her was on such a lofty level that it reduced waltzing to something pedestrian and insignificant. Surprisingly, the waltz kings, Strauss father and son, now became accomplices in my amorous strivings. For Christina reacted to my frustration on the dance floor by consoling me; somehow this opened her deeper feelings, and my desire to make love to her was met with a noticeably weaker "no."

I remembered a Russian saying: pity is the beginning of true love.

One afternoon in mid-January I took the train to her spa. Christina met me at the station, and we walked for several hours in the vast park ringing the hilly town. After reaching the highest level where a statue of Beethoven overlooked the surrounding vineyards, now covered with a dusting of snow, we gradually descended on serpentine paths to the center of town. At every bench provided by the tourist office we stopped in a kissing embrace, talking sweet, foolish stuff, and planning a dinner in one of the cavernous wine taverns. It was at such a bench that Christina, moved by my amorous pleas, at last consented to spend a night with me. She made me swear not to make her pregnant, and never was an oath more joyfully delivered. I was on my knees, worshipfully, until she raised me up and we sealed the oath with a kiss that was lost in time.

I was beside myself, filled with starlight and music, and the rest of the evening became cloudy, enveloped in a magical haze. We drank too much of the tart local wine, and it wasn't easy to get Christina home. The front door of her house was locked, and she had to climb over a fence, ripping the silk stockings I had brought along as a present. She reported the next day that her stepfather, a local doctor (and as it turned out a prominent underground Nazi), had forbidden her to see me again.

"But I'll keep my promise," Christina said, "because I love you too much to deny you, and of course we'll go on seeing each other, especially after you know what…" And she blushed.

A few days later, reality outshone all fantasy as I was bidden to lift the veil from the goddess. And gazed, awed, at the flawless creamy skin revealed before my half-blinded eyes. The sensation was so exquisite, so arresting in its shocking beauty that I was struck mute. It was an epiphany. It happened in a small hotel in Vienna's fourth district, on the night of my nineteenth birthday. With tears in her limpid blue eyes, her golden hair on a crested pillow, Christina surrendered to me her virginity. Like the romantic opera fans we were, we enacted the final scene of Richard Strauss' "Arabella". From the same glass we drank freshly drawn water, then smashed the fine crystal goblet I had provided so no one else would ever taste the fountain of our love.

Less than a month later, in March of 1938, a triumphant Hitler occupied Vienna, and I learned of my Jewish ancestry, kept secret by my father who'd raised me a Catholic. Crushed in my identity, I was suddenly confronted with issues of morals and loyalties, a fragmented mind trapped in sinister darkness. My heart was torn from me as I divulged the news to Christina. We sat in our favorite coffee house, and I looked in confusion at the shiny Swastika button pinned to the dark blue jacket of her elegant suit. We struggled to understand that this was reality, the end of our love. And blindingly aware now, the terrifying ending of my dream had become the far greater terror of a brutally ripped bond.

Over the next three months, Christina visited me in secret at my house; there was much shared pain, but she was already under the collective spell of the thousand-year Reich. The three or four times we'd made love since my birthday were talked about with sadness and longing, but events had torn us apart. When I flew to Italy in mid-June, Christina swore she'd come and visit me in the fall.

The oath was false. Seven years went by until I, now an American Officer, saw her again at Christmas in the rubble that was Vienna. She wanted to marry me then, but the Danube was no longer blue, and "Arabella" no longer in the repertory.

Peter Lynn

MARCELLA

There is much noise: hissing, and short blasts of a whistle. Smoke, too, reaches my senses. Coal burns. Gradually, my vision clears. I am at the Stazione Termini in Venice, the end of the line for all trains. I see steam engines, huge and monstrous, connected to arriving and departing trains. They account for the hissing, and there is a conductor blowing his whistle, authorizing our departure. Our train, on platform fourteen, is preparing to leave. Signs on its cars say Ferrara, Bologna, Firenze, Roma Termini. The conductor is slamming doors shut; he is raising the red signal baton in his hand, the whistle clamped between his lips. There's Marcella, a white frock dancing around her legs; she is waving madly, and with seconds to spare we climb aboard the same car. We are in a second class car, secondo classe; the seats are wooden and bard, but our embrace, laced with juicy kisses, could not be softer. The giant hands of the illuminated clock in the rapidly vanishing station stand at midnight.

The train crosses the long trestle bridge to Mestre. Marcella is asleep now, her bead on my shoulder, legs tucked under the white skirt. Her shoes have fallen off; they peek out from under our seats. Suddenly, we're in Pescia, a small town famous for its carnations. A flower market is in progress, fragrances waft through my dream, and an old woman, grandmotherly, drives by on her mule-drawn cart.

We go to her farm where it is spring or summer. We are in a rustic room now, with a wide bed and plump pillows. Lambs and goats wander outside our window, and the smells of the woman's cooking seeps through the ancient floor boards. I shake Marcella awake to greet the morning. We go downstairs where tbere's fresh bread and coffee, soft cheese, and we walk out into a meadow of blossoming apple trees: I want terribly to marry Marcella, and she says, "Yes, yes, my darling, I'll marry you", but she dances away toward a cherry tree, all pink like the skirt she's now wearing, and I slide down into the soft grass, looking up into the improbably blue sky...

I was nineteen years old and Marcella, who was thirty, had three small children and a husband fighting Mussolini's war in Abyssinia, had promised to elope with me. We had known each other for six months, living in Padova in the same house. I'd been dispatched to this Italian city by my father who was waiting in Nazi-occupied Vienna for his exit visa, expecting to join me in Italy.

I remember the night in Marcella's apartment when we hatched the details of our getaway. The whole thing had been Marcella's idea: to go away to Tuscany for a week. Her kids were taken care of by a friend, and never mind the gossip in the building where everybody was thinking of her as a tramp anyway because she had taken up with a handsome boy from Vienna. In the overripe romantic joy of being in love with an older woman, I'd thought of it as an elopement. I was homeless anyway, with no plans for a future I didn't want to think about, so a village in Tuscany, with the Maggio Musicale in Firenze in full swing, felt like paradise. And with Marcella, celibate since her husband had gone to war two years ago, finding herself obsessed with my youthful sexual capacity, what more could I hope for?

It was Marcella who introduced me to oral sex, an art form I had not yet experienced in Vienna. She was terrified of getting pregnant. "I would immediately acquire a fourth child," she would say whenever I wanted to make love to her the way I had been taught in Vienna. In fact, she would not permit my erect penis anywhere near her genitals, though she took its ever-present readiness as a great compliment. Having once seen sperm under a microscope, she thought these wriggly things could fly; that they were entirely unpredictable in their behavior, and, who could be sure by what means these creatures could get inside her? In the early days of our lovemaking she had confided to me her ignorance as a bride. She did not understand how she got pregnant three times in quick succession. Another quirky thing was her determination not ever to let me see her naked above the waist. "I have baby milk," she'd say, and I had a hunch she was still nursing her two year old son. But oral sex was Marcella's heaven. Mind you, I'm talking of having been the giver, not the receiver, Reversal of this pattern would only occur upon my urgent request, and even then she preferred her hand while I was yearning for her mouth.

Still, who was I to complain? Her very insatiability made me feel eminently desirable, irreplaceable in fact, as she never tired of assuring me after I had loved her the way she wanted to be loved. "But where have you learned how to caress a woman?", she often wanted to know. Michael, the great lover, would only smile mysteriously.

Language of course was the official version why Marcella and I were being seen together. My Italian was fluent, but, alas, in operatic terms only. While I could converse easily as Don Giovanni, or Rigoletto, Otello, or even as Lt. Benjamin Franklin Pinkerton, U.S. Navy, this peculiar talent was not suitable for attending the venerable medical school, the oldest in Europe, which I was supposed to frequent. Thus on instructions from my father in Vienna, my hosts, busy professionals, whose apartment I shared across the hall from Marcella's, were looking for someone competent to make me proficient in the vernacular. I don't doubt that in recruiting Marcella they were having frivolous fun. My friend Renzo, who was slightly older and lived two floors below, did his part by introducing me to the lush bordellos of the city: a terrifying experience for the man of the world I pretended to be. Renzo's gorgeous sister Laura, who was my age, did not think me worthy a second look, since a titled man called on her every evening in his red Lancia convertible. Their mother, Signora Augusta Antonini whose husband was rarely around, would now and then pull me aside, warning me about young matrons who behaved like hussies.

So it came to pass that I fell happily, proudly, madly in love with Marcella. She was tall and slender, had black hair and blue eyes, and usually wore black as a sign of grieving for her absent husband in Abyssinia. She also wore seamed silk stockings, held up by a black garter belt which would slip occasionally; then she would quickly yank them up – a gesture I found irresistibly sexy.

Still Renzo, the young man about town, persisted in acquainting me with the elegant houses where the world's oldest profession was practiced with discreet charm and high-fashion allure. Not far from the Cafe Pedrocchi, everyone's favorite hangout, stood the dark mansions to which Renzo, a regular visitor, would entice me several nights a week. And until my affair with Marcella took wing, I would put myself through the terrors of meeting these beautifully dressed women who knew the secrets of their ancient art. Concealing my anxiety by professing an interest in their personal lives, usually resulted in an early exit. The high priestess who collected money in scented envelopes would call for Renzo to please shepherd me out the door; I was causing a loss of trade. Calling down from the first floor balcony to the doorkeeper, "the gentlemen are leaving", she would admonish an exasperated Renzo to please not bring the strange young man along the next time.

Eventually, however, I did graduate, but only because of Elena.

These days, a scent of carnations arises occasionally from my pillow, intoxicatingly sweet, driftwood of memory. But unlike my dream image,

Marcella did not appear at the station in Venice, ready to elope. Years later however, I saw her again on Venice's Lido where I was vacationing with my wife and small daughter. Now in her fifties, she was still shapely and beautiful, standing by a cabana on the beach and wearing a black one-piece bathing suit. There was instant recognition in her eyes, but she turned away, and I really didn't want to know why she had broken her promise.

It was the second time in my young life that a woman I loved had left me.

Peter Lynn

ELENA

I had climbed to the top of a rock-strewn mountain. Three Greek-looking temples were spaced randomly among the shrubbery of this lonely plateau. I was Paris, a hero of the Trojan war, commanded to render an awesome judgement. The three supreme goddesses, Athena, Aphrodite and Hera, had chosen me to pronounce which one of them was the most beautiful. I felt proud but anxious, for I knew the task to be dangerous. In a stately procession, three women appeared, each taking her place in front of one of the temples. But they were not the goddesses I had expected. On my right stood Christina, my first love in Nazi Vienna; in the middle was an unknown woman who wore a silver robe on which the phases of the moon were embroidered: and on my left, relaxed and informally leaning against her temple, was a young woman whom I recognized as someone who worked at the elegant bordello I had visited so unsuccessfully several times. I knew her name was Elena.

I was urged to proceed with the judgement. I chose the one in the middle, and when I said so, the silver lady became Elena who now stood alone, facing me with a crooked little grin which I remembered was the way she looked in reality. She came toward me and kissed me.

My life in Padova was somewhat indolent. You wouldn't call it lethargic, really, but it was perfused with a kind of somnolent routine. I was in a low-grade depression, due no doubt to my uncertain future. Unaware when the next turn in the road would come and where it would lead, I was treading water. My hosts provided comfortable shelter and excellent meals, and for nocturnal amusement Marcella's apartment was a mere ten steps away. Dutifully, I had matriculated in the prestigious medical school, though my presence at lectures and in laboratories was at best sporadic. One day, in professor Battista's anatomy class, Moira, the goddess in charge of our destiny, decided things needed enlivening. She intervened.

"Ah, no, no. questo non è una clavicola! Lei ha studiato medicina a Vienna? E non vede la differenza fra una cavita articolare e un osso calcinoso?" Professor Mario Battista was furious. Not to know the difference between a collar bone and a calcified socket? And this young man had studied medicine in Vienna?

I said I was sorry and pleaded a prolonged *cattarale,* a cold, which had prevented my regular attendance. Seated a row above me in the huge aula, a young woman raised her hand, and very sweetly told the lecturer that she could verify my claim, and would be glad to tutor me until I'd caught up. Professor Battista was mollified, and chose to overlook the smirking faces of some of the other students.

My own face was crimson with embarrassment, for I had identified the young woman as one of the ladies who worked in Contessa Orsini's elegant mansion to which my friend Renzo had taken me on several occasions. Her name was Elena Manzoni. I'd been attracted to her, but had always asked for one of the older love priestesses from whom I could quickly flee under some phony pretext. As it happened, Elena had overheard two young love girls, Claudia and Rosetta, making fun of my shyness, and she didn't like it.

After Professor Battista dismissed his class, I wanted to thank Elena for supporting my fake story, but she had vanished. Eventually, I found her at the Bursar's office. *"Ma io pager6 il resto domani* – I'll pay the rest tomorrow," Elena was saying. I touched her shoulder and motioned her to a far corner. It turned out that she had a stipend, but owed some extra tuition for a lab course. I offered to help, but Elena would not hear of it. "Didn't you tell Professor Battista you were going to tutor me?" I demanded. And without waiting for her to argue, I pressed fiftythousand lire into her hand which felt warm and delicate. "This is for helping me with anatomy." We stared at each other until we started to giggle. Elena paid the Bursar, an elderly lady who had watched the transaction with evident suspicion, thin-lipped; her eyes followed us as we walked into the sunshine. We were headed for the Cafe Pedrocchi.

"I live in Venice with a dear aunt, *cara zia,* and I come to Padova only for classes, and three nights a week for the Contessa." Now Elena was blushing. We ordered espresso. Tongue-tied, I kept glancing at Elena. She wore a green sweater and a white skirt, I noted that her eyes were gray with an iridescent shimmer, and that her short hair was the shiniest black

I had ever seen. She was as tall as I, her face a little angular, and her figure very slim, almost boyish. The whole package was striking in a way no one would call beautiful, but it radiated a kind of erotic energy, which seemed at odds with her looks.

"Why don't you come with me to Venice? I'll stay with my aunt overnight; she has an extra room you can have, and I'll show you around."

Although I was quite familiar with the city, historically referred to as the Queen of the Adriatic, both from my earlier trips and my present stay in Padova, I accepted immediately. "I've been in love with Venice since I was six years old when my father took me to the Lido for the first time, but I've never been taken on a tour by a native."

"Oh, but I'm not from Venice," Elena exclaimed. "I was born in Bologna and I lived there until I was eighteen. My parents died in an automobile accident when I was fourteen. It's ten years ago, *son'un vecchio gatto.*" She smiled as she called herself an old cat, and I thought her smile defined her face even more sharply, and a little loopy, but I grinned at her and said, *"Sei bella cosi* – you're pretty as you are."

We took the train to Mestre, and boarded a *vaporetto* which chugged to the Giudecca, a very old part of Venice, where Zia Gilda lived in an ancient house. The lagoon lapped at its little front door from which three steps led into a dim hall, and another steep twenty to the apartment of Elena's aunt. *"Sa niente della Contessa,"* Elena whispered. I winked, indicating that her nocturnal doings were safe with me, then bowed to the overdressed woman who opened the door. She looked like Laura, the wife of a sixteenth-century Doge, Alvise Badoero. I happened to know the Tintoretto painting which features this Doge and the wife he's about to poison at a grand reception for a Venetian explorer returning from the Orient.

Gilda nodded to me and threw her arms around Elena. She looked ageless, and wore a dress that could have been copied from the very same painting. I commented on it.

Elena explained. "My aunt lives in the history of Venice; she and a group of ladies try to preserve the ancient traditions." Gilda remarked on my fluent Italian and offered espresso, but Elena said we'd go to San Marco, eat something and then return. "I like medical students," said Elena's aunt. "I have so many ailments and the *medici* are so helpful in telling me what I should not do." She cackled about her joke, and waved us off with a blessing.

Sipping Campari at the Piazza San Marco, Elena told me an unusual story. "I'm very serious about becoming a *dottoressa,* but I can only study part-time, so it will be another six or seven years before I finish. And then I want to specialize in psychiatry. I know many people go into that field because of their own problems, and I think I'm one of them. You see, I work at the Contessa not just for the money."

Elena hesitated, but I supposed that my relaxed face encouraged her to go on. "I have never told this to anyone, but I like you, Michele. I like your shyness when you come to the Contessa. It makes me think you adore women but want to respect them." I was ready to get embarrassed again but my curiosity was aroused.

"After my parents died, I lived with my mother's brother in Bologna, going to school as before. But then something happened that changed everything. I was fifteen, becoming a young woman with strong sexual feelings. My uncle who was in his forties and very good looking, seduced me. No, no, that's really the wrong way to say it: **I** was eager to learn about sex, we talked about it, and I was very willing to let him introduce me to the god." She smiled her loopy smile and said, "I mean the god Eros."

"I found I liked making love, so he was my lover for three years until I was eighteen when I entered medical school in Padova. I had some boyfriends, but nobody I was in love with. Still, I enjoyed sex more and more, and that's how I came to the Contessa. "*Finita la cantata,* "said Elena, quoting Tosca.

I had never heard such a story. No woman had ever talked to me about her most intimate life. And to hear this interesting woman, five years my senior, describe why she wanted to become a psychiatrist, to find out why she liked sex so much, was extraordinary.

I didn't know what to say. I looked across the piazza where a million stories were being enacted just beyond my range of vision, a stream of humanity in motion, weaving back and forth across one of the grandest spaces architects had ever designed. Elena was looking at me expecting a reaction. Unaccountably, I found myself close to tears, having no idea why I was so moved, but I reached for her hand, which held the Campari, and removed the glass. I put her now open palm over my eyes, partly to hide my emotion, but also to let her feel my closeness.

Elena broke the mood. Reclaiming her Campari, she smiled her crooked smile and said, "Maybe you misunderstood me, Michele. I don't obsess about sex – *non sono una nympha.* I just enjoy the feeling of a man desiring me, and unless he's repulsive or crude (and the Contessa knows not to send those to me), it makes me desire him too. And there is this wonderful feeling, *come si dice,* how do you say, of a union as if the goddess of love had come to me, and I respond to her presence with my whole body. Perhaps I'm just a pagan," she said wistfully.

I could only nod. I paid, and we walked down to the Rialto, not saying much, then doubled back to Santa Maria della Salute. Elena took my hand and led me into the Cathedral. I suddenly recalled my Catholic school days when attendance at Sunday mass was mandatory. On one such Sunday I had decided that looking at a pretty girl and thinking how she might look naked could not possibly be a sin. Then and there I had resolved not to confess such thoughts any longer. Elena crossed herself, and with the hand I had used to hide my tears, she touched my face with holy water. We knelt at a side altar dedicated to Mary Magdalen.

Elena said, "Do you remember the adulteress in the Bible whom Jesus blessed? I'm not like her, nor like the great whore of Babylon, but I feel my love for being with a man in a union is no sin, and Jesus would bless me too if he looked into my heart." She smiled mischievously. "Of course the old priests wouldn't understand; but there's a young one who sneaks to the Contessa to see me, and I always help him not to feel guilty."

It was dark and we were getting hungry. We shared my favorite dish, *Fegato alla Veneziana,* thin slices of calf's liver, sauteed, with lots of onions, then made our way slowly on foot and by boat back to the Giudecca. Elena had keys, but the apartment was empty; there was a note from Gilda, telling her not to wait up.

Looking at me with that peculiar grin I was beginning to find enchanting, Elena asked, "You want me to review the skeletal system for you?"

My mind was a jumble of gondolas, canals, and now suddenly the face of Professor Battista, the anatomy teacher, loomed before me. My onion-flavored tongue was stuck against my palate, impeding speech. What in the world was the matter with me? After all, I was a Viennese, able to converse in three languages, an intelligent young man who knew his music, his art and history, not to mention his love for Venice. Yet here I was in this old stone building, guided by Elena into a room dimly illuminated with electrified candles, which threw the shadowy outline of a massive bed against a whitewashed wall.

Suddenly Verdi's great choral outburst, the "Sanctus", sounded in my brain. "Are you related to the great poet for whom Verdi wrote his Requiem?"

Elena Manzoni shook her head. "I don't think so," she replied as tiny stars flickered in her gray eyes. She leaned her head against my shoulder. "If you would rather study the details of the female form, I wouldn't mind that at all." This, shyly, in a whisper close to my ear. "But I need to feel that you really desire me."

Given my age, my experience with women was not inconsiderable. I had deflowered Christina, my first great love, and had slept with two older women before that momentous occasion. Yet, here on the Giudecca, with this fascinating woman who studied *medicina* and worked three nights a week in the Contessa's elegant bordello, I felt like a little boy, confused about what might be expected of me.

Elena said, *"Buona Notte",* and left the room. I couldn't move. Dazed, I sat down on the bed, took off my shirt and trousers, and stretched out in my underwear on the silken coverlet. Daunted by the prospect of making love with so experienced a woman as Elena, I wrestled with my ambivalent feelings.

A small window, set high into the wall and covered with iron crossbars, revealed a sliver of the moon. I stared at its deep honey yellow until my eyes lost their focus and glazed over. I may have been in a kind of half-trance, but suddenly there were three women on the moon, lunar goddesses, and from them flowed an amber stream of carnal longing down to my throbbing tumescent self. A bolt of silvery sex shot from the moon, right through that tiny window, creating a surge of energy and confidence.

I leaped out of bed, stumbling through an unfamiliar corridor. There was a crack of light behind a door. Pushing it open, I literally fell into another bed in which the naked Elena was reading a physiology textbook. I didn't ponder the intrusion of the gods and the unveiling of the sacred in my daily life. Instead, I started kissing Elena, rapidly, as if she might vanish if I wasn't fast enough.

Elena stopped me, stroked my hair, and kissed me back, languidly. My tongue had become unglued, and in the course of the next couple of hours it was applied in different ways; words and caresses becoming interchangeable.

In hurried phrases, I told Elena my dream. I sensed that she took in my images as if they were her own, and softly caressing me she caused my desire to come rushing at me. Her own desire for me was palpable and it filled the small room like a perfumed mist which condensed into soft pink clouds. My need for her began to overwhelm me, and she pulled me into herself, her arms around my neck, holding fast. Trying to catch her breath, she murmured, "Please don't move." To me, she'd become a woodland nymph caught by the great god Pan. Surrendering to the ecstasy he promised, she inhaled my embrace as if it were a scent of herbs and flowers, and the kisses we exchanged tasted of golden honey. *"Michele, sei dolce miele, carino, ti desidero tanto!"*

I heard myself called sweet honey, and that she desired me very much, and I felt her moving beneath me in a rhythm of her own. Content to let this love goddess, who had changed from a dream to a woman on whose pillow lay a physiology textbook, I rode with her toward paradise.

Elena came very suddenly, trembling in great spasms, and I pulled out quickly. Still feeling the aftershocks of her *terremoto,* her earthquake, she bent down and drank my love as if it were the nectar of the gods. "Thank you for dreaming about me," she whispered. "Did you really judge me the most beautiful?"

"If you're not the love goddess herself, surely you serve at her altar," I breathed back. "And I worshipped there tonight."

In the morning, Zia Gilda made us coffee, and I went out to get Elena's aunt a great bunch of pink roses. It being Venice, this mission involved a boat trip to San Giorgio, but I didn't mind. In an extravagant gesture, I suggested returning to Padova via the Brenta canal, and Elena consented happily. Arms around each other, we stared awestruck at the grand Palladio villas gliding past our creaky tourist boat.

Arriving in Padova, Elena went to a chemistry class, and I to my room, there to study the kind of anatomy I hadn't discovered in a young Venetian woman's bed.

That night I had promised Renzo, my ever horny friend, to accompany him to the Contessa's mansion. I felt ambivalent about this enterprise, but Elena had extracted a promise I was determined to keep. While still floating on the Brenta, she had insisted I try my newly acquired skills with Claudia who had earlier made fun of my shyness. It was Elena's night off, and she planned to study. I'd said I'd give it a try, but when evening turned into night, I was anything but confident about making love with Claudia. Renzo arrived, confessed to three Camparis, and we raced off in his tiny Fiat in search of the prettiest girls among the Contessa's ever-changing gallery.

While Renzo was welcomed as a valued customer, the high priestess in charge of assignments barely acknowledged my presence. Renzo selected a new arrival, blond Mimi from Ravenna, while I overheard the high priestess whispering to her assistant, a pert redhead nicknamed Cricri, *"Questo Micbele è un zero, partirà pronto, te lo promesso."*

Angered by the put-down of being a zero who was going to leave soon, I suddenly felt a rush of excitement as I remembered the moment when Elena had applied her lips to my cock; still dark from her own pleasure, her grey eyes had widened in the joy of drinking me dry. I turned to the keeper of the lustful gates and asked to see Claudia. The dragon smirked, but gave Cricri instructions to fetch the lady I wished to see. To embarrass me, she reversed policy, and demanded ten thousand lire in advance. I paid, and was shown to a room I knew well from my previous visits. Mission not accomplished, those visits had always terminated in an embarrassing premature departure. Claudia appeared, wearing a diaphanous blue gown, her high breasts and dark bush accented by circular bands of luminous white. She was a buxom girl, with long chestnut colored hair, still quite young, but heavily made up.

"Please scrub your face," I said with surprising authority. "And come back quickly, I can't wait to make love to you." Raising her thick eyebrows in astonishment, Claudia did a mock curtsy and complied. What followed upon her return caused Claudia, who was not used to clients interested in pleasuring her, to moan, gasp and finally scream as I carried her to two sexual peaks. Not pausing after her first orgasm, I stayed inside her, and continued my caresses until she screamed again as I poured the milk of Pan, that randy goat-god, into her.

As custom demanded, Claudia went to make her ablutions. In those days, they consisted of vigorous douching with diluted hydrogen peroxide, a useless and burning procedure, which in no way reduced the chances of an unwanted pregnancy. She returned to find me dressed, casually puffing on a cigarette, the mark of a man of the world. She was flabbergasted. I merely shrugged, and said her beauty had so turned me on that I wanted to see her again very soon. Totally confused, Claudia broke into the accent of her native Calabria which left me uninformed of her precise meaning. But there was no mistaking her pleasure. She hugged me tightly, taking my hands to her breasts for a final caress. Without giving the high priestess a glance, I left the Contessa's palazzo, and walked straight to Elena's dorm. It was past midnight, but she was up, the organic chemistry textbook in her lap. My grin must have been as crooked as hers as I held both her hands, lovingly kissing each finger. Elena stroked my hair and teasingly tapped the front of nay pants.

"Hai fatto bene, lo so," she said. And I agreed; I had indeed done good.

Elena Manzoni became a *dottoressa* of the new psychiatric branch of sexology. She never married, but had many lovers about whom she wrote to me long after I'd moved to America and become *un dottore psicoanalitico* myself. I knew Elena had ratified her inner knowledge of herself as a love goddess, or at least as one of her acolytes, and the world had certified her as such.

The image I retained of her was of the girl with the crooked grin to whom my dream had awarded the prize of supreme beauty.

Peter Lynn

AMANDA

I hear the sound of gurgling. A man, indistinct, is turning on a faucet. No water flows out, but there is belching and rumbling, merely air escaping. There is also laughter: a laughing chorus of male voices. Suddenly I realize that I am in a bathroom trying to pee. Young men surround me, some bandaged, one on crutches, all laughing. At some distance, there are a few women, trying not to be seen, but nonetheless watching the show: female peeping Toms. Lieutenant Mary Callahan, U.S. Army Nurse Corps, pushes through the crowd. She grabs my penis and gives it a rough shake. "Oh, how the waters flowed at Lahore," I think in my dream, seeing a happy Molly Bloom finally able to pee. The crowd applauds.

Where had I been? With Lieutenant Callahan? Of course, the dimpled brunette who used to change the dressing on my penis. There was always the inevitable erection, but Mary dealt with it swiftly: a sideways kick with her hand would cause an instant collapse. She never smiled, was all professional as she repeated this procedure every day for about a week until I was discharged, and we went out on a date in the garden city of southern Germany, Wiesbaden.

But this is not the story of nurse Callahan, but of Amanda Dunbar, the daughter of the Commanding

General at the Army's General Hospital, Fitzsimmons, on the outskirts of Denver, Colorado. For it was Amanda who had inadvertently caused Lieutenant Callahan's unseemly treatment of my easily excitable member. A couple of years ago, I had taken up residence in Pittsburgh, pursuing my medical studies. Shortly after the outbreak of World War II, I enlisted in the U.S. Army. There it was revealed that my I.Q. was in the stratosphere, but when it came to mechanical aptitude, I managed to score lowest among six hundred men. To this day I like to boast of this extraordinary accomplishment.

I was assigned to basic training in the medical corps. The camp was located in Texas where the heat and humidity were legendary. Having always disliked any form of physical exercise, I was astonished how easily I met the strenuous demands. There were obstacle courses under live ammunition, forced marches of twenty-five miles with forty pounds of gear on my back, in weather conditions which often exceeded one-hundred degrees. I became a tough GI. After completing the seventeen weeks' course, I got a lucky break. From the heat of the Texas desert I moved into the crisp air of a Colorado spring, assigned to take a laboratory course in tropical diseases.

I, Corporal Michael Stone, had been transferred to this lovely post because someone had scanned my records and discovered the credits of my premed courses. A lab course in tropical diseases was given at Fitzsimmons, and the war in the Pacific urgently required technicians who could identify them. I had no illusions of what awaited me once my stint in the

Denver lab was over. Still, after the deadly Texan heat, three months in the crisp mountain air of the Blue Spruce State was cause for celebration, especially since the Denver girls loved to open their patriotic hearts and arms to the medics prowling the downtown bars every evening.

Lieutenant Colonel Maurice Zuckerman, in civilian life a doctor from Brooklyn, was the instructor in identifying tropical diseases. I liked both the Colonel and the subject matter, and was soon spotted as the bright kid in class. After the rigors of the Texan training camp, Fitzsimmons was a cushy place where military discipline was treated very casually. Other than reveille, which I habitually overslept, there were no military formalities. On a bright Sunday I decided to forego cruising in Denver, and ventured instead to church. After the service, I talked with the Chaplain, Major Jeremy La Fontaine, a Baptist from New Orleans. It turned out that the Major had just lost his organist, and I speedily volunteered for the job.

Thus it came to pass that I, solemnly playing the introit to cue the pastor's entry, caught sight of a vision in the first pew: a dark-haired girl of perhaps twenty-five who could have stepped out of a Goya painting, was sitting next to the widowed Brigadier General Chester Dunbar, the Post Commandant. She was dressed in white, and her looks so stunned me I forgot to release the pedal holding the mighty C-major chord. Due to the continued distraction of the organist, the musical part of the service proceeded in fits and starts, earning me a mild rebuke from the Chaplain. But when I confessed the reason for my sloppy playing, the good

Major was all smiles, and of his own praised his lovely parishioner. But when I pressed him for an introduction to the General's daughter, La Fontaine became cagey, and mumbled something about the difference between enlisted men on temporary assignments and the post's permanent personnel. It sounded as if the unmarried Chaplain might have an interest in Amanda Dunbar, which exceeded his spiritual duties.

I went to my teacher and mentor, the Colonel from Brooklyn. "The General has open house on Wednesdays," Zuckerman confided. "If you play the organ, I guess you're okay on the piano too," said the bacteriologist. "I'll see what I can do."

The following Wednesday I presented myself in class A uniform at Zuckerman's quarters. Doc Flatbush grinned, and said, "The band needs a new piano player." At the General's reception, I became the newest member of "The jolly Fitzes", a motley group consisting of a fiddler with the rank of Sergeant, and a mean looking kid on drums who was a Private from Pittsburgh. "Hey," said the kid when I told him I lived near Schenley Park. "Guess what? I live on Munhall Road." The band hit the popular songs of the war, with the fiddler doubling as a pretty good vocalist, crooning "Long ago and far away."

During a break, Colonel Zuckerman managed to introduce me to the General. Bored to his bones, General Dunbar twitched slightly when he heard I was a premed student from Pittsburgh. "My other daughter, Lorna, is married to a doctor there. The codger claims to be unfit for the service. You know Carl Nichols?"

Hardly believing my luck, I said, well, the name sounded familiar, sir, but I couldn't be sure. "Talk to Amanda," said the General, "she writes to her sister every day." Doctor Dunbar, now a General, didn't bother to return my salute.

My head spun. The fiddling singer beckoned, it was time for the Kentucky waltz, and I banged into the piano in a frenzied attempt to discharge my emotion. "Talk to Amanda," the General had said, just like that.

At the next break, I introduced myself to Amanda who was playing hostess with the same lack of enthusiasm as her father had displayed. But when I hinted that I might know Dr. Nichols in Pittsburgh, her face reflected the sunrise over a Spanish landscape. That was my image as I looked at her oval features, her jet-black eyes and her shoulder-length dark hair.

"You remind me of a painting" I began, my heart beating in my mouth. Amanda interrupted. "Don't tell me about the Spanish stuff, I've heard it too often. It's not a good line any more." I was dumbfounded but she continued in a more mellow way. "You actually know my sister?"

I back-pedaled quickly, but managed to keep up a running tale about life in Pittsburgh. I was actually afraid that my eyes would burn holes in Amanda's dress, but she chose to ignore my stare. She offered me some punch.

"I'm so attached to my sister," Amanda said dreamily. "We're twins you know, and I write to her almost every day." She went on to describe her activities: supervising the General's mess, hospital visits, charities, relations with the civilian officials of the city of Denver. "Maybe Lorna isn't all that interested in my little gossip, I don't hear from her that often, but it makes me feel good to write to her, and isn't that what life is all about?"

I agreed, and volunteered some information about my course, but tropical diseases were not a topic Amanda cared to explore. (Just about a year later, I remembered this conversation, when Mary Callahan dealt another blow to my inevitable hard-on, as she changed the dressing on my surgically altered penis.) My duties at the piano terminated this first chat with Amanda Dunbar. I was bold enough to ask if I might see her again, to hear more about Lorna's life in Pittsburgh, of course, and Amanda, all gracious hostess, invited me to call on her whenever my studies permitted.

Pouring on old-world charm, I began to court Amanda with poems and flowers. With the benevolent assistance of Doc Zuckerman, I finagled an occasional jeep from the motor pool, a means to take Amanda, unrecognized, to the movies in Denver. One day I arranged for a fancy picnic basket, and proposed a drive into the mountains of Pikes Peak. Amanda said yes, and a fast spin took us into a field of corn flowers and masses of alpine blossoms neither of us had seen before. On a regulation Army blanket, we munched elegant sandwiches and ripe fruit. About a week prior to this mountainous outing, I had taken Amanda to the Post theater where Deborah Kerr and Burr Lancaster burned up the screen in a most torrid love scene. Taking her home, I'd succeeded in kissing a very responsive Amanda. Now on the mountain meadow, there was promise of ecstasy as Amanda permitted the removal of her blouse. I made passionate love to her breasts, and she put a tentative hand on the outside of my trousers. She'd confided that her virginity had gone bye-bye when she was seventeen, and now, eight years later, was not at all averse to making love with me. She described me as "so European", and therefore "sexy". However, the Army blanket, Amanda insisted, was too much of a mental deterrent.

"Let's wait, Michael," she said, still fondling the hard-on in my pants, "I'll find us more comfortable quarters." I was forced to agree, and reluctantly buttoned up her blouse, but not without breaking contact with her lips, which kept yielding, suggesting urgent needs. She clung to me and things might have progressed despite the Army blanket, but a sudden rain squall made us race for cover under a majestic oak tree. Back at the Post, I politely helped the General's daughter to dismount from the jeep, and was rewarded with a furtive kiss on my nose.

As I returned the vehicle, I was intercepted by a Private who worked in the Adjutant's office. "They want you on the double," the guy said. "Orders from Washington."

Months ago, while still sweating in Texas, I had written to an old friend of my father's who was stationed in the Adjutant General's office in Washington, pleading to pull strings to get me out of Texas. I'd stressed my fluency in languages, hoping for a transfer to military intelligence. Now at Fitzsimmons. I stared incredulously at the terse order to report to Camp Ritchie, Maryland, no later than in five days. This was a big break because it made my presence in the Pacific most unlikely. What beckoned instead was the war in Europe, and as I was presently told, completing a course at Ritchie could mean a promotion to officer's rank. Terrific, I thought, feeling grateful to the string-puller in Washington, but of two minds regarding my current situation. Not only did I genuinely enjoy the study of tropical diseases, but now there was the delicious promise of love with Amanda. I took my orders and called her.

Like any woman wanting something badly, Amanda offered to do a little manipulating: if she could persuade her father to release her from hostess duties, a civilian assignment in Washington for General Dunbar's daughter would be a cinch to arrange. I was impressed with her resourcefulness, and delighted that she wanted to be near my new post.

Early the next morning I was taking my leave of Colonel Zuckerman. He grumbled a lot about this unexpected turn of events, when Amanda walked into the laboratory where the Colonel kept his deadly bugs. Pretending casualness, she informed us that she'd been assigned to the Navy Department in Washington, in a capacity yet to be determined. Zuckerman and I were speechless, but his recovery was swift. "You lucky son of a gun," grinned Zuckerman. "I hate to lose you, but our Amanda has got more balls than I." Amanda had the grace to blush prettily.

I liked life in the Catoctin mountains of Maryland. The course was extremely strenuous: language classes and interrogation techniques in the mornings; eerie maneuvers at night when I and the other members of my team would be taken blindfold to some field, given a map in a foreign language, then told to find our way to a predetermined spot within thirty minutes or else. The or else referred to the feared demerits, which could put the promotion in jeopardy.

Weekends were out, but every ten days candidates were given twenty-four hours off. Whenever possible, I was on the phone with Amanda in nearby Washington, and every ten days we spent the night in a little inn in Hagerstown, the shack-up village of the intelligence crowd. On these occasions, I would show up with roses and some fancy lingerie for which Amanda had a not so secret yearning. She loved frilly underwear, and delighted in modeling it as part of our intimate games. She never tired of yet another lacy bra, a silken half-slip, an embroidered nightie, or the most transparent panties I could find. Pirouetting around me in these flimsy nothings, I would call her a cream puff, a term that made Amanda feel she might hurtle over the brink. She would go into a rigid psychic suspension, fantasizing what I would do to a cream puff lying sweet and sticky on my dessert plate. I didn't disappoint her.

All this shopping and getting to our cozy inn left little time for relaxed sex. The twenty-four hours raced by, and even one minute late in camp counted as a demerit. This absurdly tiresome time pressure was the fly in an otherwise delicious ointment.

Another fly, discovered much later, would eventually lead to Lieutenant Callahan's palmar broadside. This particular fly started life when I happened to walk unannounced into Amanda's

Washington apartment. The scene shocked me. Amanda and her roommate Lucy, a girl who also worked for the Navy, were in bed, naked, and a junior naval officer was in the process of putting on his uniform. The lieutenant, a blond kid from Kansas, slapped me on the shoulder and said, "What a couple of beautiful chicks! And how they love getting laid? The Navy guy laughed and departed.

Quite unruffled, Amanda introduced Lucy, then pouted about my being so busy in this secret camp that she got bored, and occasionally joined Lucy who adored threesomes. "Come join us," said Amanda, "we're still very much in the mood. The lieutenant was a fast shooter."

I was at a loss, thrown for a loop. I poured myself some Bourbon, and looked at the two girls who were nuzzling each other. At a revealing moment, I verified that Lucy was a true redhead. This was both an unusual turn-on, but elicited in me angry feelings as well. Sentimentally, I'd fancied myself in love with Amanda, and was now compelled to change gears mentally. It was very unsettling.

"Come on," said Amanda. "Don't be such a stick in the mud!" Lucy chimed in. "Yeah, take that stick out of the mud and let me see it." The girls cracked up laughing.

I poured myself more Bourbon. Diplomatically, I said, "You're awfully pretty, Lucy, and I've never seen a naked redhead, but I have very little time, and I'd like to be with Amanda, if you don't mind." My disappointment increased.

Lucy got pissed. She jumped out of bed, and planted herself in front of me. “Well, take a good look, soldier, because you’re never going to see this pussy again!” She got dressed in the bathroom and left, rolling her eyes at Amanda as if to say, “This boring guy you’re in love with?”

With Lucy gone, Amanda’s mood changed. “I’m really sorry, sweetheart. This was in bad taste. Forgive me, honey?” Naturally, I did and we made love, but somehow there was too much Bourbon around, and I couldn’t tell whether it came from my lips or Amanda’s.

Two weeks later, I was commissioned a second lieutenant in the Army’s Intelligence Corps, and after an Atlantic crossing on a shaky troopship, found myself on the French-German border near a town called Thionville. The war was going badly for the Germans, and when it was finally over, my team was cozily quartered in a little spa town in southern Germany, boasting the quaint name of Bad Schwalbach.

It was there that Lieutenant Stone awoke one morning with a stinging pain in his penis. The doc on sick call, Captain Mendel, was another physician from Brooklyn. He diagnosed a wart-like infection, sexually transmitted, and ordered an admission to the Army’s General Hospital in Wiesbaden. There I was informed that a circumcision was the treatment of choice; it would prevent the spreading of my genital warts.

“These things take a couple of months to incubate,” said the urologist in Wiesbaden. “You must have picked this up some time ago.”

I flashed on the threesome in Washington. My dick hurt, but I couldn't help chuckling at the fact that a grown man needed to be circumcised.

Thus it happened that when surgery was over, Mary Callahan was put in charge of dressing the now skinless penis of Lieutenant Stone. She was a very pretty Army nurse, and my erections during the daily procedure were an unavoidable physiological reflex. I learned to expect her lateral blows with a kind of sexy anxiety, and Mary, along with some other nurses became the secret spectators when I demonstrated my hollow gurgling sound which happened any time I needed to pee. My unusual bathroom performance drew curious patients and medics from other wards, chuckling, and asking when the next show would go on. This game lasted until my discharge two weeks later.

I took Mary Callahan out a couple of times, but the nurse was no pushover. She wanted to remain faithful to her fiance in New Jersey. "Moreover," said Mary, as we tasted Apfelstrudel in a local coffeeshop, "I've handled your erections too many times to get turned on by them. No offense, Michael, you're a cute boy." And nurse Callahan gave me a very sweet kiss.

A couple of letters to Amanda Dunbar at the Navy Department in Washington were eventually returned bearing the postmark, "No forwarding address available."

KATYA

Rich, voluptuous images are moving past me. I am in a church, looking down a vast nave, the high altar at its end. Light filters through stained glass windows, all is red and gold. In the pews are men and women wearing rustic clothes, the women with babushkas on their heads. I'm dizzy with the sense of so much color. Now organ music, deep and resonant, comes to me, chromatic chords moving up and down the scale. Fast and unusual, but not unpleasant. I walk down the center aisle toward the high altar. Still some distance away, I stop in wonder. Kneeling at the altar is Katya dressed in a red peasant blouse, a wide red skirt, and lace everywhere. A white veil is pinned on her long dark hair. She turns toward me, urgently beckoning me to join her. In front of her stands the patriarch, ornately garbed, holding high a ring, a wedding ring, and I suddenly rush toward them. I kneel at Katya's side, the priest kisses the ring, and Katya and I extend our hands as he slips the ring, miraculously, over two fingers, one of mine and one of Katya's. I know this is impossible, but our hands have become one. He pronounces us bound in sacred matrimony.

When I met the great Swiss psychiatrist Carl Jung after the war in Switzerland, I decided on my profession. After years of training, I settled as a psychoanalyst in New York and became relatively well known. My patients included stars of stage and screen. Several women walked in and out of my life, but I had not yet met the great love I yearned for.

Sunday in New York's Central Park. I had a date with Katya, a woman who'd recently come to New York from Russia. We'd met at an improvised night school where I had volunteered to teach foreigners some basic English. I needed a change of routine and found the idea challenging. On a bench, watching the goalie of a junior soccer team miss every ball that came his way, we talked about love and sex in Russia. Katya told me she'd been a virgin when she married at twenty-six. "l have known one man only, my husband," she said, bravely articulating every word.

The midday sun threw sparks off her red hair. "You know much sex?" she demanded.

I smiled, looked into her green eyes and said, "I do." She looked younger than the forty-five she had admitted to, and she carried her trim shape well. Her legs were crossed, the grey skin chastely covering her knees. A gentle swell under her sweater whispered of small, soft breasts. Her husband had died in a car accident, and a distant cousin had enabled her to come to America.

I decided to make a bold move, to let her know how attractive I thought she was. Stroking her hair and lightly brushing her neck, I said, "The best way to learn a new language is in bed, having an affair."

Katya professed shock, but I knew she was secretly pleased: she had already seduced the teacher. "You're too fast," she said, but her eyes went dark with what I fantasized was Russian desire.

I went for broke and kissed each finger of her left hand, giving her pinkie a little suck. Katya, a virgin at twenty-six and a one-man woman for some twenty years, attempted an idiomatic sentence. "I am sick and tired to not know sex much."

In my apartment, she became shy, went to the bathroom and came back wearing my robe. We hadn't kissed yet. I offered to make some tea, and we went to my small kitchen. The water simmered, came to a boil, and, turning, I saw Katya's tears in full flow.

"No man make tea for me before," she sobbed, as I held her tightly, lifting her face and kissing her on the mouth, lips salty with tears.

"And no man has kissed you like this either," I said, hoping it to be true and yet half-regretting the boast. Going the extra mile on my claim, I parted the robe, breasts were revealed, and my lips planted themselves on the space between them. Her skin smelled of an herb garden, lavender perhaps.

Katya smiled through her tears, softly pushed me away, and tied the robe. "Please, let's have tea," she said, grammar intact.

As it happened, Katya's sexual expertise did not grow, not just yet. After tea, three full cups, the bathroom scene was reversed, and she emerged fully dressed. Her face had the suffused glow of a woman who'd been to bed with a man; someone who'd traveled with her through a volcanic eruption, polarities fused, hot lava now cooled down to a tranquil river.

Baffled, I stared at her. Now she flirted. "You make magic tea, Michael. I warm all over."

As a humble student of the mysterious temple rites of which all women are guardians, I was moved by her playful tea reference, yet slightly embarrassed, as if some male essence had been stolen from me, leaving me without the conquest I had planned. Had it already happened then?. Did I make love to her by serving her tea?

Katya wanted to go to the movies. "Another way of learning new language," she said mischievously. We were watching an old Marx brothers flick, "A Night at the Opera". Katya was in stitches, clutching my arm. In the famous "Two more hard-boiled eggs" scene where dozens of people crowd into a small ship's cabin, Katya shrieked, then rushed off to the ladies' room. "I wet pants," she confided upon returning. "Took off altogether." Was this an invitation to make out like a couple of kids? But no, she held my hand, snuggled against my shoulder.

At Burger King, we gorged on the promotional fare, Double Whoppers, ninety-nine cents. Katya's vocabulary increased. "I so much like film, food, and you; I am having real wonderful time."

At a subway station, I took her face in both hands and kissed her lips with an unexpected rush of emotion. I sensed a tentative response, then she ran down the steps, nearly tripped, and was swallowed by the dark tunnel. Just the underground train or our unconscious minds?

In the English class the next evening, Katya claimed the spotlight. She told the group of her outing with me, holding back nothing except that she'd undressed in my apartment. The class was enchanted with the story of the tea, the movie and the burgers. I remember feeling embarrassed, but smug and happy. Another Russian woman, older than Katya, demanded that I tutor her privately. At that, Katya's fury erupted. Russian epithets criss-crossed the room and in the ensuing melee, I escaped.

Katya found me on the stoop of the old brownstone where my class met. "You chicken," she fumed, displaying knowledge of the vernacular. "Russian men fight for lady, why not you?"

"Will you be my lady?" I asked her quietly. Katya looked away, aware of the slight tremor in my voice. The moment was tense with anticipation, storm clouds threatening a possible thunderclap. Will the goddess consent? Or had I failed the test that would admit me to the temple?

A lifetime later, Katya looked at me. Admission denied, her eyes signaled.

Bidden by my Russian wedding dream, I entered the small classroom the following evening. Katya was not among the dozen people eager to learn the language of this new land. Disappointed and in an intolerant mood, I gave the hapless immigrants a hard time, terminating the session early. From the registrar, I obtained Katya's address. She lived on an obscure street near the waterfront. Why was I here? I wondered, skulking about in this abandoned area where her house looked like it was waiting for the wrecking ball? Was I waiting for Katya to be mugged so I could have fought off her attacker and become her hero? Was that the dream's intent? Upset and disoriented, I remained rooted to the proverbial spot. Katya's name was on one of the rusty buzzer plates of this dreadful building, but pressing it brought no response.

Suddenly headlights appeared in the distance, zooming down on me. Katya stepped out of the cab, one leg on the pavement while the other was still bent inside. She fished in her purse. Slowly, all of Katya emerged. Her broad Slavic face took in my uncertain stance at her front door. Her eyes danced.

"You found my castle," she said. "Now I will make tea for you."

Peter Lynn

LISA

I am in a junk shop. The store is in the basement of an old timbered house. I'm walking down on wooden stairs, which creak loudly. I feel apprehensive. The basement is quite large. In bins is a mix of different objects, haphazardly thrown together. On one table a pair of elegant ladies' shoes, studded with gems, protrudes from a heap of silken lingerie. Next to it lies a woman's bathing suit, black and frayed. On long bars hang all kinds of dresses, many of them colorful. I become aware that all items in this store – is it a pawnshop? – are for women. I'm wandering around, aimless, unsure of why I'm here. I come upon a tall etagére, black, with glass shelves on which stuffed animals are lined up. One of them, a sleek brown cat, comes to life and jumps on my shoulder. I'm startled.

Suddenly I am in a jewelry store. Brightly lit glass cases display precious stones, bracelets, rings. A man offers me a cloudy looking drink from a golden goblet. I'm not sure if I sip from it. The man is bald and wears a red goatee. There's something dark and unsavory in his demeanor. He leads me to a back room. There, on a wall, is a huge panel covered with midnight-blue velvet. On it is mounted a pair of pearl necklaces. And next to them, dangling from a large nail hangs a black rope. The man smirks and asks, "Are you sure you made the right choice?"

When I awoke, Lisa's face was before me, and I closed my eyes again, commanding my heart to slow down its rapid thumping, or at least muffle its agitated sound.

Memories cascaded back, fragments of feelings tumbling over each other. I had been in my fifties when Lisa came to me as a patient. She was in her early thirties, a dance teacher who was also involved in esoteric rituals designed for the empowerment of women in a patriarchal world. A second marriage had recently ended in divorce and she needed to deal with childhood traumas that had been rekindled in the wake of that event. Lisa was tall and raven-haired. Her upturned nose, which had been fractured years ago, gave her perfect oval face a pert mischievous look. It belied the depth of her psyche, which one might have guessed from the deep pools of her black eyes. Though she dressed casually, mostly in jeans and sneakers, her high breasts and generous hips radiated quintessential femaleness.

She remained my patient for two years, finding easy access to her unconscious. We were both pleased. Then something catastrophic occurred. The word's Greek origin does not refer to disaster: it means "overturning", a precipitous change of course. When I had first met Lisa, nothing alerted me to the fact that all the women I'd ever known would coalesce in her; nor that with her arrival the goddess had come to claim me. Nor did I suspect that our dreams would mandate a shared life of unspeakable joy. Obeying that mandate, we terminated our professional relationship. Lisa went briefly to another analyst, but returned to me as my lover. The bond our dreams was forging was to last for ten years. When the decade was over, irreparable heartbreak ensued. Lisa left, and with her departure the goddess returned to her temple while I agonized for a year, mourning a loss so vast I didn't know how to endure and survive it.

To gain some perspective of the cosmic forces that were engulfing me then, I have decided to record this story no longer as the narrator, but as the observer who by stepping away from his ego-defined position hopes to gain a larger, more archetypal viewpoint.

One

In any language, words are desiccated, flat and limping substitutes for the images assaulting a man to whom the goddess appears in the guise of a mortal woman. Poets, novelists and playwrights have tried to breathe life into an ineffable character which touches us with elemental force, freeing emotions which had only been abstractions.

Michael's professional persona, shielded by years of experience from the pitfalls of countertransference, did not feel the presence of the goddess until two years after Lisa had become his patient. He was used to her showing up twice a week, had noted her exquisite taste in clothes, but the eye destined to see past the clothes, past even the body beneath the clothes, the eye that could behold the invisible luminosity, the moon's crescent around her face, the mark of the sacred feminine… that eye remained shut. This kind of blindness defends us against facing a loss of reality, the destruction of the fabric that has kept us safely in a cocoon. It can only be healed (if that is the right word for so shattering an experience), when a dream, unbidden, rips the veil apart: the third eye flies open, is blinded again by the exploding supernova, but can now see, in joy and terror, the creation of the universe.

Late on a spring evening, Michael strolls down Bleecker street. At the corner of Grand and Mercer, a Calypso band gently shakes the air with a seductive reggae beat. Though sated with rigatoni and creamy lobster tails, he stops to buy a cone of raspberry sherbet. A dark-skinned girl breathes throaty sounds into a hand held mike. Michael steps closer, a few feet away from the man on drums who dreamily wields his sticks, on the far left of the girl. Holding the last note of her song, her face turns left and her eyes take in Michael. The small crowd applauds, the band takes a break, and Michael and the girl walk toward each other.

"My name is Maria," she says. "And I've seen you in my dreams, many times." Michael nods, offering her the now half-empty sherbet cone. "I come from Martinique, and my mother is a priestess, a great healer, in the interior of the island. She has taught me about dreams. What's your name?"

Michael told her. "Please remember my face and my name, Michael," said Maria. "Sometimes I get a look of the future, and in my dreams you've been splashing in the ocean, the warm waters of my island, like a playful dolphin. But last night I saw you again, and you were hurt. In the eye, I think." She turned abruptly. The band started up again, and Maria took up her little mike. The empty ice cream cone lay at her feet.

Michael walked back toward Bleecker. He sat down on a bench, which faced a modern building whose entrance seemed to be around the corner. He glanced up at one of the lit windows, then took out his small appointment book to check on the next day's schedule. Lisa would come at ten, Hans at eleven, and Katherine at twelve. The afternoon was free. At the back of the daily diary he kept a list of his patients' addresses and phone numbers. It didn't really surprise him to discover that he was sitting in front of the building where Lisa lived, nor that the window his eyes had fixed on was probably hers.

But his encounter with Maria, the Calypso singer whose gift of foresight he didn't doubt for a moment, frightened him very much.

Michael's sleep was usually deep and untroubled. He routinely recorded his dreams in the morning, and meditated on them while he showered and shaved. But there was nothing resembling a routine at four o'clock the morning after his stroll in Greenwich village. There was nothing nightmarish either about the dream that awakened him; but rather a sense of immediacy and urgency, as if a trumpet had sounded, a clarion call to receive a messenger from the lands beyond normal vision, for the message would announce the removal of a veil which, had been blocking his sight.

Michael had been sunbathing on a beach fringed by olive trees. A woman was swimming toward the shore. Emerging on the beach, she was nude, except for a golden necklace clasped by three silver doves. Foam seemed to envelop her like a greenish blue mantle. Three other women came down to the beach; they carried a robe, with which they proceeded to carefully dress and groom the woman who had come out of the sea. When they had finished, they offered her some honey. Michael was observing the scene, casually leaning on his elbows.

Looking awesome yet soft, the woman approached Michael. He jumped to his feet, as she bent down, whispering, into his left ear, "I will come to you, and you shall have me, but you must not hold me, for I am who I am." She took his face in her hands, and kissed him once on each eye. The doves on her necklace were touching his chest. She turned away, and disappeared into the olive grove, a shimmering, luminescent trail being the last image Michael saw before be opened his eyes.

The image had not faded. Staring at the ceiling, he could still see the woman, clearly hear her whispered words. Outside his bedroom window, a crescent moon surrendered, vanishing, to the pale dawn of the late spring day. And Michael knew the goddess had come. And he thought of Maria's dreams, and of the woman from whose window the light had shone, and who was scheduled to be in his office at ten o'clock this very morning.

"Aphrodite, foam-born goddess of honeyed love," Michael said to the ceiling on which the image of the woman lingered. "You will come to me, but you will not stay, and I must not hold you," he continued speaking to himself. 'I've waited for you all my life; now at this late stage you're blessing me? How long have I got? And have you blessed Lisa yet?" He got out of bed, and walked to his office two rooms away. The red light on his answering machine blinked. "Michael," said Lisa's voice, "I had the most intense dream ever; I know I'll see you in the morning, but the dream woke me at four o'clock, and I just had to tell you. Bye." The machine clicked off.

Michael sat down and wept; deeply, convulsively, gripped by a joy and a sadness larger than any emotion he had ever felt in his entire life. The goddess had come in his dream, and had now spoken to him in her mortal form. His question had been answered, and he would give his all, the purest essence distilled from his long life, to make the promise of the goddess a journey worthy of her divine gift.

Two

When Lisa walked into his office in the morning, Michael tried, not quite successfully, to hide his surprise. His newly opened third eye had expected some sort of apparition. He smiled at his own innocence, foolishly confusing the concrete with the symbolic: and after all his years of experience! He shook himself, and said good morning to Lisa. There was nothing in her appearance that anyone could call divine: she wore jeans, a white tee shirt, and a dark green sweater, which loosely covered her shoulders. White socks and sneakers completed her outfit.

But as they faced each other in the familiar setting of two easy chairs, he became aware of a subtle difference. It was uncanny, but Michael felt as if he'd never seen this woman before. Her eyes were opalescent pools of the deepest black in which ribbons of other colors flickered curiously. Her long hair was piled high on her head, glowing with a dark sheen, and her hands which clasped her dreambook looked strangely warm, as if invisible steam were rising from her slender fingers. She wore three rings on her left hand.

'I'm sorry about that message last night," Lisa said, "but I really couldn't contain myself; I hope it didn't disturb you." Looking at Michael who held her gaze, she did something, which swept away all the professional encumbrances they had observed for the past two years. Reaching up, she unfastened her hair, which tumbled down almost to her hips, a thick lush mantle now covering her torso.

Lisa blushed scarlet. "I don't know what made me do this, Michael," she stammered.

"I didn't know what to expect," he replied. "But I knew it would be out of the ordinary, and I guess it's tied in with your dream. Perhaps you released the image when you untied your hair?"

Michael was no longer surprised. The goddess had to reveal herself, and Lisa's hair was the unconscious gesture her dream had imposed. With the blinding clarity his third eye now provided, he knew that her dream would match or complement his.

He breathed deeply and closed his eyes. "Tell me your dream, please," he murmured, letting himself go slack. "And don't be embarrassed by what you just did. There's meaning to it."

"You and I were in a small boat," said Lisa, and there was a soft, purring undertone in her voice. It struck Michael as almost hypnotically seductive, but he willed himself to be fully open to the message of the goddess, to understand and interpret to himself and Lisa the secrets her dream was about to unveil. "It had an outboard engine," Lisa went on, "and we both got it started. The coast we left behind was mountainous, and we headed for the open sea. It was sunny and the sea was calm. We stopped at an island where jewels were brought on board, mostly golden rings and bracelets, but some larger gold pieces too. As we took off again, I noticed I was wearing a long robe of heavy fabric, and some of the jewels were on my arms and around my neck. We came to another island. A woman asked me to step ashore, and she took me to a stone building. There were high columns, it was dark inside, and she took me to an inner courtyard. There were many women working on honeycombs, pouring the honey into little jars. I was given one jar, and told to go back to the boat where you were waiting. We both tasted the honey, and then you kissed me, or perhaps I kissed you first." Embarrassed about the intimacy of the sentence, Lisa stopped herself. The opal in her eyes now shone in calm blue. When she continued, there was an urgent, agitated undertone in her voice. "But it wasn't the end of the dream. We took off again, but the scene changed to a wide square, and a man challenged you to a fight. I gave you some of the gold to make you strong, but the man was ready to kill you, not by force, but by some trick. I pulled you away, and we were suddenly in bed together, making love, and I came so hard, it woke me up." The opal in her iris now shimmered pink.

"I looked at my alarm. It was four o'clock, but between the luminous hands of the clock the face of the trickster stared back at me. That's when I called you."

Michael sat motionless. His eyes were still closed, but he heard Lisa getting up and pacing the room. "I'm scared, Michael." Lisa's voice was shrill, all purring gone.

"Please say something!"

Michael realized he had to open himself to the mandate his and her unconscious had issued simultaneously. The power of the matching images didn't brook any opposition. He couldn't resort to transference and other rationalizations; he simply had to trust their inner truth, for if Aphrodite were denied, her fury could be monstrous. Unpardonable mistakes could be punished with impotence and frigidity, disgust, even madness.

"Sit down, Lisa," he said, his heart beating a drum,roll in his throat. "I'm going to tell you what I dreamed last night. At four o'clock, to be precise."

And Michael talked. Carefully, gently he spoke of the worship of the love goddess, weaving his and Lisa's dream together into a shiny, brilliant tapestry which now hung, visibly, in what used to be just an ordinary office, transformed by their respective images into a sacred space, a shrine where Aphrodite demanded to be honored. He spoke of the incorruptible essence of gold, and explained that Aphrodite's priestess was charged with collecting the honeycakes which were the sacrificial offerings the goddess demanded. He spoke of the honeyed kisses which lovers blessed by Aphrodite exchanged as tokens of their self-renewing sweet love. And he spoke of the golden sex of the goddess, interpreting why Lisa's dream had ended in the spasms of love: that the spiritual life of the Aphrodite woman was linked with her sexuality; that a sexual encounter with the man she loved was for her the most profound of human experiences, a primal revelation of her own depth, her inner knowledge and her deepest joy.

"What about the man who wanted to fight you by trickery?" Lisa demanded inaudibly. Her hands cradled her head and she sobbed softly. Whether they were tears of sorrow or joy, Michael could not tell, but he thought of his own dream when the goddess had said he couldn't hold her, and he suspected that both, joy and sorrow, were part of the journey.

"The man who wanted to trick me?" Michael repeated. "There is a price to pay for gifts the gods bestow; I don't know what it is, maybe I don't want to know, not just yet."

Silently, in her sneakers and white socks, Lisa and the goddess walked over to Michael and kissed him on both eyes. Then she embraced him, and they exchanged the first of many thousand honeyed kisses that were to follow in the next ten years.

Three

In her daily life, Lisa was a dancing teacher. At thirty-five, she had long studied Flamenco with some of the great masters of the art. Well acquainted with its origins and history, she was now well known as one of New York's foremost practitioners of that ancient Spanish dance. But Lisa had another life too, more nocturnal and otherwordly. Once a week she was the officiating priestess of a nameless cult where women learned the secret rites by which to worship the Great Mother goddess, in the service of restoring the power which the Apollonian age, the patriarchy, had taken away from the feminine. Powerful white magic was invoked in ceremonies to which no man was admitted.

Two years ago, two issues in Lisa's life had brought her to Michael's office. One was the dissolution of her second marriage, which had caused painful childhood traumas to be reawakened. The other, even more strongly motivated, was the need to connect consciously with the dreams and images which were inundating her as a result of delving deeply into the magic rituals by which the mother goddess could be propitiated. Her analysis with Michael had been successful. Energies, previously bound up with her cold and immature mother, had been transformed into a deeper relationship with the nurturing feminine. Yet nothing in her unconscious material had hinted at a sexual attraction to her analyst.

Thus when the double dreams of Aphrodite's arrival invaded their relationship, Lisa and Michael were swept into a boundary-shattering constellation for which they were wholly unprepared. Alarmed but receptive to this explosive breakthrough of numinous imagery, they could not help but submit to this awesome responsibility.

The goddess was well pleased. She showed her delight by infusing them with physical sensations, which opened a vast new space of erotic pleasures. With humility that soon turned into impulsive abandon, they embraced the sudden presence of the honeyed goddess in their lives. It was as if they'd come together after a separation of many lifetimes, and were now fused into a bond of ecstasy in body and soul.

A sleek chestnut-colored cat was Lisa's familiar, her mystical companion. Being of the gentlest disposition, this feline beauty was inappropriately named Sekhmet after the wild lioness goddess of Egypt. Sekhmet took her time to come near Michael. She would explore his presence with exquisite caution, often circumambulating him at a distance, then gradually contracting her circling motion until she practically hugged his leg. Attempts to touch her would make for an instant hissing retreat. Lisa watched these maneuvers with mixed feelings. And Michael sensed that he would have to connect with the cat before Lisa could surrender to him, removing the invisible veil that shielded her. The goddess herself would have to lift it so they could openly worship at her altar.

Then Michael's unconscious took over.

He was on a boat, chugging up a broad river. The land was flat and muddy. There were palm trees. As the boat rounded a bend, pyramids came into view, and a man pushed him overboard. "Swim to her," he yelled. He found himself in a vast temple, standing before the statue of an Egyptian goddess. In his hand was a cornstalk, which he placed at the foot of the statue.

Michael awoke to an insistent purring. Sekhmet had wedged herself between him and Lisa, one silken paw resting on his neck. Lisa's open eyes were limpid pools from which tears of happiness rolled down her cheeks.

"We've now become true soul mates," Lisa would marvel some time after their initial enchantment. "I have never been so happy, so fulfilled in my life." And Michael, hardly ever short on words, would nod, and silently kiss the face he had come to love so ardently. Though rooted in the physical delights of the body, their lovemaking was to him a fusion of psychic layers, spanning his entire life, an ever-renewing cycle of being born, and then dying in Lisa's arms after they had exchanged their magical fluids at cataclysmic summits. Without volition, their lovemaking was like an on-going mating call: entwined like two rose bushes sharing a common root system, Michael and Lisa made love almost night after night. They knew that the goddess had taken over their bodies, directing the erotic ebb and flow according to her divine laws, exchanging identities as to who was who, who was being possessed and who possessive, yet maintaining their exquisite polarity which kept releasing floods of orgasmic fulfillment.

Lisa had confided that for her the experience was a journey to her innermost depth, an immense source of self knowledge; that when Michael entered her, and she felt his soul stretched to reach that very center of her trembling self, a deep voluptuous darkness was descending on her, the feeling that ancient clefts of nature were opening to clasp and receive his very essence. It was like the rich mulch, Lisa would say, which eventually gave the rose its dewy glow. And the glow enveloped her like the pink foam surrounding Aphrodite when she steps moist and shiny from her bath in the blue sea.

On a mundane plane, they continued their respective professional activities, Michael seeing his patients, and Lisa teaching her flamenco classes. In her women's group, her priestly role had become more grounded and secure, yet at the same time there was in her an urgency to explore some of the more arcane and secret rituals. These she kept researching with different adepts whom she met through the grapevine of esoteric folk. One such man, Chris, a physician with a reputation for questionable sexual practices, led her to the writings of Alistair Crowley and the Hermetic Order of the Golden Dawn.

This secret society, flourishing in the late nineteenth century, concerned itself with sexual magic, and had produced a ritual, The red Lion and the white Eagle, whose aim was the creation of a so-called Magickal Child. The doctor who made his illegal living as an abortionist, provided Lisa with the secret texts of that ritual, written in alchemical code which she had no difficulty in deciphering. Initially taken aback by the prescribed procedure, she had come to believe that a Magickal Child might serve a purpose in the rites she was exploring in her women's group.

Though quite unusual and involving obscure sexual intimacies, the ritual was fairly straightforward. It required a spiritually committed couple, wishing to achieve success in a specific cause. To that end, they would engage in intercourse in the exact manner prescribed in the texts. After the usual preparations such as creating a sacred space adorned with candles and incense, the couple is instructed to invoke mentally their respective god and goddess, building up the form of the deity and imbuing it with life as they engage in sexual congress. At the moment of orgasm, which must be simultaneous, they imagine their own bodies blending into one with the divine essence, and must hold fast to whatever image imposes itself on their minds. These images will indicate the future of their creation, the Magickal Child, a powerful astral being, and its success or failure with respect to the cause they wish to influence. The combined sexual fluids of the couple are then extracted, mixed with wine in a specially consecrated chalice, and consumed in a slow libation. This mixture of the fluids is called the Elixir or the First Substance, and symbolizes the life blood of the Magickal Child. According to the texts, the power of the Elixir is virtually limitless, and certain historical events are said to have been influenced by the proper execution of the ritual.

The description of the ritual affected Lisa in a way she found difficult to explain to herself. There was a curious pull, but there was fear as well. And for reasons even less clear, she didn't mention it to

Michael. The golden honey of Aphrodite was still very much present in their lives, though not all was harmonious.

Four

One time, which threw a long and ominous shadow, occurred on a trip to Ireland. It began auspiciously enough.

"We are spiritual beings having a human experience," Lisa said, as she and Michael sat in the warmly lit living room of an old mansion near the town of Mallow in County Cork. Tiny sparks flew up in the fireplace as the hollow log gave out its final crackling sigh before falling apart as hot embers.

They had come to this gracious inn for a brief summer holiday. Their relationship was all so very new, and yet with each passing day their nearness to one another didn't seem near enough. Michael thought of it as a psychic adhesive, giving each of them just room enough to breathe separately. Lisa's images of their fusion were far more esoteric: colored layers of an indefinable fabric were being woven around them, both transparent and solid, and in their dark depth, two hearts were beating in different contractual rhythms.

It was Lisa who had suggested their destination. Attracted to Celtic magic since she was a child, she craved a first-hand experience. An article on the Druid worship of trees was dancing in her mind, especially the mystical connection between the White Bull whose blood was used for divination, and the sacred Oak

Trees on whose branches the magical mistletoe grew. Michael would have preferred to go to Lake Como in northern Italy, but when Lisa invoked ancient Irish legends of numinous power, he readily agreed.

Waiting to be seated for dinner, Lisa said, "I feel I've come home. It's as if I was on an I.V. drip, an infusion of ancient magic that I've known existed somewhere, and here it is." Her moist eyes longed for a deeper connection with these forces, and Michael, although less sensitive to occult energies, felt himself drawn to them as well.

An enormous flock of black birds was assembling in an ash tree outside the dining room window. Rain fell steadily, and in the darkness the birds looked like a featureless mass. "They too have come home," whispered Lisa, "come to greet me." She began to shake and gripped Michael's hand. "You know, the Morrigan, the Great Queen who was Morgan Le Fay, King Arthur's sister, appears as an oracular black bird, a raven, delivering sinister messages. Let's go out for a moment!"

She rushed past the astonished diners and stood in the rain under the great ash where the birds were congregating. Michael followed her and saw her embracing the tree, trance-like, while the birds overhead made a hellish noise. Through her sobs, Lisa was smiling. "It's all right," she said, "they're not bearing misfortune. They only wanted me to return their greeting." Used to her otherwordly channels and their impact, Michael stood for a while with Lisa under the tree, trying in vain to get a reading of his own on the arrival of that dense chattering cloud high up in the ash. After a few moments they went back inside.

The dinner was delicious. Lisa radiated happiness, and Michael found himself enthralled by this new powerful, erotic and spiritual partnership, content to share her presence in this magical land.

After a week they moved on to the lakes of Killarney in County Kerry to a town called Kenmare. Their first day began promisingly enough. Driving down the winding road leading to the Tork waterfall, Lisa stopped the car, and pointed to a small weather-beaten church high on a hill, next to an abandoned parish house from which the Killarney lakes would have presented a spectacular view. “If this property is for sale,” exclaimed Lisa, cheeks aflame, “I want to buy it. This is where I belong!” She gazed at the speck of a church in her familiar half-trance, which always indicated to Michael that part of her unconscious was transmitting a coded message she might later translate for him. They proceeded to the famous waterfall where they took pictures. When developed, one showed a circle of light around Michael’s head. Unaccountably, Lisa appeared upset over that particular shot, but didn’t elaborate.

At dinner that evening, she informed Michael that the moon was full, and she intended to follow the account of an old Irish legend. “On a night like this,” said Lisa, “there’s the chance of meeting the sacred bull, an encounter with the deepest magical level of the Self. I’m anxious about this, Michael,” she added, “but being here is an opportunity I can’t disregard.” Michael offered to accompany her, but Lisa declined.

Later that night they argued. Hysterically, Lisa denied that Michael had ever made the offer to accompany her. Had he been with her in the field where she met a white bull but ran from it in terror, his presence would have given her the strength to face the fear, and thus meet the power she was seeking. However, as it went, Lisa accused him in near-manic agitation, his failure to be with her had prevented the encounter she craved.

Michael was hurt beyond words. Refusing to join her in their room, he spent the night walking in the vast parklands of the hotel. He felt wrongly accused, scapegoated, and deeply wounded; Lisa had questioned his loyalty, had in fact accused him of lying to her face.

There was no reconciliation the next morning, for each stuck to their own version of the truth. In time, the incident was forgotten, the hurt and mutual sense of betrayal deeply repressed. On the flight home, it occurred to Michael that the arrival of the ravens that night in Mallow had been a bad omen after all. But as he would learn later, not nearly bad enough in view of what was still to come.

Five

Michael and Lisa had been together for ten years. The decade was filled with twenty-two trips: nine summers were spent in Europe, fall and spring found them in the Caribbean or their favorite island, Bermuda. Aphrodite's honey was perhaps a little less viscous, thinning out a bit, and losing some of its sweetness. There were fewer epiphanies, which probably threatened the continued supply of the sacred ingredient. And when the catastrophe occurred, it was as shattering as the arrival of the goddess had been. This time it was heartbreak and sorrow rather than joy which washed over them like a giant wave, a tsunami, destroying the beach and the shore onto which the goddess had stepped ten years earlier.

It is said that parting with Aphrodite is more of a trial than absorbing the shock of her arrival. When she comes, she brings the golden gift of honey, tasted in the sweet enchantment of her sensual bed. When she leaves, desolation takes the place of secret love, and we no longer smell the intoxicating scents of her lush garden. Flowers die in the frozen solitude as the soul, ripped from its mate, drifts again among the galaxies in search of the Other, the one that can heal the hurt and restore one more time the sight in the third eye, the beat to the crippled heart.

When their world collapsed, it was Michael who first felt the change, foretold in Lisa's dream, which had roused her to greet Aphrodite's arrival. After drinking the nectar of the goddess in that little boat, her dream had exposed a man who was going to kill Michael by trickery. On a warm night in May, Lisa was leaving a meeting of her group. Still feeling the emotional impact of the service she had just conducted, the worship of the goddess transmuted to become the flesh of every woman, she heard her name called.

A man from her past, long before she had met Michael and whom she had left because he'd insisted that she abort his child, was crossing the street. Like two stones amid the eddying stream of people, struck dumb, Lisa and Timothy had stared at each other. At last they said, "Hi", and decided to go for coffee to catch up. "It's been twenty years," they said at the same time, sizing each other up. Had they aged? No, they looked better than when they'd been married, had done acid, and cheated on each other. Exchanging phone numbers, they agreed to meet again, for old times' sake. His number was unlisted, protected by the government agency he worked for.

With some excitement, Lisa told Michael about the encounter. After dinner, Michael and Lisa walked in Central Park. By the lake near seventy-second street, they sat on a bench, watching ducks. Lisa kept talking about meeting the man she'd been married to; what touched her, she said, was that he had called her name from across the street. And that this had taken place right after she had concluded her priestly function in her group. Michael heard her say, I've been summoned, and a summons left unheeded violates my sacred devotion. At the time, this powerful statement left him curiously unaffected, and after stopping for some ice cream, they went home. Later they made love, but Lisa suddenly disengaged herself from their embrace, and began to weep.

Unable to respond to Michael's tender questions, she got out of bed, leaving him bewildered and, quite fleetingly, afraid of wanting to know more. Eventually, she returned, and snuggled up to him. To Michael, it didn't feel like snuggling; Lisa was holding onto him, seeking protection from something that suddenly frightened her.

Several days passed. Then, one morning, as they were having breakfast, Lisa said, “I’ve been invaded by very powerful dreams the last few nights; they seem to beg me to find a deeper meaning in this chance encounter with Timothy. Can I tell you?”

Michael put down his grapefruit, and took her hands. “Haven’t we always shared our dreams? And any other outer or inner event that touched our lives?” He got up and kissed her eyes. This caring gesture caused a flood of tears.

“Oh, Michael,” Lisa sobbed, “I’m so afraid that something will hurt us! Last night I dreamed about two necklaces. One was shorter than the other, and it was for me. The longer one was for Timothy, and a voice said something about my having to act. And the night before, I was reminded of the sacramental debt I might have incurred when I left him; it was his child, which I aborted against my deepest feminine convictions. And again I was supposed to look for the meaning why he’d summoned me, call me to account for something I might have neglected to do.”

Michael heard the words, and though he believed himself to be tuned into this woman with all his faculties, he failed to hear her secret voice, urgently, intimately telling him that a new mandate had arisen in her unconscious, demanding an accounting for whatever it was she’d not done in the past. The possibility that she might become intimate with this man from her past was not even on the dimmest frontiers of his awareness. Very much later he remembered her words, as they were sitting at an outdoor cafe, "Timothy keeps coming on to me." Again the words flew past him. Nothing jarred Michael into consciousness. The most obvious questions remained unasked, "Do you want him? What are you planning to do?' For once in his life he was unconscious of the threat hanging over them, unconscious even of what he'd remembered long before Lisa had been summoned: that there would be a man who was out to kill him by trickery.

And then it happened. A message on his answering machine asked Michael not to wait up for her. She was going to a late dance show at a small place in the Village, and would see him in the morning.

What Lisa confessed the next day, after a dinner fraught with grim silence, was the beginning of his slow descent into hell. They sat in their living room, and Michael didn't ask, "How was the show last night?" Instead, he took a defiantly male, confrontational stance and asked, "Did you sleep with him last night?"

For ten years she'd been straight as a golden arrow in matters of truth. Now Lisa was evasive. She did a little dance around his question: no longer guileless, like a child, she answered instead with a question of her own. "What do you think?"

Suddenly aware of the enormous pain squeezing his heart, Michael suspected that his love was moving away from him. The utter trust he'd offered Lisa had cracked, poisoned by the sinister force that had engulfed the woman who'd been Aphrodite's honeyed gift to him for ten years. And the goddess had offered herself to Lisa as well. Was their time up? Was the goddess truly leaving?

Michael was numb. He felt he had two options: To take her in his arms with all the immense tenderness he had for her and offer his understanding that she was obeying an inner reality; that he was ready to forget and forgive, provided she'd never saw Timothy again. Or, he could explosively vent his green-eyed monster, show his hurt and his rage, and tell her that he never wanted to see her again.

Michael took neither option. Too stunned to assess his true feelings, he threw some kind of childish tantrum – which had a brief effect when Lisa, suddenly overcome with guilt, said, "Will you take me back?" But things deteriorated quickly into a screaming match, and weeks later she denied ever having asked such a question.

The core of Lisa's confession that evening was the revelation that in sleeping with Timothy she had invoked the secret ritual of The red Lion and the white Eagle. The same sexual rite which she had discovered years ago. The intimacy of the ritual, and its purpose to create a magickal child with Timothy utterly destroyed Michael. It became obvious that she had intended to build a container for a new committed relationship with this man from her past, the new man who had summoned her, and that she no longer felt committed to Michael.

He was devastated. Knowing rationally that it was going to end some day, that this had been one of the goddess' warnings, was no help to his emotional breakdown.

Lisa left, moving to a small apartment not far from where they had feasted on the divine honey for so many years. In the months following her departure, they kept hurling accusations at each other, both of them devoured by pain, anguish and rage. Michael refused to understand her obsession about wanting to be with Timothy; and she had no further explanation of why indeed, other than her necklace dream. This so enraged Michael that he wished he had a necklace with which to strangle her. She forbade him to come near her physically, shouting something about a visceral reaction if he attempted to embrace or kiss her.

When he found out, a couple of months later, that Timothy had dropped Lisa, fed up with her obsessive demand for a committed relationship, it gave him little comfort. Like fairytale lovers, separated now by a cruel witch, they were utterly alone.

Lisa endured the humiliating rejection by the man whom she'd thought she truly craved, and continued with her dancing lessons and her women's group, but spent her nights alone in the virginal forest of Aphrodite's sister, the dark lunar goddess, Artemis.

Six

And Michael? Depressed beyond imagining, he saw his patients, and sought the counsel of friends and colleagues. Until he could stand it no more, and escaped to a fancy resort on a Caribbean island. Very much alone, he swam a lot, but pursued by the furies mocking him for being cuckolded by Lisa, he found no peace, until a minor miracle became palpable reality. Descending in the hotel elevator one afternoon, the doors opened on a lower floor and a young woman stepped in. She was clearly Latin, petite, wearing a knotted halter of peacock colors and sky-blue shorts. Her thick black hair fell in waves to her shoulders, and when she briefly glanced at Michael, he smiled, and nodding at her hair, which she was shaking out, he said, "Gorgeous."

The woman smiled back, and said, "Thank you", and then asked where he was from.

"New York", Michael said, as they reached the lobby. She smiled again, then rapidly walked away.

He saw her again later that same afternoon. They sat by the pool, which had seven waterfalls at one end, reachable only by swimming the length of the pool. This time she wore a one-piece bathing suit, fiery red, with diagonal ivory-colored stripes. Her hair was high in a bun, and she wore sunglasses, which covered nearly half her lace. She motioned Michael over, and he remarked on her suit and glasses; her skin was so delicate, she said, she needed as much covering as possible. Her name was Maria, and she lived in a nearby town, but could use the pool whenever she wanted. She spoke in a light banter, but Michael's intuitive nose twitched: she must have come out of a room when she entered the elevator, and if she wasn't a guest, how come she'd changed her clothes?

Maria read his mind. She gave a little nod and looked straight at Michael. "Do you mind? Are you disappointed?" There wasn't a trace of guile in her questions, and he shook his head firmly. A great smile was his reward, and then they swam the length of the pool, standing under the waterfalls, and Michael felt better than he had in months. The water pummelled his back but the mist prevented him from seeing her swim away. He discovered her in a deck chair, shaded, her hair now open and dripping. Sitting down next to her he found himself mute.

Maria took off her glasses and looked into his eyes. "Why is there such deep sadness in your eyes?" she asked. Michael fumbled, saying he wasn't sure he wanted to talk about it, and it would be a very long story anyhow. Her own eyes were hazel, and she said matter-of-factly, "Look Michael," reading his name off his bracelet, "there is a man on the fifth floor who is waiting for me, and he's probably making a fuss about where I am, but he fell asleep, so I went for a swim. He shouldn't worry," she added, wrinkling her nose, "he hasn't paid me yet, so why would I run away?" Again she offered this without a trace of self-consciousness.

She rose, vigorously rubbing her hair with an enormous yellow beach towel, and somehow words came from deep inside him as he said to her, "If you really want to know about my eyes, I will tell you tonight in my room," and he gave her his room number. "I'll be there at nine," Maria said in her lilting accent, "and I'll knock once, pause, and then two times very quickly." She was off, leaving Michael dazed, but feeling a quick streak of joy like a shooting star in high summer. He lay back in his chair, pondering the fact that he'd never had commercial sex in his life. It seemed foolish to refuse a remedy that might help the sadness in his eyes; in fact, he argued with himself, it wasn't any different than buying aspirin for a headache.

When the coded knock came, a few minutes after nine, Michael was wearing pajamas, and putting a bottle of champagne back into the ice bucket. Maria walked in, her hair open as he had first seen it in the elevator, wearing a short white dress, cinched at the waist. On her feet were sandals, and around her neck lay a choker of little golden crucifixes, a most unusual piece of jewelry. Her skin was nearly translucent, and her thick black hair made for a mysterious textual contrast.

They sat at a small table near his balcony, and Michael poured champagne. "Are you rich?" Maria asked, in the same casual innocence, which belied what he took to be her full-time profession. Michael laughed (how long had it been since he'd laughed?), and said he wasn't, but that he wanted to treat this as a very special occasion, and then told her why.

Maria looked thoughtful and said, "You're not the type to buy sex," and then, like a child springing a surprise on an unsuspecting adult, she added, "Who says you're buying it now? I just came because I wanted to hear the story of your sad eyes."

With that serious pronouncement she took her glass, put it on the left nightstand of his kingsize bed, slipped off her sandals and her dress, and said, "I like to hear bedtime stories, so come to bed and tell me." All she was wearing now were white panties and her crucifix choker, the crescent-shaped earrings, which he hadn't noticed before, went the way of the sandals and the dress.

Michael took off his pajama top, turned the air conditioner down, and joined her under the sheets. "Get your glass and the bottle," Maria said. "I don't want you to jump out of this bed every five minutes." He complied, and when he returned, she lifted her face to his and kissed him sweetly on the lips. Michael took her face in his hands and kissed her eyes, her nose, her chin, and finally her lips, which yielded instantly. As she extended the tip of her tongue into his mouth, his own tip met hers, and that's as far as they went before they disengaged. She raised her glass, spoke some kind of a toast in rapid Spanish, and then snuggled up against him and said, "I want to hear the story of the man with the sad eyes," and then repeated the sentence in very slow Spanish, wanting him to understand. And slowly, but with increasing intensity, Michael poured out his story, the story of Lisa's betrayal, withholding nothing except the magic sex ritual. Maria did not interrupt him, watching quietly as he tried to keep back the tears.

She disengaged herself from the crook of his arm, stretched out on her back, and said softly, "Please make love to my breasts." Driven by his pent-up feelings of loss, he did, but very tenderly, covering her breasts with kisses and gently sucking her erect nipples, which were dark, almost black, reminding Michael of the blackberries in the woods near Vienna where he was born. And as he sucked, energy flowed into him, he felt his penis engorge, and Maria must have felt it too, for she removed her panties, took his hand to her damp pubic hair, and then down to her secret lips, and that place was as moist as his tears.

And she came on top of him, put his hardness into herself, and they were joined.

She moved slowly, giving Michael time to control his growing excitement, and after a while she bent down and started to kiss him, saying, "Please keep your eyes open when you come, and I'll do the same." And then they said nothing for some time until she sharply bent forward, rubbing her clit against his pubic bone, and with a keen cry and wide open eyes Maria came, and he followed almost immediately, looking into her hazel eyes which glistened, the lids fluttering briefly. Their eyes stayed locked, and Michael read a silent command in her dilated pupils. The meaning escaped him.

Maria became very serious, and said, "You haven't told me the whole story; why are you keeping something from me? When there's such sadness in a man's eyes," she continued, hesitantly, "there's more to it than an unfaithful woman, or even a woman he's lost for good." As if opening a door that might slam back in her face if what she was about to say would be disbelieved, or even ridiculed, she said reluctantly, "You see, Michael, I come from the interior of this island, and my mother is a very great witch, a good witch, what we call a Great Mother, and she knows potent magic. She taught me many things, and I know from your eyes that there's magic somewhere in your story, but you kept it from me."

As if Maria had touched a secret button, Michael's inner eye opened wide. He saw himself on the corner of Mercer and Grand streets in Greenwich Village, where a Calypso singer named Maria had told him to remember her, that she had dreamt he'd be hurt some day when he was no longer frolicking in a warm sea. He shivered, but was suddenly filled with enormous gratitude that this new Maria—or was it the same?—had come into his life.

She turned away and went to the bathroom, perhaps to give Michael time to absorb what she had said. But the synchronicity was scary, and he remembered his fear about the Calypso Maria's prophesy. Here was this girl who had not only divined that there was magic in his story, but whose mother operated on a psychic level not unlike Lisa's, and who was in fact something of Lisa's Doppelganger.

Michael nervously anticipated her return. When Maria came back, she stopped a few feet away from the bed, inviting him to look at her nakedness, to look fully and with great concentration. And her thoughts came to him, "Look at this woman, man with the hurt eyes, take her into your soul so that you may be healed, knowing that some of us are true and pure of heart. We look like members of the oldest profession, and that is true, for we serve a great goddess; we're her priestesses, keeping her temple sacred. Sometimes we make mistakes as I did this afternoon: the man on the fifth floor was not hurt in his soul, he was just angry that his wife had left him. My instinct failed me there. But my heart opens to him who seeks the blessing of the goddess; she can right the wrong that one of us has inflicted on his immortal soul, causing the deep despair and grief I see in your eyes. She who betrayed you no longer serves in the temple; her misguided magic aroused the anger of the goddess."

All this Michael heard without Maria speaking a single word, but remaining still, offering her body to his eyes, and it was beautiful, and yes, it was holy. And so he told Maria about the ritual, and she listened intently, as Michael held her in his arms, burying his face in the rich lushness of her hair, and breathing the scent of her sex, which smelled of sandalwood.

At last she looked at him and said, "Judge not the woman too harshly; she truly believed it would give her back the child this man ripped from her, not a real child, you see, but something of his fertilizing power she craved."

Michael shook his head, the thought of not wanting to be a father at his age pounding in his temples. Did it all come down to the twenty-five years, which separated them? He'd loved Lisa so totally, given her all he had, including what little he now knew of what the magickal child represented. Should he have married her? Would that have guaranteed Aphrodite's staying? Recalling his dream, he knew the goddess could not be detained; but did that fully absolve him?

Maria's words broke through these ruminations. "Pity her instead," said the young priestess, "she was hurt very badly herself: hurting you was not her intention; her instinct in going to the other man led her astray. In her deep need, she didn't see him for what he was, that he had nothing to give her, an empty shell of a man. So her loss is great, perhaps as great as yours. But she cannot go back to you, her shame is too great, and she's a strong prideful woman who will not beg forgiveness. You both must bear the pain of this immense loss. I will do all I can to make it a little easier."

Michael listened to this as if in a trance. This young woman spoke to him with the voice of a seeress, commanding him not to disbelieve her. More than that, she offered to help him bear the loss, even pleaded he be merciful with Lisa who herself had been punished severely. And even if Lisa were to humble herself and ask to be forgiven, his feelings would never be the same again. It was best, then, to spread the mantle of time over these cosmic disasters, and let Maria do her own brand of magic on his eyes. What could he say to that, in his fancy hotel room, a half empty bottle of champagne on his nightstand, and this serious, beautiful woman next to him in her glorious nakedness?

So he said nothing, but kissed her again, and they made love again, crying out as they came, clinging to each other, and Maria caressed his eyes, murmuring lilting Spanish sounds, praying for the divine healing balm.

And now it was midnight. Maria got dressed, kissing him once more full on the lips, and walked out the door. Michael had not dared mention money. Seconds later, the coded knock was back, and when he opened the door, Maria said simply, "I'll be back tomorrow at nine, but in the afternoon we could swim together, if you like." Michael's eyes brimmed over, he nodded wordlessly, and long after she was gone, he sat on his bed, offering his thanks to the force that had arranged this extraordinary therapy session.

For the next two afternoons, he frolicked with Maria in the pool, and on two more nights she came to his room, healing his eyes in ways too mysterious to understand. The third time she stayed all night and they fell asleep entwined. When Michael awoke, she was gone. On her pillow lay one of the tiny crucifixes from her choker. Michael kissed it, and back in New York he found an amulet for it; attached to a silver chain, the talisman cradled his neck, releasing a faint whiff of sandalwood.

Seven

He knew he wasn't fully healed. There were moments when his passionate hatred for Lisa squeezed the very air from his lungs and he feared to suffocate; then the reverse would occur: he was possessed by the most desperate yearning to make love to her. His memory, like a strange veil of surgical gauze, shimmering and opaque, was rendering his life with Lisa into an improperly sutured incision from which drops of blood occasionally oozed into his consciousness. But somehow there was always Maria, and if he began to weep uncontrollably, he would touch the tiny crucifix inside his amulet, and he found he could endure his fate. Months passed. Maria's amulet kept sending out its healing vibrations, but the effect began to wear off gradually. Vampire-like, Lisa's image refused to stay buried, and he relived once more, obsessively, the days of her betrayal. The demons resorted to the imagination's oldest trick: what if? What if he had intervened at point a, point b, and on and on through endless points in his torturous alphabet? Occasional phone calls with Lisa ended with screaming accusations, she not asking forgiveness just as Maria had predicted, and Michael ranting at her for not doing so. Yet he knew he wouldn't want her back.

Still, her living presence ate at his brain like a malignant tumor for which there seemed no cure. And his psyche, his dreams? Psyche, that unpredictable butterfly, which had found Eros only because of the grim trials imposed by Aphrodite, had shown no mercy for his suffering.

Friends advised dating. Michael met half a dozen women, some of whom were witty and entertaining, even physically desirable, but he could not conceive of getting close to any of them.

Not knowing what to do, he chose a path guaranteed to keep him suffering. It was summer, and he fled to Austria. Several of the women he had met showed an interest to accompany him, but he declined. He went to a place he'd gone to with Lisa, four glorious summers in years past. The resort was near Salzburg, that magical city where southern Baroque holds the promise of nearby Italy.

The owners welcomed him graciously, and he poured out his pain to Murli, the retired grand lady of the hotel. They sat on the terrace overlooking the lake and its backdrop of mountains, and Michael saw Lisa's apparition flitting to and fro in front of his tear-clouded vision. Womanly-wise, Murli counseled patience. She'd been very fond of Lisa, and reminded Michael that Lisa was not replaceable, that his seeking diversion with other women would make the loss more painful still. In her words, Michael recognized echoes of Maria, the young priestess in the Caribbean who had offered similar advice.

He visited the cemetery where Lisa had once taken a picture of a wooden Christ erected over an old grave. The Christ had been embraced by a profusion of red climbing roses. Now the Son of God was bare, His wood beginning to crack, the grave abandoned. Michael bought a single red rose, pinning it with a rusty nail to the Godhead. For the millionth time he tried to bury Lisa's image in that very same grave, but even as he was hammering in the rose, the soft, siren-like breeze floating over the cemetery announced the arrival of the sorceress. Like Tannhauser, whose pilgrimage to Rome ended in despair when a stubborn Pope would not grant him absolution for having dwelled in the grove of the love goddess, Michael's stay at the Austrian lake resort ended without granting him relief for having loved Lisa, the incarnation of the love goddess herself. But unlike Tannhauser's goddess who wanted him back, Lisa had expelled Michael from her love by giving herself to another man, who briefly exploited her and then lost interest.

And why in the world did he consent to go with Lisa to Bermuda? True, the trip had been planned long ago, but she was now in the midst of her affair with the new man, and still they went to the island that had been their favorite love spot for so many years. And there, to Michael's shame, he had acquiesced to her "don't touch me" condition, even though she charitably opened her favorite sexual pathway to him, to be pleasured by him one last time. Recalling that moment, Michael's breast-beating became a drum roll driving red waves of shame to his face.

All this fed his despair as he kept constructing alternate universes, nailed to the unyielding cross of his fate. And searching his deepest intuition for the truth, there remained only the dreadful suspicion that his clock had stopped, and without Lisa's wanting to rewind it, his time had run out. But whether it was the trip to Austria and Murli's advice to be patient, or Maria's amulet which he still wore, or simply time, that mysterious healer of all wounds including psychic brain tumors, Michael eventually found relief in a source which he'd trusted all his life. At long last, his unconscious offered up a dream, which pointed in a new direction.

Michael saw himself as Pimen, an old monk in the story of that unhappy Czar, Boris Godunov. Pimen spent his days in a cell, recording the bloody history of imperial Russia. But Pimen was also endowed with prophetic foresight, and he recorded future events as well. As Pimen, the dreaming Michael was not in a dark monkish cell, but in a sunlit room resembling a modern library. On the desk before him lay an ancient folio, the pages looking like illuminated manuscripts.

When he awoke, the dream's point rang a loud bell in his mind. What he needed to do was record his time with Lisa, either as his own memoirs, or as a story in which past, present and future would blend with the voices of other characters throughout the ten years, thus creating his own magickal child.

And Michael started writing. Astonished and grateful, he realized his creative stream was flowing again. And there was a promise, faint and barely discernible, that Aphrodite might visit him one more time, briefly perhaps, but that he couldn't hold the goddess captive by taking her for granted.

ALLEGRA

Crepuscular storm clouds race before a sliver of a moon. A heath? A moor? Macbeth's witches? I feel disoriented. I'm leaning against a tree when a car drives up. It is an unusually big car, painted silver. A woman gets out, followed by three children, two girls and a boy. Even though it seems to be night, her face is illuminated and I see that her eyes are iridescent dragonfly blue. Then an old man appears who reaches for her hand; but I see the snake coiled in her hand, and grab her by the wrist so that she falls to her knees. I realize that I am protecting both the old man and myself from the woman's snake. I walk away.

Suddenly I am in a street. Shops line the streets. There is brilliant sunlight. I am standing opposite a store whose sign reads "Women's Centering". I watch several women going in. Suddenly the snake woman is here, too, elegantly dressed. She too wants to walk into the store but then I am inside the place, shoving her back, shouting, "You can't come into my temple." I shut the door in her face. She throws the snake at me, but it only hits the window.

"Oh, Allegra," I said to myself, coming out of a deep sleep. "You were a witch on my heath, and from your fancy car you wove snaky Medusa spells. I fell for your witchcraft spell very hard. This is how it went…"

One

"Just imagine," gushed the woman in the sickly green dress at the next table, "she found him through the personal ads in New York magazine; and they're getting married next week!"

Michael shot her a killer glance. The restaurant was crowded, and he'd had to endure the shrew with the shrill voice for the past half hour. Already in a dark mood when he'd walked in, he had hoped the filet mignon would restore a sense of modest contentment. But the nugget of beef was not dainty and delicate as the word mignon promised: it wasn't done the way he liked it, the sauce Bearnaise lacked scallions, and the woman at the adjoining table was the last straw.

Unreasonably annoyed, he threw some bills on the table and left. Whatever made him order steak for lunch anyway? Walking past Lisa's apartment building, he looked up at her window and saw the familiar spider plant on the sill; beyond it, all was dark. He walked on. A bench in Central Park looked inviting, and Michael sat down, trying to sort out his emotions. His writing had been a powerful compensation for the pain Aphrodite's departure had inflicted. While his higher self had bowed in grief over the loss of the honeyed goddess, his earthbound male ego was still occasionally choking in fury over Lisa's treachery and her secret deception. In a rash gesture of vindictiveness, he had returned to her all the gifts she'd given him over the years, wanting to deny that the decade had ever existed, wrathfully wishing that they'd never met. The saner part of him knew he was spurning the deepest friendship he'd ever had, but on the plain physical level he could not bear the thought of seeing her again.

Michael felt terribly alone. In his dreams, there had been glimpses that the feminine was busying herself in the background, engaged in domestic chores like dusting his books or cooking simple meals. He understood that she represented a calming sense of the caretaker, and part of him was grateful for her silent presence in his unconscious. From the dim past he recalled a saying: when ensnared in Aphrodite, the wise man should return to Hestia, goddess of home anti hearth, there to wait patiently for the return of summer, when a soft fragrant breeze might, just might, announce the arrival of the buzzing bees. Michael left the park and walked west on seventy-seventh Street. He passed a junior high school, kids milling around. They were kids, barely in their teens, but they kissed.

The girl was blond and petite, wearing a school-type wrap skirt, fastened with a large safety pin, a sweater and running shoes. The boy's face looked unshaven, his hair hanging to his shoulders, tight stonewashed jeans and trainers with no laces completing his outfit. He towered over her. They kissed, but could not quite make their lips fit together. It was awkward.

Michael glanced at them, taking in the school behind them, the whole block full of youngsters. But only these two kissed. The woman's voice from the restaurant was suddenly in his ear. "The personal ads," she'd said. Would he ever do that? He looked again at the boy and the girl who were still brushing against each other's lips. Kissing, yes, it was kissing he missed most. "What the hell," Michael said aloud.

The text for the ad typed itself on the keyboard behind his blue eyes. "World-class osculator, handsome 60's, seeks younger sensual counterpart. Photo a must." He grinned to himself, looked once more at the young kissers and silently wished them luck in practicing osculation.

The ad appeared in the PERSONALS of New York magazine and drew a huge response. Two weeks after publication he had received fifty-two replies. Michael found this astonishing since his two lines, a lark really, had revealed nothing about himself, except his expertise in an extremely narrow field of human interaction.

Sifting through this pile of women eager to meet a man who displayed his erudition by using a Latin term for kissing, was a strenuous task. Those who confessed needing a dictionary were ruthlessly discarded. Telephone chats eliminated many others. Finally, he met in person with six of the remaining fifteen. One was an attractive psychologist, but she mostly talked about her analyst who specialized in visualizations and when she kissed him goodbye at a subway station, all saliva and no lips, she was speedily eliminated. Another respondent, a truly beautiful Welsh woman, turned out to be a fundamentalist whose sensuous nature glowed visibly beneath her bible-pitching exterior. She was fun though, and they met several times.

Meanwhile, more replies poured in. One envelope, bearing a strong handwriting in deep blue ink, revealed a letter which arrested all other action, not unlike an operatic diva launching into Butterfly's famous aria, "*Un bel'di vedremo* – One fine day we shall see."

The letter carried a faint scent, which instantly activated his pheromones, a deer lifting its head in a sunlit meadow, suddenly alert. The enclosed picture showed the writer with a grandchild. The photo was not flattering. Though 5'6" tall according to her letter, she looked hunched over, apparently playing with a cute baby in the water. What she wrote, however, was intelligent, informative, funny and faintly teasing.

"I am mortified to be responding to a personal ad but my friends insist that I do it once. How embarrassing if you should call. What in god's name would I say! Why am I doing this? It is difficult to talk about myself. What I would like in a soulmate is someone who is energetic, handsome, warm, giving, expressive, ready to make up for the first fifty years of life by living the next fifty years one day at a time and to the fullest. Laughter is essential. Does this sound like an osculator? I only ask for semi-perfection in a man, and to be able to trust someone, which, of course we know from life experience, rarely exists. Who of us is perfect, anyway? I don't even know if this is what a responsive note is supposed to say. I've just decided to do this once, only once, perhaps out of curiosity to see if you are what you really say you are in the ad. I love red wine, walking and biking."

The letter further explained that she was writing a book and working with an editor in New York, having recently relocated from St. Louis. She had three grown children and four grandchildren whom she adored. The bold signature said Allegra.

He called her immediately. The voice was clipped, business-like, but the timbre of the silent subtext was a soft vibration of sensuous curiosity. He briefly described his appearance and they arranged to meet at Lincoln Center three days hence, at five p.m.

Looking back at their first meeting, he saw it as a magic ceremony, a stealthy hunter circumambulating the rarest of preys, the sacred Unicorn, but was prevented from a direct approach by his shyness of the ineffable totem animal, the mark of the goddess. In mundane terms, he noticed a stylishly dressed woman, standing aloof in one corner of the vast lobby of the concert hall, two large shopping bags on the floor nearby. At last he broke through the invisible barrier his mind had erected around the woman in the beige suit.

"You're not Allegra, are you?" he managed to say. A faint smile washing over a face with the bluest eyes he had ever seen acknowledged that it was indeed she. He failed at first to take in her incandescent beauty. This was not surprising, since she was the first woman in the ad game whose looks exceeded his expectations by a distance, which separated an early cubist sketch from a portrait by Caravaggio.

Over Cappuccino, he sneaked a closer look. It was difficult, for those huge luminous eyes acted like on-coming blinding headlights on a dark country road, the make of the car nearly indistinguishable. Still, he took in the lush black hair, worn in a curious fashion whose mechanics escaped him; the, full figure tapering off to a tight waist and long slim legs.

They chatted easily, she seemingly far more relaxed than the world-class osculator. At one point he wondered about her name. "It's my favorite musical notation," said Michael. "Frothy and spirited. Are you like that?" Allegra laughed. Silver bells, Michael thought. Like in The Magic Flute.

"No," said Allegra. "I'm mostly dark and somber." She grinned. "But my mother was a musician."

Michael said nothing. Allegra signaled the waiter for another to Cappuccino. When it arrived, she aimed those sapphire eyes at him and said, "You know, Michael, I feel I've lived a dozen different lives already. Trying to be a writer is my latest incarnation."

His senses fine-tuned, Michael listened to her story with growing interest. Some years ago, Allegra had met an older woman, Julie, who moved in many social circles, enjoying a certain cachet of knowing everybody. Her career began as a pathologist's assistant from whom she learned what people died of. Pouring her energy into holistic health, she soon became an articulate speaker on conditions in mental health institutions. Politically astute, she was on close terms with Mayors and Senators, and even enjoyed the personal graces of his holiness, the Pope himself. When Allegra met her, she had decided on yet another career, that of literary agent; she was going to see to it that Allegra's book be acquired by a first class publisher. And Allegra, flush with the excitement of having completed her first novel, had entrusted the manuscript to Julie. She was in awe of Julie's reputation, and lavished on her a friendship which had a curious reciprocal effect: riddled with cancer, Julie had willed her New York apartment to Allegra but was determined to live long enough to see her book become a bestseller. Admiration and unwanted responsibility were the emotional see-saw on which Allegra was balancing herself, especially since she was sharing Julie's apartment, redecorating it with her own furniture. Julie retained one bedroom from which the nightly sounds of someone requiring special nursing care were a constant reminder of the double bind Allegra found herself in.

"Well, what about you?" the blue hyacinth eyes demanded. "You were giving me some bare bones about your life; would you care to put some meat on them?" She glanced at her watch. "Good heavens, I've got to run." Collecting her shopping bags they walked to the exit of the Mozart Cafe. There they shook hands and Allegra walked away. She hadn't taken ten steps when she turned and waved to him. Michael hastened over. Again those blue beams flamed at him. "Look, Michael, I'm sorry I had to rush, but I'm giving a small dinner party next week. Would you like to come?"

Of course he would. Watching her disappear on the crowded sidewalk he felt like holding a winning lottery ticket, but that it was by no means certain he'd ever get to claim the jackpot. The date was the third of October.

Two

The dinner was scheduled for Saturday, seventh of October. But if she'd expected not to hear from him until then, the two dozen pink roses delivered the very next morning unequivocally stated the case for his courtship. Another metaphor, developed months later, compared these first roses to a racehorse at the starting gate: "The stallion of Eternity was mounting the mare of Time." Two lines accompanied the flowers: "Allegra, finding you, a needle in a haystack? No, more like beholding the Hope diamond!"

At the dinner, Michael met her editor, a waspish woman of major professional reputation but with a bland, turn-offish personality, and a Frenchman who claimed to own an original TV idea. Allegra looked ravishing in black and her easy way to lay an affectionate hand on Michael's shoulder was bewitching. When he left, her lips brushed his cheek and he went home with her scent on his face and poetry on his mind. The poem, accompanied by more roses, was consigned to the doorman one day later.

"The sourcebook says; she is most rare.
A water lily, wondrous fair
The night reveals her rose-white sheen.
For only then her bloom is seen.
A sweet enchanting moon-born flower
Nocturnal like Titania's bower
She now grows roots on CP South
Bewitching him whose lips and mouth
She touches with her fragrant kiss

Pink clouds descend, a wordless bliss
Pursues his dreams, a heartbeat feel…
My God, Allegra, are you real?"

"EVE's BLOOM", an exotic solitary waterlily, having a single, rose-white nocturnal flower, slight crescent-shaped shiny leaves.

From A Compendium of the World's Rare Flowers, *London, 1857. Publisher unknown."*

Three

On the twelfth of October Michael took her to lunch at the Ritz. In great, horrifying detail she spoke about her life with the man who had physically abused her, vitriolically demeaning, and sexually violated two of her children. Her novel was a fictionalized account of these nightmares, which had been played over and over in her dreams and been fruitlessly dragged through the courts for years. He could hardly bear listening to what this beautiful, composed-looking woman recounted. It was the first time he caught a glimpse of her capacity to endure, a survivor buffeted by mental storms of such anguish and magnitude he had never before encountered. And he, the experienced psychoanalyst who thought he had seen and heard it all, was shattered.

"I don't know why I answered that silly ad," she said suddenly. "I've made so many wrong choices about men in my life." She made the familiar signal for having her coffee refilled, and looking past Michael she said, "I don't mind telling you that you've touched me in a place that I'd thought off as protectively dormant, a place I'd wanted closed off. And it disturbs me."

Michael touched her hand and the luminous eyes rested on his face. "I want to tell you about my four marriages. Perhaps that will clear the air.., for both of us. Either way," she added enigmatically. Launching into her past she revealed that the first two marriages were harmless errors, each producing a beautiful daughter. The third had been the child abuser with whom she had a handsome son. And husband number four, a man she'd married for security who had gambled away her money was now a sick and broken ruin. That marriage had been good in many ways, but looking back now she realized what she'd wanted from him was actually what she'd lost in her father – security, unquestioning love and stability. But it was a love that felt more like gratitude. She didn't love him really, but thought gratitude for loving her was called for. Divorced from him for two years, her latest attempt at a relationship was a lawyer like herself. Not long after they'd become intimate, he callously dropped her, disparaging of her body and lack of wealth. Undaunted, she followed the advice of trusted friends and answered the ad of the man facing her.

"I've been a survivor for so long," said Allegra. "You want to know about the most hurtful rejection?" Michael thought he detected a tear and nodded. Her next sentence made him realize that the tear had been an illusion. Her eyes were blue steel. "My father, a well-known scientist, called me into his office and said, 'Now that I've divorced your mother and am remarried, I can no longer love you. My new wife needs all my love.' I'd been sixteen."

Michael couldn't conceal the emotion welling up in him. But Allegra continued in what now sounded to him like an obsessive confession. "And ever since I've been searching for the one man who will heal this terrible hurt. And what have I found?" she asked rhetorically. "More grief, more disappointment. Except for my beautiful children and their children I am deeply alone, fearful of committing to any man, and yet craving the warmth and safety of someone I can finally trust. But now I've got my book, maybe it's a hit. So I'm still an optimistic survivor at age fifty-three." She asked for more coffee. "Albeit an exhausted one."

Perhaps it was at this point that Michael's horse, having slowly trotted away from the starting gate, was beginning to canter, set on a predestined course from which there was no turning back.

"I told you that I find you disturbing," said Allegra. "Now I'll go a step further. I don't know what compels me to look at you, trying to figure out your expressions. But I feel you're winding silken ropes around my neck. And I don't know if some unseen hands are pushing us closer together. You seem to be charging into my private space, not aggressively, I can tell, but you're wrapping me in a mantle of exquisite sensibility. The touch of your fingers feels like you're holding my heart in the palm of your hand." Her mood changed abruptly, as if she wanted to erase the intimacy she herself had created. "Some story, huh? But I bet you hear that stuff all day long anyway."

Michael didn't feel like talking but her hand in his spoke directly to what had passed between them. A day or two later, she flew back to St. Louis to defend an indigent woman who wanted justice from a system which had so far protected her abuser by the same legal maneuvers which Allegra was painfully familiar with.

Four

On the twenty-sixth of October she returned to New York. They met at her apartment the night she came back. Her new living room furniture had arrived; the fireplace was working, and over several whiskies she urged Michael to tell the story of the woman he had loved for ten years. Reluctant to open a wound, which, after a full year of intense depression, had formed a solid scar, he haltingly told her how his writing had yielded some of the energy that promised a return to life. Now, miraculously, his feelings seemed to flow once more toward the soul-image of a woman he had given up for lost. And so,lying on the carpeted floor of her living room, illumined only by the flicker of the burning logs, Michael spoke of the great love Lisa and he had shared until she had betrayed him with another man in the guise of a secret sexual ritual her unconscious had supposedly demanded. Confident Allegra would understand, his story flowed easily. But she had questions: why had they not lived together?

Had only seen each other daily and gone on so many trips together? Was he perhaps afraid of contaminating this great romance with concrete household chores? Would the goddess have been trivialized by such domesticity? Michael thought her questions were astute, touching on things he had never clarified for himself, but a complete and truthful answer eluded him. Briefly, he wondered what marriage meant to her: why had she married so many times? Surprisingly, Allegra easily opened up about her own sexuality. It had been difficult for her to enter this mysterious realm, but she had gradually discovered what gave her the most intense pleasure. The intimacy of the moment was forging a bond of mutual recognition, and Michael took her in his arms like the soulmate he hoped she was, and she let her trust flow into their embrace with a confidence she didn't know she still had.

"You know, Michael," said Allegra, her back to him, staring into the embers. "When we first met I didn't find you appealing. But I wasn't looking for anyone just at that point in my life. I had been drowning in my own quiet desperation and had not yet allowed myself to come up for air. I saw you had character and charm, and when your eyes found mine I knew there was something unsettling about you… and me."

But it went no further. Secrets had been exchanged, but acting on them would have to wait until mutual desire, and perhaps love, would eventually indicate unquestioned trust and commitment. It was to be a long road.

The first two weeks in November witnessed a fast moving, telescoping cluster of events. In that brief period before Allegra left again to spend Thanksgiving with her family in St. Louis, they saw each other on ten separate occasions. It was not just the rapid increase in the number of rendezvous that made for a breathless anticipation of what was going to happen next. True, Michael's canter was speeding up, approaching almost a gallop, but her own horse, the "mare of time", was now leaving the gate, following the timeless laws of instinctual energy.

He had invoked the blessings of Aphrodite and the goddess was beginning to respond. The energies, which flowed from her were as fluid as the water from which she was born. It is equally difficult to restrain water as it is to restrain Aphrodite's energy, for they both find their way through the smallest fissure, always seeking to flow freely, evading every obstacle.. The two horses carrying Michael and Allegra were committed to the track eternity had laid out: union through desire meant the preservation of life and coupling the most powerful paradigm of this fundamental unity, without which there could only be death, desolation and hostility between men and women.

They talked about these things at different restaurants, and at her home when she once ordered Chinese food to be delivered. Another time, when such matters were not up for discussion, she cooked dinner for him and the formidable powerhouse of the woman in charge of selling her book. This terrifying person, bloated with her terminal malignancy, slyly insinuated that Michael was a poor risk for a relationship since he would soon become terminally ill himself. When Allegra related this to him, he referred to Julie as the Angel of Death and refused to meet with her again.

Five

On Saturday, eleventh November, they went to see the movie *Carrington.* The film was a gripping portrayal of the tragic life of the young woman painter, hopelessly in love with the gay writer Lytton Strachey. Afterwards, they went to the Oyster Bar. The place was Allegra's favorite spot for an appetizer. Michael had wondered how she got along on so little food. Thin-crusted pizzas were the main staples of her sustenance, as was red wine, champagne, and her evening Scotch.

The oysters were on a downward slide over her pink tongue, past her palate and tonsils, and her eyes lit up. "You know what they are supposed to do for you?" Allegra asked.

Michael didn't answer. It was one of those moments when her beauty was filling him with an intensity that made his heart race. It was as delicious a sensation as it was unsettling. He watched as her tongue was searching for a morsel of oyster on her lip. She had put limits on how close he could come to her physically, and he knew she must not be pressured, for the larger issues of her life concerned her deeply. The sensible part of his mind wished to respect her pleas, but his yearning to touch and caress her was a constant threat to his resolve. Allegra had accused him of being too needy, had warned him about her "bad track record" where men were concerned, but her words became meaningless when his eyes found hers and held. The part of him he couldn't control was performing a ceaseless erotic dance around her countenance; he was powerless to stop it.

Allegra repeated her question about the effect of oysters. In response, Michael leaned across the table, his tie brushing Rockefeller's mollusks in her deep dish, and held her face in his hands. Their lips met, the briny taste lingering for the briefest moment, and then all he felt was the fullness of those lips, and he knew if everybody in the Oyster Bar tried to pry him away from them they couldn't do it.

The promise of such a kiss, where would it carry them? He wanted an eternity of kisses, kisses that only she with whom he was now sharing appetizers could allow and return: delicious, he would forever be addicted to them, addicted to her who at this crazy moment was kissing him back.

Michael finally let go of her mouth. Her face was flushed and she looked around, expecting collective disapproval. Instead, a roar of applause thundered through the restaurant and he, ham that he occasionally was, took a deep bow. A giant plate of cold seafood arrived. "Compliments of the management," said a blushing young thing. He tipped her generously, then gallantly kissed her hand. She ran away to more applause. It was as if Eros, Aphrodite's son, had come to the Oyster Bar: even elderly ladies daintily pressed their gloved hands together in approval of the arrow which so obviously had pierced his heart.

And what about hers? Had Allegra's been pierced too? "Michael," Allegra said, "it seems there are unseen hands pushing us closer and closer together. And now, in front of all these people, I returned your kisses. I'm making a total fool of myself.I should run before it's too late. I have too much on my plate, too many things to worry about, a job, money, my children – how can I deal with your desire? You'll be possessive, jealous, angry if I don't give you enough of my time." The tone was bitter, a touch angry. "Yes, they're familiar rationalizations. I know them only too well – but there you are.

"I remember a phrase by Anais Nin: that true kissing is irresistibly magical, and that the mind is no match for magic," she said. Dreamily now. As they left the restaurant, Michael's arm was protectively around her shoulder, drawing her nearer to him; there was more applause. From nowhere a single rose was thrown at them. He retrieved it, broke off the long stem, and stuck the flower into her dark hair. It was early evening, unseasonably warm, and he walked her home. The acacias in the park greeted them with their sweet intoxicating fragrance. "These people applauded you, the hero on his charger. And I know just what kind of verdict that jury would bring in. They would want me to make a commitment."

They took the elevator to her apartment on the ninth floor. She led him into the warmth of her bedroom. But once again she hesitated. And he did not force things, for he knew what a crazed battering ram had done to her in the past. He wanted her to reach out for him, secure in the conviction that he had earned her trust and she was responding out of the fullness of her love. He couldn't guess that this shaky issue would be tested the very next night.

For now, Michael went home, whilst Allegra confided her feelings to her computer, the way women had always entered their secrets into hidden diaries. This is what Allegra typed:

"My heart felt as if it was beating to some strange inward drum – pulsating and pounding uncontrollably through every fiber of my body. When not with him, I'm aware that he has pervaded my every conscious thought the way a virus can take over each vital organ of the body. When with him, I'm aware of his every gesture, and aware simultaneously and helplessly of my own movements as I respond to his erotic dance. Our coming together is not so much what happens as we touch and caress as it is the music that results – the notes and melodies, which produce some unique harmony that even we are unable to recognize at first, but which is rapidly becoming an opiate to each of our beings. We have been given a gift and we are both floundering around with the significance of it – unable to verbalize – unable to grasp the ups and downs of… dare I call it that? …our love."

And against all her resolutions she faxed Michael the page. He stared at the piece of paper rolling slowly out of his machine. His mind struggled to absorb the golden promise Allegra was revealing. Sharply, he pulled the reins of his horse, which wanted to jump the next hurdle, trembling with anticipation. He put on a record of *La Boheme* and drowned himself in the love duet between Rodolfo and Mimi, "O *soave fanciulla*"

Six

On Sunday, twelfth November, the city was hit with the fiercest rainstorm in years. Around nine p.m. Michael was overcome with such longing to see Allegra that he rang her bell unannounced. Wearing no make-up, only a white tee shirt and men's pajama bottoms, Allegra was speechless. Her hair flowed uncombed to her shoulders. He was soaked to his skin, but took off only his coat, jacket and shoes and then stretched out on her bed. The TV was on, Allegra was working on her computer, rewriting and editing.

When she joined him, tense and exhausted, he offered her an ancient remedy: inner balance could be restored if she were to let him exert quiet pressure in her most intimate place. She consented, and soon her breathing became regular, deep and relaxed. She was centered.

Then, very slowly, things escalated. Sexy whisperings crisscrossed the pillows. They kissed, caressed and explored, bathing in delicious sensations, yet alert not to drown in them. Once again they were at the edge of the cliff. Michael knew she would not resist the ultimate connection were he to ride his horse into the gate of jade beyond which there was dark lubriciousness, warm as a freshly baked donut dipped in syrup. But it would have been a transgression. He wanted to be invited into the hay and straw of the mare's stable, where she would bid him welcome, whinnying in delighted anticipation, He imagined a tiny voice saying, "I don't see how you can leave now." But he heard the subtext more clearly: it wasn't the voice of the lover desirous of her beloved, but rather the voice of power and seduction which would have slammed the door in his face the next day.

When Michael emerged into the night and the rain lashed his face, he felt happy. He knew Allegra needed more time, but he shouted his love for her into the squalls of water which wrapped him into turbulent wet sheets, whipping his body about in the storm. There would come a time when the jackpot would be paid out.

Confirmation that Michael's intuition had been on target came the next day. Allegra wrote:

"Look my dearest friend – about last night – I am uncomfortable. I feel overwhelmed as if I'm being pushed toward something I'm not sure I can give right now. I absolutely adore you but you are now smothering me and pushing me faster than I want to go. Maybe it was the physicalness of last night, which I'm not sure of and I'm not ready for it. I am in great need of space, of healing, of feeling secure. I can only do this myself and therefore must be allowed to find my way. I have grown to need you and love you in a very special way in a short time. I will not allow either of us to hurt each other. I don't have the track record, as you know, nor do I feel secure enough for even a small commitment other than deep friendship. You signal to me that you want much more. It frightens me although I am not strong enough to walk away. Lovingly, Allegra."

And Michael replied: "My dearest, you imply neediness. Perhaps so. But we have far more in common than that. We both have terrific minds, are gifted people, we wondrously laugh together, and for my part there is a feeling of deepest intimacy with you. I praise whatever divinities are watching over us that you 'are not strong enough to walk away'. For that would be a grave violation of our growing love. We don't know what the future holds, but I promise not to pressure you into something I hope you will reach out for when you're ready. But I cannot let you go from my life regardless of your 'track record'. The uncanny speed with which we have come together in so short a time must not be ignored. It speaks of a turbulent encounter between two souls destined to occupy the same space in the universal chaos/order of things. I treasure the feeling of adoring you, even though it makes my yearning for you a deliciously painful experience. Love, Michael."

What he withheld from her was his cry of such longing that if she'd heard it as a song, she wouldn't be able to erase it from her memory. Acting on it would be to reach inside her, aching to have her put her hands, her mouth on him. And if she did, he would make her feel the ecstasy which happens inside a woman's body, the waves, the heat, the heaviness, the scent, and finally the looseness as if, though naked, still another layer of clothing had been removed.

Seven

Michael waited for her at a far table, the large package unopened next to him on the banquette. When Allegra walked through the door, he waved and she came toward him, smiling. He inhaled her scent as if hooked up to an oxygen dispenser, and if he failed to breathe, he would die.

Allegra eyed the parcel, curiosity in her enormous blue eyes, and he desperately wanted to embrace her, right there in front of all these people and kiss her eyes, which had become the twin beacons of his life. They ordered drinks and he struggled with the parcel. Finally, from under bits of straw and newspaper, a statue emerged. She blushed when he presented it to her, her eyes darting to neighboring tables. Had people seen it? He explained that the two figures were Shiva and Shakti, the Indian deities of the highest sexual and spiritual love. Shakti's open legs were wrapped around Shiva who towered over her, smiling beatifically as if already embedded in her warm, moist folds.

Protected by the overhanging tablecloth, Allegra overcame her shyness and lovingly stroked Shakti's callipygian behind. Then she gave Michael a parcel of her own. In it were his pajamas which he had asked her to wear for a few nights so that her scent would be with him during her impending absence. They both ordered Piccata but the food did not hold their attention. Unobtrusively, they touched and caressed each other, exchanging little butterfly kisses and lightly stroking their pinkies. The talk was erotic, charged with fleeting jolts, as each wanted to know what the other's pleasure was when they climaxed. Was he noisy? Did she scream when she came? Or were her sounds stifled moans until the spasms overtook her, lips glued, bleeding?

He told her about the effect their talk was having on him, and wanted to know if there was reciprocity elsewhere other than on her glistening lips, full and deliciously moist. By way of a reply, she ordered a second glass of wine, pointing at the liquid. He was in heaven.

For two hours they made verbal love. Then, carrying their respective packages, Allegra went south on Broadway, Michael north.

Eight

On the seventeenth of November they had dinner at a bistro on the upper West side and then went to see "The Love of Three Oranges", a charming fairy tale by Gozzi, set to music by Prokofieff. Their seats were way down in the orchestra, about five rows from the stage. Allegra was wearing a black velvet gown, cut quite low, with a bra, which gently pushed up her full breasts. The sight excited Michael and he was tempted to bend down and kiss her there.

The tuneful show was beautifully costumed, the sets imaginative and somewhat risqué for an opera which was high *Commedia dell'arte* and intended primarily for children. On one set, a man's hand was reaching for a woman's half-exposed breast about to touch her nipple. But the man in the fifth row was so engrossed in Allegra's physical nearness that she had to mischievously point out the painted drop to him. Whereupon he leaned even closer to her, hoping for a revealing glimpse down her cleavage. Though she wiggled a little, the bra held fast. At intermission, they leaned on a wall pressing against each other. Allegra teased him about taking another woman out during her absence – just so that no stone would be left unturned, she said, before their commitment to each other became truly serious. It was the first time he'd gotten upset with her: the idea was preposterous, it didn't merit a reply, and his eyes flashed in momentary anger. But when their eyes locked, his anger dissipated instantly for love shone in her face. Still, Michael understood her fear, her ever-present tendency to run though her eyes begged him not to let her go. And he knew he wouldn't.

After they resumed their seats and the story of the oranges played itself out on the stage, the couple in the fifth row started a sexual dance with their hands. Exposing the cleft between her thumb and index finger, Michael moistened it, and began a slow up-and-down motion with his own middle finger. In both of them the sensation became so intense that Allegra pleaded for a fifteen – minute respite. He complied, but shortly resumed his erotic strokes. She tried to immobilize his hand but he wouldn't let go of her. Michael suddenly saw a fleeting movement under her fur coat as she squeezed her thighs together. Eros had triumphed.

Michael glanced over at her. She was dabbing at her eyes with her hanky and let go of his hand. She moved away from him, to the far side of her seat, and pretended to follow the intricate plot of the puzzling oranges. A tiny red dot had appeared on her left cheek, pushing through her makeup. His whole being wanted to kiss that little dot, the secret sign that she had answered his mating call.

The show over, they walked toward Allegra's building. She did not want to go home where the Angel of Death waited for her, so they stopped at a familiar bar. The bartender fixed her an herbal drink to soothe her tummy and other organs, which had been drawn into a recently activated energy field.

She took him to the rooftop of her building, a warm enclosed space, inaccessibly safe. They looked out over the sparsely illuminated Central Park and she hugged herself deep into her fur coat. She spoke of her concern about her own future and theirs as well. She confessed that the urge to run away had consumed her during the intermission at the opera, and that her teasing him about another woman was a defense against the powerful desire to fall – and stay – in love, this time for real.

Michael listened to what she poured out with joy and a terrible ache in his heart. How could he comfort her on issues that were beyond his intervention? He spoke softly to her and she began to sob, just a little, burying her fragrant hair in his chest. He kept telling her he would never let her go, would be there for her even though his reassurance would add to her confusion in the months to come.

Allegra relaxed and kissed him on the lips with a rush of intensity. And suddenly, without conscious volition, the goddess spoke through her: "Please center me again," she whispered. "I need to feel connected." They stayed entwined, motionless. He did not want to be aroused, wanted only to let her feel secure in this deep physical bond, wanted her to draw strength and confidence from their union. Then they went down to her floor: she to face the dragon, and he all the way down to the lobby, and then to his own bed uptown where his pajamas, steeped in her scent, invited him to spend the rest of the night filled with images of his beloved.

Nine

On the eighteenth of November Allegra left to spend Thanksgiving with her family in St. Louis. Her farewell note read: "Take care, my darling, you're very special to me. You are my soulmate."

Michael replied: "What I feel for you is the kind of love that I experienced only twice in my long life. It is a love that wants to hold you, reassure you, make you believe in yourself even more than you do already, and give you the warmth, care and affection I feel when I'm with you and even more when we are separated. We have come together at a crucial intersection of ourselves, our paths have crossed at midpoint between the time the traffic light goes from red to green: we met at yellow or amber, and if we don't go for the green, the red will return and this segment of our lives will remain unlived. And that possibility scares me more than I can say.

"We have nameless things to give to each other which will enrich our lives, in unpredictable ways, but overflowing with unlived energy. Having said all this, I will not let you love me the way my body yearns for you, not until you can open yourself to my love, on all levels where our feelings can reach a true confluence. Stay safe, my darling. Michael."

She'd only been gone for a day, yet his Sunday was as triste as the November drizzle outside his window. Michael yearned to hear her laugh, to play sexy word games with her, kiss her to his heart's content, make love, and then settle down in front of her fireplace and throw ideas around for their new book. The Merlot would be on the floor in front of them, providing Bacchanalian inspiration. By seven p.m., having come up with a couple of funny ideas, they'd get hungry and would order in. As always, she would eat little, while he attacked everything on his plate and on hers as well. He had to have his sweets but they'd forgotten to order dessert, so he started on another source of sweetness, a place which exceeded anything a chocolate mousse could have provided. These images helped him over that first day of her absence, but how would he deal with the remaining twelve or thirteen days he knew she was going to be away?

A card with lots of cats flew to St. Louis where her three Siamese had welcomed her with a torrent of feline affection. It said in verses:

"Oh, Allegra, how unfair!
Pussies, pussies everywhere!
While in NYC I freeze,

Three seductive Siamese
frolick in between your knees!
In frustration he just begs:
'Let me purr between your legs!'
You've got three, no, three plus one!
But poor Michael he has none!"

Thirteen letters and poems were speeded to her during her Thanksgiving stay. He also sent a small gift book of kisses, inscribed, "To Allegra, who had answered an osculator's cri de coeur." Photos of an Austrian hunting lodge to which he hoped to take her in the summer were dispatched as well.

At seven Allegra called. When he heard her voice, the onrush of his feelings surprised even him. She said she was exhausted, yet her bubbling spirit zipped through the ether like a graceful gazelle running rings around her young. She related some tidbits of her life, and they agreed that the midpoint in her absence had been reached. He told her about the thirteen pieces of mail coming her way and she stunned him momentarily by asking why he was doing this. He didn't react fast enough, just said this was his way of staying connected to her. Why would she ask such a question? Didn't she know how her absence affected him? Or was this the well known "not so fast, please" defense? But he made her laugh several times, and she showed curiosity about the hunting lodge and that made him feel she was hugging him one thousand five hundred miles away and was even offering her lips to be kissed. They bantered a bit about her four cats. Four, she said? And he made a pointed remark.

She claimed number four was asleep and he had sugarplum visions how he was going to play with that sleepy feline, making it purr and stretch languorously. He smelled her scent on his hand while her voice described the spa treatment she was going to get the next day. The triple sensation made his head spin: her voice, her scent and his image of her being massaged at the spa, he giving her the treatment, first back, then front, from her toes to her earlobes, with warm scented oil. He would turn the light off and leave her alone to absorb the way her body had been enveloped. In the dark, she would think about him, wishing he had stayed. Ultimately, the fantasy would make her collect some of the oil frown her body, on the tip of her middle finger. She'd slide it under the sheet he had covered her with and touch her folds, flirting with herself for a while. Her desire would mount and she'd go to work in earnest. Just as the waves would break, he'd return…

"I'll see you for breakfast on Tuesday," Michael was saying.

"No, no," came the quick reply. "I'll call you."

"Soon, please?"

"Yes, of course."

"I love you."

Pause.

"Me too. Bye."

"Bye."

One thousand five hundred miles apart, two handsets were returned to their respective cradles. On both, her perfume lingered for a brief time.

Ten

Allegra returned on the fourth of December. That day, Michael went to Saks and bought her a black negligee. Then he got her a set of her favorite scent, complete with body wash and body lotion. It was almost obsessive how he wanted to clothe and perfume her in ways close to her skin. They went for dinner to a French bistro. Again, as in other places, the best table was made available for her, as she lavishly dispensed charm to the owner and the bartender alike. Whichever restaurant she walked into, a flow of good cheer emanated from her and she was made welcome no matter how crowded the place. Though his persona made him look like an extrovert, Michael was really quite shy, and thus he marveled at the ease with which she made everyone like her.

There was no question Michael was in love. Smitten, infatuated, all his senses awash with Allegra's very being. He longed to look at her huge blue eyes, to touch her skin, and inhale her, hear her voice, that elegant Boston accent overlaid with a warm mid-western timbre. Michael was consumed with feelings he had not known in years. At night, he couldn't wait to slip into his pajamas, which were sprayed with her perfume. Thinking of her, he was astounded how similar their taste and interests were, how they laughed together, wittily picking up on each other's puns, making fun of people and the world at large. On all counts, Allegra was the kind of woman he'd dreamed would once more enter his life, the goddess blessing him one more time.

Oddly, there were no dreams. Michael's unconscious was mute. His sleep was sound and refreshing, but the dreams, the source he'd been connected to all his life, the spring that always fed his conscious mind, wasn't even trickling. Each morning, he saw with astonishment the blank pages in his dreambook. But in his exuberance, his full orchestra playing a ceaseless fortissimo, he failed to notice a lone oboe playing a mournful tune somewhere in the silent woods.

Their love had not yet been fully consummated. But unusual physical intimacies had been exchanged with passion and joy, and it was Michael who respected Allegra's reluctance to commit herself sexually. Her innocence in that area amazed him. She had no idea that a woman could experience many orgasms if her body were properly worshipped. Still, her signals of being in love with him were unmistakable, but the weighty issues on her plate demanded resolutions first.

For one thing, there was the man in St. Louis from whom she'd been divorced for two years, but with whose life she was still connected by guilt, taxes, and the alimony he was no longer paying. For another, there was her book, still being edited and the ambivalent relationship with Julie, whose pitiful condition Allegra watched helplessly while counting on the sick woman's connections to sell her book to the highest bidder. Then there was her family. Her two daughters and their babies demanded attention, sometimes to the extent that Allegra would fly to St. Louis just to baby-sit. All this with pride and joy, of course, for she had the strength to take on all obligations – or so she thought. Being a survivor of four disastrous marriages was a theme she sounded often, like an invincible jungle animal pounding its chest.

Michael registered all this, but more with his professional ear, which could easily enough be plugged up by his emotions: relentlessly, they shoved, pushed, and drove him into her presence.

At her apartment, Allegra gave him a set of Nick Bantock's mysterious correspondence between Griffin and Sabine. The books fascinated Michael: enchanted with the story and the artwork, he got the uncanny feeling he could have written this himself. It was a complex Jungian tale of a man and his anima, and what it took for them eventually to merge, overcoming fearful obstacles, almost drowning in the process. Three wonderful, magical books! Unexpectedly, he recalled that she had liked his profile the other night as they walked through a drizzling rain to a French bistro. The thought made him feel foolishly happy. Once again, Michael realized how completely he'd been taken over by Allegra's very existence; it held him hostage, imprisoned, and he loved every painful moment of it.

Eleven

Their next lunch took place on the twelfth of December. The moment Michael spotted her, her tenseness burned him like a live wire. He looked at the wine in her glass and imagined tiny wavelets rippling across its ruby surface, set in motion by the agitation she exuded. He understood that this time her plate was not merely full, but spilling over in all directions. Though she claimed not to be angry, he could feel the heat billowing inside her. Of course, he would be one of the targets of that heat because she so desperately wanted to be alone and finish what she had labored over for so many years.

And yet she was not alone. Michael was with her. Moreover, the two women most immediately connected with her project, Julie and her editor, were frustrating her at every turn. But there was still more on her plate.

A lover from the past had unexpectedly turned up, pleading his case on a single sheet of yellow legal paper in a small, mean-looking handwriting. And Allegra was so moved she gave him several hours of her precious time. "Because we have a history together," she said, pretending to overlook the circumstances under which he had dumped her some five months earlier. Which dump, of course, was the cause she had answered the ad of the man now sitting with her. A stranger two months ago, Michael was now so captivated by her, it made him choke.

He was profoundly shaken by the reappearance of this man and told her so. They spat at each other like two hostile cats, his jealousy sending up little puffs of the steamy fish stew they were eating, stinging his eyes and nose. It seemed to him the restaurant was showing signs of an impending earthquake. For her part,

Allegra repeated an old line, accusing him of neediness.

It was their first real fight. Allegra even challenged that theirs was a relationship at all. Michael swallowed his anger because he felt the depth of her frustration and was in fact quite worried for her: her book, the apartment, her alimony, her Rolls-Royce possibly impounded by the tax people in St. Louis. It all looked like gigantic tasks to be tackled. There was the unbroken instinct for survival, but this time she was hanging on by her immaculately groomed fingernails.

In between these angry bouts, her wonderful smile came back for a moment or two, and his hope returned that all would go well. They went to her house, arguing when to exchange Xmas gifts and finally agreed to meet late that evening. He was grateful when she cancelled the Saturday lunch with the man from her past, and offered to meet instead with Michael who was burying his face in her hair, whispering an endearing four-letter word, which she promptly ridiculed.

But it didn't matter. They'd made up and Michael was too deeply, too irrevocably in love with her and that was going to be not just his problem, but eventually hers as well. Predictably, the planned coffee in front of her fireplace did not materialize that night. Allegra was far too involved with her deadline, but called him around midnight, giggling a lot, and so overtired she thought she'd lost two chapters somewhere in the bowels of her computer.

Michael told her what the other man's handwriting revealed and she was generous enough to admit he was right. Small-minded. He felt a lot better, it almost made up for the missed fireside chat. "Call me," he begged. "Of course," she said.

His glasses were rose-colored again. True to her word, Allegra called the next day, inviting him over for Friday evening, the fifteenth of December. And, Michael asked anxiously, were they still going to meet Saturday for lunch before she left again?

"Of course," she said again. And his heart jumped.

They met in her apartment to exchange Xmas presents. Julie had managed to go out for dinner and Allegra was trying to relax. The accumulated stress had caused an infection in a tender area, so the champagne Michael had brought was a no no. Anxiety over her project had been increased by the possibility she might lose the apartment, but the survivor carried the hour. Later that night, the sick man in the far city threatened to kill himself if she didn't come back to stay with him. Though divorced and generously permitting him to live in her house, illicit guilt washed over her. "They'll say I abandoned him, heart attack and stroke, and think me a bad person."

Michael gave her two presents. A pair of sexy handcuffs, which made her laugh, and a jewelled butterfly pin which glowed on her, pregnant with Psyche's transformations. In addition to little loving gifts, Allegra treated him to a Xmas tradition in her family: every year she'd read aloud the story of the Xmas Tea, an ancient fable. Dreamily, he listened to her voice, a *viola d'amore,* weaving a soft lullaby.

As he left, he spotted a poem in magnetic letters on her fridge. He begged her to fax it to him and she did:

Watch over me... please...
Would you?
And I will love you.
Stop the ache and crush me
Beneath your shadow,
You are my only friend
We will be sweet together as one
In the storm.

For a while, they played fax games, then she signed off, for the Angel of Death had returned and she pretended to be asleep.

Twelve

Saturday, sixteenth of December. Allegra would leave this afternoon and fly back to where the sick man waited for her. At lunch, she told Michael of the sick man's breakdown and his heart contracted in fear she might cave in to being manipulated, now that her future in New York looked black. 'Telling Michael news they both preferred not to acknowledge, now carried its own stage directions: her head turned left; a far-away look indicated she was thinking of how best to put it while he anxiously stared at her elegant profile. At last she'd face him, determined to be truthful.

Michael used all his powers of persuasion to make her see the trap which would catapult her back to the city from which it had taken so much courage to escape.

"My darling, I cannot bear the thought of being without you." The phrase ran obsessively through his mind, realizing the sick man was using the same argument. Not as a love call, to be sure, only as a cry for Mommy not to leave him, even though he had irresponsibly caused the money mess she was now facing. And he hadn't even touched her in years.

At the table, Michael was trumpeting his love call and Allegra promised to fax him frequently, advising which date might possibly permit them to go to a Caribbean island for a brief vacation, His mind flashed back to her poem, and he thought of the story of Amor and Psyche and all the trials poor Psyche had to endure before she could surrender to him who had wounded her with the arrow of his love.

Allegra kissed him good-bye, kissed him hard, and he rallied, almost ready to face the three long weeks he'd be without her.

Thirteen

What happened in St. Louis around Xmas time, Michael recorded in an exchange of faxes.

Allegra: "This is craziness – beyond the call – kids all day – no work on book – no time to think – full house tomorrow and Monday – take care, tomorrow long fax follows – love – A."

And on Xmas eve: "Well! Everyone's been sick all day – sitting around watching TV and doing nothing.

My Dad helped me cook the clam chowder that we make each year for Xmas eve and all the stockings are hung with care and I didn't get to read the paper or take a nap – but so what. Everyone comes at six-thirty except Dad's date just called to say she was sick – and I have to tell him. That I will do after this. Hope all is well with you! I've been listening to Xmas music all day to keep my, spirits up and suddenly broke down thinking about how much I miss my mother. I'm no 'Allegra' now, more like 'A*dagio pesante con tristezza'*. I wonder if Santa Claus is coming tonight and I've been a good girl this year. Do you think he'll bring me a present? Ah Well! *C'est la vie. Je besoin de toi – I* need to be centered. But, I'm alive, aren't I????????? Love and merry Xmas, A. Ho! Ho! Ho!"

And Michael replied: "Ho! Ho! Ho! to you too, triste Allegra! We all yearn for Mom when things go over the top. I don't know about the first nine months of this year, but since October third you've been a very good girl, and this Santa's deputy carries a year's worth of centering for you, renewable each Xmas if you don't stray! In the depth of his bag he has two more presents for your stocking which must await personal delivery. Right now, eleven p.m. NY time, I try to visualize you reading the Xmas Tea story to everybody… though you can barely hold the book without your eyes falling out… but you're alive aren't you? Love and merry Xmas, M."

Allegra on Christmas Day: "I got up at five-thirty a.m., after four hours sleep from cleaning up Xmas eve party, and cleaned some more, set the table for fifteen, stuffed the turkey, made marinade for the roast beef, did the potatoes, cut the carrots, and set places for breakfast. I've never felt so alone and here I am in the midst of many people – family – who love me. What is off here? Is it perhaps that I want someone to care enough for me to share these chores with – I don't mind the giving. I'm tired. I want someone's arms around me. I want to have someone laughing with me at five-thirty in the morning, insisting as we labor that I have a glass of champagne, hugging me, stuffing the turkey with me, setting the fire, and listening to Xmas music. Then, grabbing the paper, another glass of champagne, jumping back into bed until at least eleven to read the paper, cuddle, and dream, I'm such a hopeless romantic. Bah! Humbug! This is not what I want my future Xmas's to be. I've done this for thirty odd years and I'm tired. And so alone in a house full of life, cats, and people. How odd. Merry Xmas, my love. Changes are a'comin… at least on my end. Me, I just got the newspaper, wrote you this letter, and made myself the biggest vodka and cranberry/orange juice, turned the Xmas music down low, snuck into bed and may get two or three more winks if the vodka works and my tears stop.

"Love, yes, I'm feeling maudlin and sorry for myself. It is only momentary. Allegra *vincitor!* (Do you know your "Aida"?)."

Michael's reply: "Xmas Day. My darling, I hope you survive this one as well, with some reserves intact I mean. I've had the most vivid dream last night. I was in this city, supposed to be St. L. trying to get to your house. No one was helpful, kids sending me on wild goose chases involving old-fashioned street cars.

Finally, a little old lady came along, a true fairy godmother, in a silvery gleaming model T-type car. She drove me to your house, which was a sprawling affair on a hillside. It was springtime, vast sloping lawns, and I was a guest in your house. The house was very modern, many bathrooms, you introduced me to lots of people. Next scene was early morning, in your bedroom, sunlight streaming in. You were alone, in crumpled sheets, on your knees, your head buried in pillows. I sat on the bed and gave you all the faxes I had sent you. You told me to get dressed for breakfast, I took a shower next door, then could not find my way downstairs, went down floor after floor on stairways. It was now a modern hospital, rooms full of patients, a kind of Swiss sanatorium for rest cures, no one was sick. Finally, I emerged on the bottom level, walking out into a blossoming meadow, had to climb up a long hill back to your house. You stood in the door with a bouquet of flowers in your arms, wearing a long blue denim skirt and a peasant blouse and said, 'I've been waiting for you, breakfast is ready.'

"I woke up with wonderful feelings, lovely image isn't it? And so obvious in meaning."

Michael paused. Was it really so obvious? A clinic?

Allegra: "That was a beautiful dream – some sense of peace there except for the searching – wow!! Thanks."

He paused again. Something was amiss. It was all coming from his head. Wishful thinking? Somehow his heart was staying out of this conversation.

But as Xmas day drew to a close, Michael knew that what Allegra had written to him some six weeks earlier was going to come to pass. Vulnerable and anxious, she'd nevertheless confided her feelings.

"And then slowly, very slowly, things began to change in both our lives and we began to struggle with what was inevitable – the seriousness of the commitment to each other a heavy burden that each of us had to bear and that we were powerless to change. 'I will not let you go,' he said once to me when the urge to run had consumed me once again.

"I will not let you go,' I said to myself, knowing deep inside that whatever was to happen would be decided in the months to come.

"'Please, don't let me go,' I said to myself, knowing that it was far easier to run than face the obstacles ahead and yet wanting so desperately to finally let go and truly love as only we could love each other. I felt that I would, must, go with him. We were that inseparable. Yet, I wanted to give him all the freedom that he wanted, for that was the key for both of us to endure."

And Michael wanted desperately to believe it.

Fourteen

But predictably and terrifying, Allegra managed once again to put herself into a nightmare of her own making. And along with the sick man, the rest of her family, the careless, unreliable editor, she tried to throw Michael out with the garbage. He'd warned her about her editor, not once but repeatedly: there had been ample evidence of her not keeping promises, not meeting deadlines. He advised Allegra not to pay her until the job was done. No, she could not do that, waving a worthless contract in his face. No, she could not let her family down, had to serve fifteen dinners on Xmas Eve, ditto on Xmas Day. Superwoman.

Throughout the Xmas days, they had kept each other's spirits going as best as distance allowed. But now, on the twenty-ninth of December, the nightmare engulfing her, Allegra used Michael as just another target for the mess she had created. Good-naturedly, of course; in the service of hallowed tradition, of course; family and food first, of course.

"My own life? Way down at the bottom of the list. Warm arms around me? Hopelessly romantic! Champagne in bed? Would be nice, yes – but, no, duty first! Still, je besoin de toi."

Thus stressed, flailing invisible arms, she cried for space. "Don't call me endearing names… I'm seeing two thousand other men… this is not an exclusive relationship."

Michael's heart overflowed with tenderness and pity for her, while at the same time his anger boiled at her superwoman-unconsciousness. The badly needed few days of sunshine in Florida had to be cancelled; another sacrifice offered up, all because she did not know about time and priorities. And she was pushing away the only friend she had to hold onto throughout this senseless nightmare. He didn't take it as a personal rejection, but it was hard not to be upset, vicariously, by the scene taking place in the far city.

But there was nothing Michael could do. She had to sink or swim. And knowing her spirit and her power, he believed in her swimming. Bruised, breathless and half-sick, no doubt, but swimming. Saving her life with her book. Everything else was on hold. He could take it. Because he loved her. And wanted her to win. Because he believed in her. Believed, too, that she would someday, someday soon, see herself as who she really was – and what, and whom, she truly needed in her life to keep her centered.

But the bullets did not cease flying, they only changed caliber. Returning home around eleven p.m. on Saturday, thirtieth of December, Michael found a short fax: she had actually done it, was going to celebrate with her kids, her ex was in Florida already. And she was sorry for the angry fax. He was thrilled, and immediately phoned and faxed her. There was no answer on either line.

On Sunday morning, the last day of the old year, Michael heard a message on her St. Louis machine that she'd be in New York, eighth of January. By the afternoon, there was a message on his machine: Allegra was on her way to Palm Beach, wishing him a Happy New Year. She left no phone number where he could have wished *her* a Happy New Year, could have told her about his wishes for her, and his own New Year resolutions. Why was she hiding?

It was the worst New Year's Eve of his life.

Hoping for a call, he sat by the phone from midnight to three a.m. No word came. Disappointment changed to fury. How could she be so insensitive, frolicking with friends in Palm Beach, toasting the New Year, kissing somebody, while he sat, as alone as the Little Match Girl in that heartbreaking fairytale, unable to reach her? Was this the much-touted need for "space"? Which he would have respected, of course, had she asked him to. But to shut him out from her whereabouts was a gesture of mistrust: a cruel and unusual punishment. All throughout the Xmas period they had been in touch: she mostly despairing and angry, indulging in romantic fantasies; he supportive and present.

In the afternoon of New Year's Day there was a message from the beach: "I'm thinking of selling my house and buying one here… will call in a couple of days." Again he was barred from returning her call.

Michael couldn't believe it.

He smashed five champagne glasses, slammed every door in the apartment so that the walls rattled, and was just considering a lethal close of pills he always had on hand, when the phone rang.

Angharad, the beautiful bible-toting Welsh woman who had also responded to his osculator ad and whom he had seen several times before he met Allegro, called to wish him a Happy New Year. She was at the Plaza, and had been stood up by her date. Would he care to join her?

Indeed he would, if she promised to stop being a fundamentalist just for the day and would let him kiss the daylights out of her, only because it was New Year's Day. She giggled, obviously smashed, and allowed as how it was said that God looked the other way once a year, perhaps this was the day he wasn't looking. So they smooched for a couple of hours in a bar on fifty-fifth Street, then he took her to Penn Station where she boarded a train to her Long Island home.

As he walked home, past Allegra's apartment, his anger got the better of him again. He remembered her warning about her "bad track record." But it was no use. He truly loved that crazy woman, with her half-truths, and whatever shit she was now throwing in his face had to be swallowed, part of the hero's trials on his way to the Self.

At home, he sank into his aromatic pillows as her face mocked him to sleep. And dreamed.

A city in India. Teeming with poor filthy people. Twilight. Somewhere voices calling to prayer. Michael is a tourist wandering the streets. He comes to an open area, round, where a snake charmer keeps a cobra swaying to the tune his assistant is playing on a flute-like instrument. She's a girl, late teens, long black hair. The man keeps his eyes on the snake. People stand around and Michael joins them.

As he focuses on the scene, it seems to him that the cobra is playing the flute, the girl's face merging with the head of the snake; together they're playing the hypnotic tune; the girl's neck is really the flat head of the cobra.

The man turns to Michael and speaks. "It's easy, if you can lock eyes with the snake."

The girl-cobra's head shoots forward and strikes Michael's hand. He's not sure if it is the girl's kiss or the cobra's bite.

He woke up. His first thought was *Maya* – illusion. And his flesh crawled, not in fear, but in anger.

Fifteen

The silence from Palm Beach continued. By now it was clear Allegra had a game plan, one hatched the moment she realized she could make it to Florida after all. This plan did not allow for a man to call her there since she was trying to create the impression of being unattached. Interested and available in America's richest playground where America's richest men, two thousand of them, were always looking for beautiful women. Especially women who radiated power, who played at being the stakes in a liaison with the highest bidder. And Allegra liked wealth. "My lifestyle," she used to say. "I'd never take a bus when I can ride in a cab." The Rolls-Royce. Poor Allegra, he thought, anger and bitterness in his heart. Was she doing it all over again? Looking for wealth and security, and the hell with trust and the man who so obviously was her soulmate?

"I only ask for semi-perfection in a man," she had written in answer to his ad, eons ago. It would be easy to find out her phone number: Allegra's office in St. Louis would tell him. But he wasn't going to stoop so low. If that was the game she wanted to play, Michael had misjudged her character. It was not honorable to behave this way toward him. And if she really meant what she had faxed in anger when the deadline had been upon her, that theirs was not an exclusive relationship… why was he hanging in there?

Michael was hurting. Hurting in a way that drove home again the depth of his feelings for this woman. Tree, she had made no promises, but the signals they had exchanged over these three months could not be misinterpreted. "I'm not strong enough to walk away from you," she had written. "You're very special to me, my darling. You are my soulmate and I adore you. I will not allow either of us to hurt each other." A noble sentiment. As long as she was in control. Thus subject to change without prior notification.

Michael looked at the Xmas presents that were still waiting for her. How lovingly had he chosen them! Would they be delivered? And the list of everything he wished for her to happen in the New Year. Never sent. Access denied.

And now? Where had his trust gone? Disappointment and anger were replacing it. "La donna e mobile," sings the Duke of Mantua as he merrily seduces women, while the woman who truly loves him winds up with a knife in her heart.

What would happen when she returned to New York? Would she do her faraway-look thing while searching for the right way to tell the truth?

Michael didn't want to think about it. But he'd be damned if he was going to track her down in Palm Beach. And the cobra girl floated into his vision.

Sixteen

Late Thursday afternoon, fifth of January, Michael decided to call Allegra's New York number, hoping for a message that would indicate the date of her return.

Allegra answered the phone, sounding annoyed. Michael's bewilderment threatened to become permanent. She explained. The Palm Beachers had had food poisoning, so she returned early. The sick ex, having been informed by her that there were other men in her life, threatened a money fight. And Michael was just like her father, asking her to check in "every second", which she would not buy into.

Why had she told her ex? A sick, insecure man who desperately wanted her back? To fan his jealousy, provoking him to exact revenge in money matters? And proud of how he took it? Did she still know so little about men? All her life she'd been on the cliffs of destructive relationships, getting knocked down time and again. And picking herself up time and again.

None of this made sense to Michael. So when Allegra called the next morning as she'd said she would, he faxed her the chapters of his story which dealt with the past week, his New Year's wishes for her, and his own resolutions. He also explained how she had driven him to his paranoid projections.

If he'd expected a reaction, any kind, but specifically one of understanding of what she'd put him through, her silence showed otherwise. This was a side of her he'd not met before: no regrets, no compassion. Quit bugging me. I'm in control. After they'd communicated daily, St. Louis-New York City for more than two weeks.

Michael stewed all day Friday, sending his intuition on a fact finding mission; it drew a blank; and he felt more and more alienated from her. Then he did something he hadn't done in over a year. It threw him back to a bad place though the call girl was friendly. No blame.

Saturday morning, January six, Michael called Allegra. Proposed lunch. She was on her way to spend the weekend in Connecticut. The book? Yes, Julie had sent out letters. Cool, distant. Back on Monday.

Fuck it. A good thing he had an article to proofread. Also, a patient with acute panic attacks was coming today, probably tomorrow as well. The problems of others always helped. Monday would come soon enough. And it would be her move.

Fuck it. Michael turned to the diary where he'd recorded how he and Allegra were evolving. He had done this to honor his dream of long ago when the Russian monk, Pimen, had recorded the past and future history of Russia; that dream had led to the rebirth of his creative writing. Allegra had loved the idea; she was hoping they would soon write a book together. Perhaps about the New York personal columns. In Puerto Rico.

On Monday, he faxed her his latest chapter. The result was an explosive accusation what a bastard he was. *"C'est fini,"* Allegra replied. She never wanted to see him again. The charge list was long and incomprehensible but the gist was, no one was going to abuse her, and he had done that. His diary, she said, was the evidence.

Baffled and upset, Michael pleaded for a chance to talk face to face. "You've terminated everything by fax," Allegra replied coldly. But she agreed to meet him on Thursday, eleventh of January (for which date he had ballet tickets), provided his behavior would be civil. He assured her it would.

What had he done? His story was an accurate portrayal of everything that had passed between them since their first meeting on third October, seen of course through the eyes of the writer. And until the confusion around New Year's Eve, communication had been warm and trusting, mutually supportive. Then, because of imprecise information, he fell prey to a terrible misperception of her reality. And from that moment everything he'd written had been with the voice of the wounded heart. Why couldn't she see that? Perhaps lunch on Thursday would bring clarification. Unless it was all a tragic, albeit unconscious conspiracy of what Allegra had threatened all along: She'd rather run away than commit to something, anything, involving a man.

At lunch, reprieve was granted. After a long and painful confrontation, anger and hostility were defused, care shining from her sapphire eyes. Spontaneously, Allegra grabbed his face, her cheeks touching his. Michael's voice cracked, raw feelings on the surface. He polished his glasses, not wanting people to see his tears. Good god, how strong were the social conventions still! Had they been alone, he would not have hidden the tears her gesture had coaxed forth

– challenging the patriarchal stereotype that men didn't weep.

They went over ancient battle grounds. "You pushed me too far, I don't want it, I can't handle it"... "I can't help it that I'm so deeply in love with you"... "If you suffer, it affects me too." Perhaps there would a ballet tonight.

It didn't turn out that way. Still, Michael was slowly climbing out of the slough of despond.

Allegra gave him a copy of her manuscript and he wanted to read the final version immediately. Smiling, she put a copy of his story into her capacious case. As she was rummaging through the papers, the brochure of the Austrian hunting lodge caught her eye. It took all his will power to conceal from her the images which arose unbidden in his inner vision: the mysterious, compelling urge to bury his face in the place of the most humble smells and tastes; the quivering of flesh, the hair, the wetness. To submit to her belly, to her other mouth. It would be the most potent of sexual acts, completely divorced from biology, the most secret of acts, an act of power derived from the most vulnerable kind of intimacy.

He vowed to keep his lips sealed. She'd barely gotten over her anger and distrust of him. And he, too, needed a hiatus to connect with their new present, slowly. So the images faded as they left the restaurant, and he was satisfied to slip his arm into hers, shaken as she impulsively kissed him on the eyes and lingered on his lips, tightly. And promised to call.

At home, Michael immersed himself in her book. Was it the energizing, complex frequencies of seeing her again after four weeks which were reluctant to fade and restore to him objective thought patterns, or had the book changed since he first read it? Astonished, he found it tight and gripping, difficult to put down.

Seventeen

At seven-thirty that evening, he stood in the lobby of the State Theater, unsure what to do with the two tickets for tonight's ballet. No one he knew was available on such short notice. Not being a ballet fan, he was reluctant to go by himself. He scanned the crowd streaming in: perhaps an attractive woman would show up in search of a last minute ticket to the sold-out performance. He'd be happy to offer it to her. No such luck. He did spot a pretty girl in jeans and boots, early twenties at most. Smiling, he said no to himself: this would truly be inappropriate. But he approached her. A lovely smile and good English revealed she was Dutch, a student of classical dance. First time in New York. A friend, male, was scouting for cheap tickets outside by the fountain. With a happy heart he offered her the best seats in the house, and received a gushing thank you. She dashed out to fetch her friend, a handsome kid, probably gay. They could not get over such generosity. "Only in rich America," said the boy. Wishing them good luck, he recalled the kissing high school kids who had inspired his osculator ad.

Back home in his easy chair and sipping his Bourbon, Michael puzzled about the unacknowledged underground storms against which she defended so forcefully. He thought he understood why. So much brutality, abuse, loss of trust… all of it at the hands of the men she had lived with, whom she had thought she loved at one time. Now she was free, free to live her life one day at a time, ready for whatever would engage her mind, her talents, her professionalism.

So why should she take another chance on a new man, one who could not support her, not remove the concern about money, one who was only in love with her and who might become possessive, jealous, if she did not live up to his expectations? Hadn't he already displayed disquieting attitudes? So much so that she was ready to break it off. Now she had given him a reprieve – but a commitment, however small, however intimate? With all the unresolved issues in her life? Indulge in a romantic fantasy without concrete foundation?

All this Michael understood, had understood almost from the day they'd met. And yet his feelings for her, his desire to hold her, nuzzle her, kiss her, kept rushing over him, a ceaseless stream of images, tactile sensations – or the deprivation thereof meant that all his senses were in motion, engaged in their respective function and design, tormenting him with desire, he only had to close his eyes, and her scent came off him like an intoxicating breeze.

Michael was on a wheel, the mysterious wheel of the Kabbalah, the wheel of starclusters around the immense horse-head nebula, twenty thousand light years out in another galaxy, spinning, spinning, unable to get off, and threatened to be flung into nothingness by the gravitational force of his love's monstrous desire.

("WOW!" he said out loud after writing that last sentence.)

Eighteen

Three days later, on a Sunday evening, Michael left a message on Allegra's phone. In French, he suggested dinner on Monday, *dans mon quartier,* and then go to his place to present her with the long overdue Xmas gifts. For a week there was silence.

Perhaps she was out of town, but it was curious that she'd let messages go unchecked; and quite out of character not to acknowledge a dinner invitation.

Once again he felt like being punished. Did she enjoy making him feel miserable? The idea was absurd. Still, she knew from his recent suffering how her silence tortured him. Paranoid projections shot unbidden to the surface: was she with the lover from the past?

Allegra had been emphatic about not wanting to be treated as the twelve-year old who needed to check in with Daddy. Michael understood that fully. But this was different. His longing for her presence, or just her voice, or at least a message, stemmed from the purest desire a man in love felt when the beloved was absent: he could not help radiating it out to the universe, waiting for an echo from space, without which there was only the cosmic void, the far edge of the solar system, somewhere near the orbit of Pluto where the temperature was absolute zero on the Kelvin scale, or minus two hundred and seventy-three degrees C.

The only thing soothing his existential anxiety was to keep writing their story, even though no new data was available, However, his tormented feelings were unfailingly available: "Je besoin de toi.'

If anybody needed to he centered now, it was he. He was so far from his own balanced resting point, the molecules of his body were struggling to find their proper configuration: the pieces, which when properly aligned made up his well-defined identity – the neurons, vessels, muscles, bones – had been flung randomly across his inner landscape, tenuously strung together by her name, Allegra.

By chance, it was revealed that she'd never received his French message; Julie was suspected of erasing it. Only now, a week after their lunch, was she off to Washington, would return in four days. Rationally, the pause had been appropriate; he'd been forgiven, and returning to daily contacts would reawaken the specter of pressure. But his longing for her blew reason away, swatting it like a pesky insect buzzing around his heart. His frustration – would she call it neediness again? – led to a phone call she had taunted him with that night at the opera: Joy, the bathing suit lady, another respondent to his osculator ad, was thrilled to hear from him, and a date was arranged.

Immediately Michael chided himself. Had he so little faith that Allegra would eventually respond to his fervent courtship? She certainly wasn't making things easy. Though his awful mis-perceptions had been cleared up, she had not called him in a week. At first, he took it as penance, but with each passing day his yearning got the better of him. And images, similar to those he had suppressed before now, invaded him with ferocious intensity.

Michael knew there were rivers in her that no one had ever discovered, lands that no man had explored. That somewhere in that unexplored darkness stood a temple, surrounded by water and accessible only by a narrow, dangerously swaying suspension bridge. And if he managed to cross it, he would come upon a massive door, covered with ivy, and a hidden cleft within the climbing vines would lead him inside the sanctuary where she lay, gloriously nude, round and soft, the ancient smells of the Goddess in heat rising from her body. Why did Allegra defend so tenaciously against the wisdom of her blood? Was she so unaware how her sensuality shone in her eyes, luxuriating catlike in the fluidity of her movements? How her lips became fuller when she looked at him even though her body language was one of protestations, one hand always held up, palmside, warding him off. Yes, he knew what she had been through, how she'd been violated, her femininity ripped apart by the men who did not know they were defiling the goddess.

Michael had to make it up to her, must apologize for these brutes, had to banish the shame and fear she harbored, and impart his knowledge of her sacred vessel which must be restored to its terrible beauty so she could freely receive the offerings due her as the Queen of the Night; she who truly reigned over the dark magic of sex.

With these powerful images criss-crossing his awareness, he wondered about meeting Joy. It was a most confusing state of mind for a first date. On his way to the bar at the Top of the Sixes, a sudden thought caught him up sharp: Michael had not slept with a woman in almost two years. He didn't mean sex, but the warm embrace of a beloved body, the delicious closeness of sleeping skin to skin, entwined, entangled with the soft shapes of breasts, belly, buttocks, and most important, inhaling the fragrant silkiness of hair, burying his face. The thought created an instant, hollow pang of emptiness, as if some part of himself, some invisible lifeline had left him, floated away, as hopelessly out of reach as the fruit poor Tantalos was condemned not to reach until the end of time.

Michael remembered Allegra's body the night of the rainstorm, when he touched, caressed and kissed her breasts, stroking her open, scented hair. He shuddered at the memory which sent fiery flashes across his face, burning his mouth; and his lips puckered as if he'd bitten into a lemon.

Why was he going to the Top of the Sixes? The surface part was a puny gesture to get back at Allegra for keeping him at a distance. Childish, really. But it went deeper than that. Responding to an unknown woman who wanted to meet him was gratifying to his maleness, a test if he could still pour on the charm should he find her attractive enough to enter into the ritual dance of dating. And what if she really was attractive and indicated that he appealed to her as well?

No, he said to himself, no woman could displace what he felt for Allegra. Racing way past infatuation, it had become for him a love so intense, a desire so fierce, he wanted to be with her every day, share her bed every night, would want to marry her if circumstances allowed it. Just the thought of being in her presence elicited a rush of feelings, a desire to shower her with presents, the consuming wish to be the man in her life whom she would truly trust, and ultimately love unconditionally.

The thought of walking by the Plaza made him want to turn around. But a gentleman wouldn't tolerate such crudeness. He would meet Joy. But be true to himself. And true to her who carried his soul-image.

Nineteen

Prior to this evening's date, Allegra's fax greeted him in the morning like the sun breaking through a wall of fog: his melancholy, cloud-covered heart of darkness (pace friend Conrad!) skipped a couple of beats before resuming a powerful pumping, rich arterial blood flooding his body, the Oklahoma kind, "Oh, what a beautiful morning!" But her fax was anything but joyful: there were new troubles with the Angel of Death.

Michael met Allegra for lunch at his own neighborhood watering hole. Ravishingly beautiful as always, she exuded agitated depression. In a pathologically exaggerated fashion, Julie had lashed into her for insignificant errors in the manuscript, doubtless because her grandiose handling of the book was being questioned, a sacrilegious insult to her egomania, like doubting the holiness of the Pope. Michael squeezed her hand reassuringly, but his heart, so joyful a couple of hours ago, was heavy – once again aware how this survivor encountered turbulence wherever she went. No wonder her shoulders were always hurting. Michael wanted to kiss them and tell the little girl she refused to accept in herself that a good night's sleep would make it all better, that tomorrow would be a sunny day when she could play with her friends, and there would be no homework either.

He shook himself out of this paternal reverie, and they went over to his apartment. As Allegra walked through Michael's rooms for the first time, the sun flooded them as he embraced the woman who stood in his very own healing space, He concealed the desire to crush her until she was quiet again, and to never let her go. Her presence in his place became something religious, connecting him with the wounds from which both were bleeding: sacrifices needing to be offered and accepted, to appease the gods.

The long delayed Xmas presents were placed in her lap. His choices pleased her. "What exquisite Italian lingerie," she gushed. Coquettish. Allegra then read his latest chapters, laughing and caressing his hand, not the least bit surprised about his impending date with Joy. Instantly, his paranoia clicked in: was she hoping Joy would take him off her plate?

Nonsense. This time he felt certain she knew that he was an anchor that held. The battle over Puerto Rico continued, but in soft pastel tones; it touched on what her ex might do if he found out – though she'd told him she was seeing someone in New York. Michael felt her anxiety and tried to defuse it. More relaxed, Allegra accepted the offer of his hospitality – even liked the room that would be hers – and he could have kissed the makeup off her face.

But her literary agent was the absolute priority of the moment. Michael counted on the Dragon Lady's inflated self-esteem, which would be fatally damaged if she failed to fulfil her part of the contract. He urged Allegra to keep cool, and to stay with him, if only to escape the noxious fumes the dragon kept exhaling through her malignant nostrils.

And in three days she'd go back to St. Louis to babysit with a sweet grandchild, then drive her Rolls to New York, returning the first week in February, his Aquarian birthday month. And he was sentenced to another two weeks of solitary guard duty. Guard duty? But of course, he had to guard his love against the likes of Lady Joy whom he was to meet that very evening. He would meet Allegra for a drink Wednesday afternoon, day after tomorrow.

Twenty

The bar on the Top of the Sixes is arguably the quietest spot in town. The view makes you gasp, the drinks and snacks a class act. Joy was punctual and Michael rose to greet her. The picture she'd sent was a fair enough representation of her physical appearance except for her face, which was anything but pretty. Trim and muscular, she wore a red silk suit revealing an overly exposed cleavage. Her black hair was medium long, her eyes a color not part of the visible spectrum, the mouth slightly pinched and the voice – well, it wasn't really the voice which Michael found so off-putting. Rather, it was an extroversion of the most fearsome kind: she talked, and talked, and talked. Behind her words was the sort of energy he associated with pumping iron, and sure enough, she was a gym freak. He minced no words about her barreling down a truck lane, and it worked. She slowed down, and turned out to be an intelligent, well-informed woman in a top executive position, managing the portfolios of several prominent people, mostly movie stars. She consumed two glasses of red wine in rapid succession while he nursed an exotic rum drink whose only benefit was the attractive glass he could keep as a souvenir.

It became quickly evident that Joy found him appealing, and had the guts to say so. Briefly flattered, Michael felt like a fraud, knowing he would never want to see her again. But she played it smart, drawing him out in his professional expertise by relating rather intimate details of her dating experience. He matched her candor, told her about Lisa and Allegra, portraying the latter as a "femme inspiratrice" who mostly lived in a distant city, but led such a fascinating life that it provided him with material for a story he was writing. He inwardly apologized to Allegra, knowing that she would approve of the way he was handling himself in a situation he didn't really care to be in.

They found some common ground in movies and medicine (she'd been married to a cardiologist, her third marriage), and as they parted she pointedly expressed an interest in Jungian analysis. He replied that there was no such thing as a free lunch, and she took that well, a good sport, in good spirits. Exiting 666, she kissed him hard, arms around his neck, then jumped into a cab, athletically, heading for Grand Central.

He walked slowly west on fifty-fourth street, past the deserted MOMA building, shaking his head, and thinking for no clear reason of Allegra's long earrings and the fact she'd not worn a bra under her white sweater. And how much he'd liked that. Though Sixth Avenue was dark and cold, the wind howling from the east, he had this warm sensation that he and Allegra had been lovers for a long, long time, probably several lifetimes over, and that in one of those past lives they'd had twins, inexplicably named Sean and Mirella.

Twenty-one

On Wednesday, twenty-fourth of January, Michael waited for Allegra in the familiar surroundings of the Chandler murals. He hadn't been at the Cafe des Artistes in several years. Vaguely, he recalled a dinner there with Lisa, celebrating either her or his birthday, the owner, George Lang, toasting them with some rare Hungarian vintage. Michael was sipping a Manhattan, a cocktail associated with the 50's, his total being attuned to Allegra's arrival. The bar was still empty, and when she swept in, his heart did the usual extra-systolic leap. Time and again her beauty threw him. Of course, the anticipated image was always idealized, but when he saw her in the flesh, her eyes focused on him as she did her quick, coat-shedding movements, simultaneously touching her hair and his hand, all in the same slightly nervous fashion – then the ideal paled before the incandescent reality of this breathtaking woman. His persona remained smooth, polished, wordly. But inside him raged the kind of storm which made Ulysses beg his shipmates to tie him to the mast, else he would fall prey to the Sirens' song and stay on their enchanted island forever. Belying the uproar, he calmly inquired about the events of the past two days.

Yes, the Dragon Lady had apologized, and was given sixty days in which to make good on her end of the deal. Then, sexily curious, an iota of jealousy in the wings, Allegra asked about his adventure at the Top of the Sixes. He'd brought his latest chapter and she read it, chuckling, then laughing out loud. Her mirth made him wish that the ropes be tightened around the mast, for the lights dancing in her eyes couldn't keep him sitting sedately on his bar stool. Those dancing lights were like trembling votive candles in front of the Madonna's chapel in some old church, Italy perhaps, or Spain, and they spoke of the spiritual flame steadfastly burning in Allegra's magnificent body whose voluptuousness could easily mislead those who had not been initiated into woman's mysteries. At such moments, lasting only seconds, his love for her became a primal urge to merge with her, to fulfil a destiny that had made them come together, to create.

Allegra talked about Robbie, the man from her recent past. Michael listened, argued, questioned. Jealous, yes – how could he not be? but concerned more about her true motives: how could she dismiss the way Robbie had dumped her? Perhaps now that he'd left his wife, the dump did not count any more. And they did have a history of some intimacy. Skin deep. Like his handwriting: small, mean, pinched, an ungenerous soul. Still, this man got her where she was most vulnerable: her loyalty.., and money. Michael knew how fierce her loyalty was: for years she'd proved it with husband number four, the sick man in St. Louis; now that Robbie might have a serious illness, she was determined to be loyal to him, had in fact set the twenty-eight of February as the date when she'd say yes or no to a permanent commitment.

Michael knew better. Which always infuriated her.

"How do you know you love me?"

"Forget about our magical twins," Michael said, "though I'm convinced we're their parents, that's how an intuitive 'knows', and that's how I know that no man has ever understood you, loved you the way I do. No, I can't support you, and, yes, you may marry Robbie or someone else, even if you make it on your own – which you will – because somehow marriage has always been important to you. Remember when you said, 'Find me a gay husband and we can be lovers'?"

And so it went. They did not really fight. In fact, the more poor Robbie was being talked about and his diagnosis worsened, the more ardent, youthful and exuberant Michael became. And Allegra didn't get mad; she'd already promised Valentine's day to Robbie, but Michael's birthday was the fifteenth of February, and there was only one present he wanted, and wanted it like nothing he'd ever wanted before in many a decade. She would consider it, she said, then vacillated between yes and no all the way along Central Park West as they walked toward that fixed point in her life, the bar at San Sabato. (Why wouldn't she let him drop her off there? Oh games, games!) He was shouting his love in front of the Mayflower hotel, wanting to tear her clothes off. "Please let's rent a suite here for the night," he'd begged ages ago.

"Mail me your story to St. Louis," she said, kissing him goodbye, saying maybe again to his birthday wish, waving, waving. She promised to be in touch, and to call in case she needed a co-driver; he would love that, for there'd be many motels along the way.

Twenty-two

On Thursday she left, yet by Sunday Michael was frantic. Silence again. Though the tension between them which had accumulated since the unfortunate Palm Beach episode, had relaxed, the newly announced deadline of February twenty-eight was yet another fire and water test, the Magic Flute all over again. He was the punching bag, and she kept delivering the punches, oblivious to his feelings. "Don't push me." He had express-mailed her his story, three days ago, begging her to call.

But frantic was not how he really felt. He was getting angry. What would it cost her to pick up the phone in St. Louis, or turn on her fax, so that he wouldn't feel so cut off? Considerate of the sick ex, Michael did not want to call her. On her high horse, Allegra was the champion of loyalty. To what? To whom? Four times she had married men who were bad choices: a youthful innocent folly; a gay guy; an abusive sociopath with an "abnormally large cock"; and, finally, a father substitute, now sick and infirm, whom she'd never loved but had been loyal to in return for his supporting her in a grand lifestyle. Until he had gambled away her money, leading to divorce number four. Then last year in New York, she'd become intimate with Robbie who had been helpful with her book. This paragon had then dropped her when her body struck him as too fat, her status not wealthy enough to warrant a continued liaison.

Then she met Michael through the New York personals. Something bloomed she had never experienced with another man. Michael was different, there was truth and trust in a fast developing relationship. But once again, her power-hungry animus kept interfering. She did not want to see what Michael could do for her devastated and defiled femininity. With pretences galore, she kept holding him at bay, claiming the priorities of her book and her overflowing plate: money, job, apartment. The book.

And now, with Robbie having left his wife, changing his mind about Allegra's waistline and dangling the diamond bangles before her blue eyes, the same eyes which were holding Michael spellbound, he felt choked in his love for her. But Robbie was now sick, perhaps malignantly so. Ah, the cue: "He needs me,I must be loyal to him." Money was beckoning in the distance, fool's gold once again. From his long professional experience, Michael knew that unconsciousness could not be fought. A blind woman, especially with a power animus in charge, could not be made to see, could not recognize true love and trust when it was in front of her face, even if the blindness had reduced her to a mere survivor of four marital disasters.

Michael had to face two questions. One, why had he fallen so hard for a woman with that history? And two, what was he going to do about it? The first one was easy. He had always been the rescuer, the man who often succeeded in healing wounds other men had inflicted. His soul was warm, generous and yearning to redeem the feminine whenever she'd been hurt. With Allegra, there was the powerful attraction of having found a fellow writer, an incredibly beautiful woman with a true funny bone, who shared his vision that sex and spirituality were the essential components of a lasting relationship.

The larger problem was the second question. How long was he going to allow himself to be battered by her whom he truly and passionately loved, yet who played games of cruel ambivalence, not even conscious of how desperately he waited to hear from her? Sadistic she was not. Uncaring neither. Mixed up, yes; a full plate, yes; afraid to be pushed, yes. But why did she not jump into the very arms, which could give her the centering comfort she craved? Didn't she even know how badly she craved it? Was it all obscured by her power drive: 'I'm in control and I know what I need?" And the permanent refrain: "Don't push me."

Michael was beginning to hate her; this, he well knew, was the dark side of loving someone so deeply that the shadow was free to emerge. He was sick at heart, it felt like the end of his life. He was falling into an abyss unless she extended her hand by coming to her senses, and knowing where the real gold was. In a curious way, his heart seemed to grow bigger as the energies of love and hate were feeding on each other.

The Marquis de Sade would have relished Michael's self torture as Sunday night retreated before the wan light of Monday morning. Doubtless the Marquis would have preferred overt whipping, birch or cane, but the hot spikes Michael kept driving through his love/ hate-sick mind provided enough stimulation for any devoted masochist.

Allegra's message changed all that. Was he okay, she inquired; the kids were keeping her busy, she'd call later.

Sunlit skies swam again before his eyes. Three patients and a sandwich later, he took his coffee to his bedroom, intending to nap. But what occurred instead, was a sleepy kind of daydream in which he made love to Allegra, the details so deliciously real, it would have taken just a couple of strokes…

The locale was vague, but suffused with comfort. There were flowers, a crystal pitcher holding a pink liquid, an enormous bed, pillows, duvets, lace, all in shades of ivory. Allegra's scent, aromatic, perfumed the air, and there she was on the bed, wearing the pajamas and earrings – he had given her. Her hair was open, no makeup on her face, those aquamarine eyes looking at him, coquettishly, as if she were both very young and the mature woman she actually was. She opened her arms, an invitation to paradise, and the slowest, exquisitely drawn out kissing began. His lips touched her face, her neck, slipped into her ears. The earrings came off. He kissed her nose, her eyelids, purposely staying away from her mouth. Her arms were around his neck, she was yielding up her body, wonderfully passive, letting him love her. He unbuttoned the pajama top, drawing circles with his lips over the slowly revealing skin. His lips brushed a nipple, feather light, quickly moving away from it again. Now their lips met for the first time in the heavenly setting this incredible fantasy provided., they kissed lightly at first, but seconds later their mouths were glued to one another, tongues probing, tentatively.

He could feel that she wanted to become active, kissing his chest, but he begged her to let him drink his fill, to just receive his love which had been on the brink of overflowing for so long.

"I'd like to give you my love, too," Allegra murmured. "I'm not used to being loved without returning it."

'I know, darling," Michael whispered, "but indulge me, please, I want to send you on the road to eternity first, and then it can be your turn…"

She smiled. 'It'll be a new experience for me, I'm usually the giver, but… okay." She relaxed into the sheets, eyes closed.

Now his caresses covered her breasts. Her surprisingly small nipples responded to his warm lips, and a small moan fled from her. Her face turned sideways, into a pillow, the open hair black and lustrous against the ivory. He moved to her feet, slowly sucking each toe, swiftly moving up to grab her left hand, sucking there as well. Ever so slowly, the pajama bottom was pulled down. His lips went to her thigh, close to her mound. Time stood still as he kissed his way down her thigh, lingering on her calves. He backed up to her navel, the sacred omphalos which is the entrance to the other world, licking, licking.

"I need to touch you,"Allegra whispered, and he swung around, her hand finding his penis, holding. Without conscious volition, she opened her legs. Softly, he blew on the treasure she was revealing. The hairs glistened where a few honeyed drops had come to rest. The musky scent, mixed with verbena, was intoxicating. His tongue began to trace her lips, and they slowly turned a dark pink. As he continued to explore her, he got a glimpse of the lavender folds, his tongue reaching deep inside her, sipping the moisture, now dripping freely.

Like a butterfly alighting on a flower, his tongue flicked for a moment over her clit. Allegra gasped. Suddenly overcome, she let go of his penis and grabbed his head with both hands, pressing him into her. His tongue circled her clit, gently pushing the hood aside, sucking now rhythmically. From nowhere, he was holding a vibrator inside her while his lips continued loving her wetness.

Abandoning, surrendering, she floated into the joy, seeking the ecstasy, allowing herself to be enclosed in the rapture. Jolts of delight radiated from her center, as feline growls and little breath-catching sobs collided in her throat, struggling to escape. Helpless, trembling in her passion, the growling cat changed into a supplicating woman: "Oh God, yes," she pleaded, her head moving rapidly from side to side. Her body was no longer her own: an orgiastic power was possessing it, pushing her, spiraling upward, toward an unknown peak where she would surely die.

"Le petit mort," *he felt it. He had never known such pleasure in his life. All his senses were merging with the lust she was feeling. As her orgasm was building, he had an image of flying through the night toward the full moon, securely holding her hips, and when she came in wave after wave, melting and sizzling, he remained glued to her, drinking the nectar that kept coming.*

Recovering slowly, Allegra felt totally relaxed and centered. And she wanted to be the giver now. But Michael's mouth gave her no respite; it remained fastened to her source, and with infinite tenderness he sent her off on the next round of their erotic carousel, pausing only to switch his mouth from lips to lips. Like a composer at the keys of a newly tuned organ, he played her body, touching it like he'd been given a music score to her most sensitive secret spots, the paths to her pleasure. She couldn't believe it. But her trust was now solid, and she learned what it meant to come again and again.

"Love, my love," he breathed, so softly she could not hear him. "I shall never love again the way I love you; you are the last terminal on my lifeline. Beyond you, there's oblivion."

His alarm was ringing. The next patient was due in fifteen minutes.

Twenty-three

On the fourth day, third of February, a fax arrived.

It was a remarkable document, especially the sequence in which Allegra listed the salient points: "1 – Manuscript corrected. 2 – Robbie has prostate cancer, I'll be at his side through this ordeal. 3 – I will spend three hours with you on your birthday, eight to eleven p.m. 4 – With Robbie's help (read money, Michael thought), I'll have a new apartment. 5 – I'11 drive to New York, leaving tonight, can be reached via car phone for next three days. 6 – I'm thinking of you often as my soulmate and friend, wishing you'd understand."

Michael was not really surprised. Pissed yes, no doubt about that. But above all, feeling manipulated and used. How could she be so blind? After all the therapy she'd had, all that she went through with sick or crazy men, why was she still so horibly unconscious? Robbie drops her, she meets Michael who is different from any man she's known; he genuinely falls in love with her, matches and complements her in so many wonderful ways… and she goes back to Robbie, who has now left his wife and has cancer, as Michael predicted only a week ago! And of course, Robbie asks her to be with him and she says yes. An act of friendship, understandably. Michael didn't care about Robbie's prognosis. He cared only for Allegra. Hadn't she learned anything at all in her life? One more sick man to tend to? Did she think his "ordeal" was a one-time thing, or was she insane enough to commit to a long-term relationship, his divorce, their marriage, pre-nuptial agreements, with a man who would never again live a normal life? No doubt his wife would get involved, now that he was diagnosed. And he might go back to her, a frequent pattern when terminal illness strikes.

And Michael, the only healthy, vital man in her life, encountered through a "meaningful coincidence", who truly loves her, is now supposed to be the "friend and soulmate", hours limited, eight to eleven p.m., fifteenth of February. Is this the giving nature she believes she possesses? The kind which alleviates suffering? Indeed not. Ungenerous. Playing Vestal virgin. A crude slang term would be even more appropriate.

She was unwilling to open her arms for even one night, just to talk, to pour out her heart, trusting him who knew how to center her; to give him the loving gift of her presence on his birthday. That too would be loyalty. Loyalty to the force that brought them together. Otherwise, she might just as well send him a birthday card. It was insulting to be thought of as a time slot in her calendar, squeezed in as an obligatory gesture.

And all this huge reshuffling of the deck via fax! She hadn't phoned him in days, knowing he was home. Talk of avoiding personal communication! No doubt she must have been upset by the news. Still she didn't reach for the hand that could pull her to safety. Her inflation was monumental.

Yes, Michael was her friend and soulmate; he loved her as a man who wanted her, needed her for a profound love relationship, relishing their joint creativity, sexually and spiritually. He wanted a true, genuine love affair, which would heal the wounds she was continually inflicting on herself and on him as well.

"Wake up, Allegra," he shouted to the walls, pacing about in his room. "Wake up before your life goes down the drain!" Sputtering angrily, he continued his tormented soliloquy. "By all means, stand by Robbie as the friend you are, the friendship you apparently owe him, but love ME as I love YOU, and I will support your standing by him, will console you when he gets worse, but for your sake and mine, make a commitment to us! Come to your senses, Allegra (enter here all your married names, as reminders how often you screwed up), and don't miss out on some joy in your future! Remember the man you wanted around when you were all alone preparing Xmas dinner at five-thirty a.m.? There is such a man, just reach out and touch him, he is real!

"Surely, Robbie will be grateful for your support now that he's received his grim sentence and is counting on your well known loyalty. But for him to confuse friendship with sexual fidelity would be like a sick child not wanting his mommy to go out and do her own thing. And this goes for you in spades: do you want to put your centering love life on hold until Robbie dies, next month or two years from now, just because YOU can't differentiate between friendship and sexual fidelity, foregoing the joys of being in another man's arms, safe and protected, while simultaneously offering your devoted friendship to a dying man?

"Curiously, your February horoscope in *Vanity Fair* reads as follows: "Why must you always hook up with people whom you end up carrying across a minefield otherwise known as your life? These 'saviors' reveal struggles with intimacy, dangerous health issues, or a dozen other problems that make it impossible for you to lay your head on a breast without having to listen for the heartbeat. Jupiter is in your seventh house now, though, so that's all changed. Someone is there. Someone understands you. Someone cares deeply. The question is: Can you take it?"

Exhausted, he poured himself a drink.

By Tuesday night, Michael figured, Allegra should arrive in New York, and would park her silver Rolls in the garage thoughtfully provided by Robbie before he got the bad news. Michael would wait for her call. And pray for her sate journey. To the City. And to his heart, the road to which was marked in giant red letters. Spelling LOVE.

Twenty-four

On Wednesday, February seven, around noon, he found the fax. His mind reeled. A "Dear John" letter from Allegra.

Michael blew up. And screamed three outraged messages into her answering machine. She was back in New York, with the Rolls no doubt, and had nothing better to do that very first day than to dump him? Dump him by fax! Quite in character, he realized, just like the fax from St. Louis, just one small difference: the birthday promise, the insulting eight p.m. to eleven p.m. entry in her social calender, was reneged on. "Compassion" was replacing it. Contradictions of explanations. Duality everywhere. Madness.

To preserve the integrity of his story, Michael decided to reproduce the fax in its entirety.

"Feb seven. Dear Michael, Your story is heartbreaking, and moves me greatly. Much of what you, the author, writes is true. I am filled with compassion for this hero, for it seems to me, that he has been stricken with a deep and fatal attraction and love for this woman, Allegra, me, and that certainly she is undeserving and unfeeling, to say the least. I know that I'm struggling with lots of emotions, and that I'm giving mixed messages to your narrator which is cruel and unfair. I have great feeling for Michael, but I'm filled with guilt for the way things have progressed. For months, I've wrestled with trying to put the relationship into some sense of perspective for Michael that their relationship, from her p.o.v, is a friendship and cannot be anything else at this moment in time. I want desperately to ease your pain, which consumes me daily with such guilt that it is easier to avoid him. I'm feeling great remorse and wish I could erase your pain, but my needs are so clearly different from his that the communication between them is nonexistent. How sad! I believe, knowing Allegra as well as I do, that she hopes to preserve a special friendship with this very unique man, Michael. I think he is most intelligent, sensitive, and deserving of a great love. The problem is that Allegra is not ready, is still in love with Robbie, whether it be right or wrong, and the sad thing is that Michael's love for her made her aware of hidden feelings that she still carried for Robbie. The compassionate thing, and the thing that must be done, to preserve Michael's sanity, is for me to stop all communication with him. I cannot bear Michael's torment, pain and frustration. The sad thing is that it will be my loss. I still want badly to write a book with Michael. But more than that, I need, and this is purely selfish, peace of mind knowing that Michael is going on to be productive and active with his life, not consumed with me and my problems – my challenges – and not consumed with whether or not I am playing 'games', which I have not been doing, or telling 'half-truths' to hide my true feelings from Michael. Sometimes, letting go, regardless of the loss, is the kindest act of all. Keep writing. You have a great gift. With love, Allegra.'

And Allegra, having heard his screaming messages, replied with an icy fax, dripping with sizzling fury.

"I cannot tell you how damaging your three phone calls have been. Julie heard all of them and was furious when I walked in – thinking I've been conducting a torrid love affair here. I'm out of here. I'm staying at a hotel until Friday evening. Then a friend and I are going up to look at property in the Hamptons and on Cape Cod and visit my cousin in Boston. I have appointments to see apartments tomorrow and Friday. I am not seeing Robbie other than for business purposes. We both came to an agreement. I don't want to see you or talk to you or receive letters or faxes. I don't owe you anything other than a face to face with you as a matter only of respect for you. I will not take harassment from you and will not be threatened. I made a promise for your birthday, but after reading your story, realized that it would be inappropriate in every way. I made errors in my life. Who hasn't? I will most likely continue but it will be my choice and mine alone and I will be responsible for any consequences. I did not 'dump' you by fax. I said I did not wish to see you or talk to you, that it was the compassionate thing to do. I am sorry that you 'genuinely' love me but I do not believe that you are the only man who can truly understand me or truly love me. The important issue is that I'm not in love with you. Your threat that you won't let me go is ridiculous for no human being can hold someone in bondage. You will let me go if I wish to go or I will take legal measures that will be very embarrassing for you. If you wish to see me face to face – I can see you Friday for lunch – twelve-thirty or so. Since you will not be able to contact me, I will call you from my hotel and see if you want this. *C'est tout,* Michael. Allegra.'

Now, because of that crazy bitch Julie, Allegra is "out of here", blaming – who else? – him. He could just see Julie, playing Grand Inquisitor: had Allegra been carrying on a torrid love affair in her apartment? What if she had? Did the Angel of Death consider the place a nunnery?

But Allegra's language stunned Michael. She'd "take legal action" if he didn't let her go. Before his very eyes, her picture underwent a radical metamorphosis: this was not the loving, caring and giving woman she had professed to be all along: a vengeful fury, straight out of the "Eumenides" clawed at him in her lines. Like in classical mythology, when the gods punished some hapless shepherd because he'd fallen in love with a nymph (who happened to be one of Zeus' daughters with another nymph – Zeus was big on dallying with nymphs), Michael thought the earth would open up and fling him into Hades, the realm of the undead. But one insight from his dream blazed brilliantly: it wasn't the girl's kiss, but the cobra's bite his hand had received. Was the venom going to kill him?

He could not grasp what was happening. Here it was, a week before Valentine's and his birthday, and he had just bought her a ring, rubies and diamonds, even though he'd accepted her spending Valentine with Robbie and his malignant prostate (all changed, by the way, "we've come to an agreement", more games). Perhaps stirred by her rarely wakeful conscience, she offered, as a "matter of respect" to have lunch on Friday prior to taking the Rolls to the Hamptons in search of property. My, my. This time his Palm Beach suspicions, wrong as they were according to her version, were palpable reality. Only the Hamptons would do: they, the Rolls and Allegra would go well together, and a man to finance all this would not be hard to find, love not being part of her requirements, so either poor doomed Robbie or some other sucker would do nicely. About Friday, Michael was of two minds. For the moment, he needed to vent his darkness before it choked him and he was damned if he was going to die on her. Whether he actually wanted to see her face to face and try to defuse the shit she was dishing out, he'd leave that to his unconscious: a dream would guide him, as it always did.

And so he vented, spewing bile, not attempting to rewrite anything, just letting it flow as if he were indeed talking to her magnificent, beautiful, lying face, without having to put up with her uplifted, protesting hand. That his love for her had rekindled her amorous feelings for Robbie was not really sad, as she put it; it was hilarious in its idiocy. But in character.

Michael opened his steam valve and tile underground treasure, like priceless oil, gushed and caught fire because he refused to cap the well.

He decided to address what now looked like the final chapter of THE OSCULATOR AND THE LADY, a true-life love story, had it not foundered on her seemingly small, niggardly soul, which contained riches beyond her wildest dreams, were she to entrust him the key. That night, an image he knew well from his life with Lisa, returned in his dream.

On a beach, moving down from the olive grove, a woman with her back to him, walked slowly into the sea. Michael wanted to follow her, but she turned and faced him, shaking her head. The No was a divine command.

Michael walked up the hill to the olive trees, and sat down on ancient stone steps leading to a temple. Flutes sounded from somewhere inside, and he walked into the sanctuary. A giggle made him look back: half concealed by an olive tree a young woman was playing peek-a-boo. Michael smiled, gratefully, and continued walking toward the sound of the flutes.

On waking Michael wrote to Allegra.

"Do you ever wonder, Allegra, why you answered an osculator's ad, a man who was into kissing, not just into escorting you around? Ever think about the consequences of your actions? Apparently only after you've discharged your, venom. Yes, my story is heartbreaking, but it is only my heart that is breaking, not yours. You nimbly escape to Hampton land, the right place for your first-class lifestyle where someone will support you, just as your last husband has done, now gone to his solitary reward alter fourteen loyal years.

"How could you do this to me? To the first man who shoved the mirror in your face because he loved you in spite of the mess you are?

"And games? You're a woman whose victims litter the landscape, yet you're the most tragic victim yourself. You say you cannot bear my pain, torment and frustration, and so the 'compassionate' thing to do is to cut yourself off from me, like ripping the oxygen hose from someone whose breathing depends on it. I would have done anything for you to keep you centered. But I will not relieve your guilt for tearing up the bond we had, which was my lifeline to love and creativity. You are (and this late eye-opening feels like a vise around my heart) what the heroine of your book comes to realize about herself, 'a complete phony.' Her ex-boyfriend Adam says it well in a letter. 'I don't think you can ever enjoy an adult, intimate relationship with a male.' How prophetic! But Adam was smart: he loved her, would always love her, but got out before she damaged his heart irreparably. 'A child-woman,' he called her. Well, Michael could only agree.

"And have you changed, decades and several marital disasters later? Sadly, no. And do you recognize a possible change when one comes your way? Sadder still, no.

"But me, you have changed irreparably. My story, our story, Allegra, may be the last thing I will write. With one pitiless stroke you've killed my muse. Were you a grown woman, you'd have found another way to stay related to a soulmate, with whom you also enjoyed the deepest caress. Yet vacillating all the time about going to bed with me, wanting to, not wanting to, afraid your lifestyle could somehow be compromised. But my flame kept on burning. And for destroying me, I will not give you peace of mind. Let the bad dreams return.

"In the unlikely event that the above, written straight from my slashed and bleeding heart, should cause a light to go on in that mind of yours that can't find a center, you know where to find me. If I'm still around."

Twenty-five

On Friday, ninth of February, Michael met Allegra at the Plaza. Not for lunch, only to hand her the final chapters of their story. A love story, which ended because of a woman's lie, and a man's outraged exposure of it. Her chance for a promising bond to lighten the darkness and redeem her mistakes, was carelessly destroyed by her illusions. A woman blind to her true nature, and refusing to try on the glasses which could restore her sight. The tragedy of it struck him as cosmic, a violent spurning of what had been decreed.

In her black fur coat, Allegra stood by the little table in the lobby going through the paper, perhaps looking for apartments. She looked small and haggard. And angry. Molto agitato e furioso.

"You have hurt me terribly, Allegra," said Michael. Her response was quick and mean. "Four months can't be as bad as ten years." Nonplussed, it took him a moment to realize she was referring to his relationship with Lisa. "You've given me the loneliest New Year's

Eve of my life, and now the saddest of all birthdays," he managed to say. "Quite an accomplishment."

But the outstretched palm was already in the air, warding him off. And without another word or a glance she walked away, a small angry figure in black.

What he'd wanted to say arrived a few seconds too late. "I wouldn't want to live with your conscience." But that was water over a dam that had already burst two days ago, and the freshly roaring flood would make no difference. Funny how that woman in black, receding into the left corridor of the Plaza, in the direction of the Oyster Bar, now struck him as the incarnation of evil, man-eating and self-devouring at the same time. Still, his foolish heart, now bloodless and frozen in anger, would most likely have been transported to heaven or hell, had she decided to continue to bewitch him.

Michael was kidding himself. With all trust gone, Allegra had become a specter, neurotically sell:righteous, unlikely ever to heal herself. It would be a long time before he could see straight again. He felt like an emergency room physician who failed to reverse a cardiac arrest, no matter what resource he applied.

The patient died. Time of death: eleven-fifty-two a.m., ninth of February, the Plaza Hotel, New York City.

Twenty-six

How comfortably she could have stayed in his apartment! Safe from Julie's hassles, he would have spoiled her, softening up her stubborn "survival" label which she wore as if it were the Congressional Medal of Honor. Loved her, he would have, honoring the ambivalence she chose to place on their intimacy. They would have laughed a lot, and eventually she would have thought of this eccentric arrangement with the funny bone she possessed in such abundance.

With her car now in town, they would have spent lovely weekends in old Connecticut inns, relaxed and safe. Centered, she would have looked for a new apartment, gradually setting up her life the way it suited her. And then they would have gone to Puerto Rico, writing a hilarious bestseller on the vagaries of the New York Personals.

Still, with all the loving comfort he was eager to provide, her power-obsessed mind would have soon seen it as a prison; for love was the one thing she could not accept, though she was pretty good at giving it to her children. But with a man, it would have been Adam and the others again.

How sad! How heartbreakingly sad! On fourteenth February, Valentine's day, hearts and flowers mocked Michael in every shop window. This was the day she was going to be with Robbie. Foolish as most of her comfort-dispensing attitude was, Michael had realized that her newly unearthed "love" for the man with the malignant prostate would be offered to him in hearts and flowers fashion; especially, since he seemed to be the money man backstage, thus reprising the role husband number four had been playing for so long. For which she "gratituded" him. So with Robbie, gratitude was once again in order.

On the other hand, love, which would have been flowing toward her from Michael, was a commodity Allegra could do nicely without. Quite nicely, thank you. Who needed hearts and flowers, kisses and tender hugs, when restoring her first-class lifestyle was the top priority? And Robbie would be only too eager to pay for her supportive presence. "I only see him for business reasons," Allegra had stated in her final insulting fax. Well, money was her business now, and a woman had to show some gratitude even if the man with the checkbook had been underwhelmed with her physical assets not so long ago. Well, Michael had no idea how and with whom she would spend Valentine's day, and he tried hard not to care. Indulging his pain, he'd put Allegra's picture up in his bedroom, staring at those incredible eyes, which stared right back at him, searing his heart… weren't eyes supposed to be the windows of the soul? If so, Allegra's were the exception proving the rule. No love shone from these windows, surely not for him, as she looked out of the picture he'd taken, wearing his butterfly pin on her black dress, enigmatically withholding. No, that colorful butterfly, symbol of Psyche's transformative potential, wasn't going to take wing: its evolution was threatened, perhaps doomed, by the ice-encrusted heart beating under that black dress, sounding a dirge for love lost.

Michael should have known better, paid attention to the "bad track record". But when did reason ever prevail over a heart signaling, "yes, she's the one you've been waiting for; she answered your call, she needs you in her life?" And indeed she'd returned those very same signals over and over, in between her pattern of running away, which in the end won out. But at what cost? To her, unknown. To Michael, the agony of the silent scream. His mind wished her well, but his wounded heart wanted badly for her to stumble, finally grasping that even a "survivor" only gets a finite number of chances; and when they run out, and there are no more cards left in the deck she'd been dealt at birth…

Michael left the sentence hanging. He didn't want to be the Seeress of the Tripod whose prophesies were true but met with disbelief. Thus Troy fell. And Helen whose face had launched a thousand ships and destroyed every man who fell for her beauty, ended up a specter whose lips suck forth their souls, as Marlowe had so succinctly put it.

It was one p.m. on Valentine's day. A decision, born of despair, made Michael reach into the stack of letters women had written in reply to his ad, many months ago. Amazingly, his first call was answered: Margie, who had no plans for tonight. She remembered the note she'd sent, and they met for a late dinner in the Village.

Margie was tall and slim, with long blond hair, wearing a black dress with little golden rectangles sown into the fabric. She was a family therapist, divorced after a twenty-year marriage, which sounded just like Allegra's to her ex of fourteen years. In gratitude to him, but needing empowerment. Three grown children, grand-children, Jewish family values. Very attractive, clear soft skin, perhaps a lift, middle fifties, Michael surmised. Delightfully self-assured, relaxed, and into dating, but wanting to get married again. Thrilled to meet an analyst for a free session, free dinner.

Michael listened, made witty conversation, but feeling his anger at Allegra rising in his throat. How dare she discard him after what they'd been through together in that incredibly short time?

Margie, skilled at seeing past the surface, picked up his feelings halfway through her salmon. And Michael poured it all out. Her reaction was predictable.

"Four marriages? Your heart and mind must not have been on speaking terms with each other!" Time flew by, and it was midnight when she got into her red Italian sports car, off to her duplex townhouse in Soho. They agreed to meet next week and talk about warm climes. Her lips were ice cold. "I need a warm body," she quipped. On cue, Michael applied for the job.

At home, he looked at Allegra's picture, and his chest contracted in a spasm that made him double over. He knew it was not a heart attack, but a hurt so deep, no physical pain could match it. He knew Allegra was dead. Her grave yawned, but he hadn't buried her yet. It would be a long time before he could close her lying eyes, slam down the lid on her coffin, and dump it as unceremoniously as she had dumped him.

But that was wishful thinking, born of helpless frustration. His heart would never dump her, for she was the last love of his life, a gift however flawed, was still a present from the gods. The next day was Michael's birthday. The day she had promised to be with him.

And broke that promise. On the flimsiest of her neurotic whims. The lid of the coffin remained open.

Curiously, in a very distant part of his mind the peek-a-boo nymph giggled.

STELLA

One

I'm in a museum. High-ceilinged rooms follow one after another as if a TV camera were trying to catch up with someone just ahead. Gradually I realize that it is I who's behind the speeding lens and that I can slow things down if I want to. Now I'm standing in an immense room slowly looking around. On the walls are huge paintings, portraits of women. There are many different styles. Seated on a swing against a gaudy French impressionist background is a blonde woman wearing a pale lilac petticoat with narrow ribbon shoulderstraps. The painting next to her, in the style of Whistler, shows a dark-haired woman, haughty, disdainful. She's dressed in a long gown, deep black, a shower of diamonds on her high collar. I keep moving past the galleries of more portraits. Now I stare at a lissome nude. She has small breasts, pale as clouds, and her dark hair is falling in a glossy sheaf to her shoulders. The sheen of her body looks alive, and the expression on her face is irreverent, saucy. She exudes the authentic smell of woman. Boucher has painted her.

I'm confused about these women. I know them, but I don't. A man appears. He too looks familiar. He says, "I would like to build an opera house on a high mountain. "My confusion grows. Then I remember the speeding lens and I race through many rooms, all filled with portraits of women, going up and up until I see the night sky.

One giant star hangs next to a waning moon. The firmament looks like one big ring, a circle really.

As I opened my eyes I instantly knew who the woman was the dream had exhumed from my memory. I'd been taken to the warehouse where images of women from my past, known yet wholly unknowable, were stored. Nameless. Until the star had flashed the one name I was meant to remember. And the story came flooding back, rushing into my consciousness like the waterfall that had played a magical part in our encounter. I remember precisely how it started.

The sky above Nagasaki was full of stars as Lieutenant B. F. Pinkerton, U.S. Navy, carried Cho-Cho-San, his fifteen-year-old wife into their tiny house and a wedding night that was to end, two acts later, in a betrayed mother's suicide, Japanese style. The conductor held the tragedy-foreshadowing D-minor chord until the great gold curtain had completed its slow descent. Applause erupted as the two protagonists took their bows, the burly American tenor and the petite Roumanian soprano with a voice that had soared to the heavens in the magnificent duet which concluded the first act of Puccini's masterpiece.

I left my seat in the orchestra and made my way to the salon where crystal chandeliers illuminated the magnificent draperies. People began to crowd around the enormous buffet, piling tiny sandwiches and sweets onto fine china, then moved on to where coffee, with schlag, was dispensed from silver urns. Standing around or sitting at small marble tables, the Viennese patrons were engaged in a hallowed tradition.

Two weeks ago, I had come to Vienna. A year had passed since Allegra had walked out of my life, frostily demeaning my love, and some months ago I had managed to close the coffin and cremate her remains. Following my instinct and a series of unspecific dreams in which the cathedral of St. Stephen, Vienna's most prominent landmark, kept appearing, I returned to the city of my birth. I had no plans other than to let the magic of Vienna permeate my soul. Time was warped, of course, and as I strolled among familiar sights I was never quite sure of my age. Did I see the house where I was born through the eyes of the teenager who fled precipitously when Hitler came, or were the museums, the parks, theaters and the opera house visions from my thirties, my forties or my present age? I found it paradoxical that the vital, healthy man I felt myself to be was in real time reaching the threescore and ten mark. This was confirmed every time I met an old acquaintance: "How come you look so vigorous and youthful?" these men with whom I had gone to school would ask, carrying their paunch bellies like pregnant women. I would shrug, inwardly grateful to whatever it was that kept me fit – the genes, or perhaps my close relationship with my unconscious? I didn't know, but marveled at its reality. More remarkable still was my feeling this way after the last two relationships into which I had poured my love had ended in heart-breaking betrayal.

An aspic-encased egg salad on one plate and a slice of Sachertorte with schlag on another, I moved toward the coffee area. Two young women were in charge, black dresses and white aprons, and they coordinated my goodies on a small tray as the coffee was sending up its quintessential Viennese aroma.

In the farthest corner of the vast salon, near a window from which one could have looked down at the Operngasse had it not been covered by the grand tapestry depicting a scene from *The Magic Flute,* I espied an empty table. Balancing my delicacies I claimed the spot and sat down on one of the high-back chairs upholstered in red velvet. The love duet from *Madam Butterfly* ran through my mind: how familiar it all was! The score rewound itself, lushly, the inner tape machine not missing a bar. I saw myself in my teens, part of a group of passionate opera fans, standing night after night at the back of the orchestra where the standees adhered to a strict code: places were assigned either on the basis of seniority or if someone had a personal relationship with one of the stars of the performance. I had qualified on both counts; moreover, my absolute pitch and ability to read orchestral scores gave me additional privileges such as initiating or terminating a round of applause.

"Quante stelle!" Butterfly was singing in my mind as she looked up at the stars, gradually yielding to the naval Lieutenant's ardent wooing. The coffee cup was on its way to my lips when my reverie was interrupted by a woman, who in the polite ways of Vienna asked if the other chair at my table was taken. I jumped up, offering her the seat. She carried no food, only a small cup of espresso in a hand that trembled slightly. Small talk about the performance began immediately. I asked what she thought of the Roumanian soprano, and the woman said she couldn't remember a more beautiful voice, that she especially liked the dark vibrato which underlay her soaring lyrical top. "As if she knows the darkness that's in store for her," she said. She wore a dark green dress with a straight neckline. Her only jewelry was a single strand of pearls encircling the nearly translucent skin of her neck. Her oval shaped face was surrounded by shoulder-length hair the color of burnished mahagony. The sparkling crystal lighting prevented Michael from discerning the color of her eyes. Oddly, a dark lipstick accentuated her hollow cheeks.

I thought she looked sick, and. guessed her age at no more than thirty-five, about half my own. Her espresso drained, she rose, said that she hoped I would enjoy the rest of the opera, and walked away. I now saw that she was tall and slender, but her gait was cramped as if she had trouble straightening up. In my mind, I again heard Butterfly calling to the stars, "Quante stelle!" and Pinkerton's yearning for her, and I suddenly recalled the giggling nymph from a dream of a year ago when I had walked into a temple, following the sound of flutes, just as the affair with Allegra was coming to its cruel end.

The memory of the dream was strenghtened as the flutes and other woodwinds danced around the simple oriental tune in the prelude to the second act, teasing, waiting: how soon would the sailor return from far-away America? "When the robins do their nesting," Pinkerton had promised. The version performed that night connected acts two and three, obviating a second intermission. With the sharp dissonance of the final chord vibrating in my ear, I walked down the splendid Baroque staircase, feelings, memories tumbling over each other, the vast panorama of a lifetime inexorably bound to this city and its opera house. How often had I been in this house – before the great war with Christina, and after it had been rebuilt, with Lisa. And the time before tonight it had been a "Rosenkavalier" with Lisa when their love was still cradled in the warmth of Aphrodite's gentle fire.

At the exit I collided with the woman in the green dress. Apologizing for my clumsiness, I followed her to the small plaza where the three-cornered fountain splashed loudly in the warm June night. Adopting the polite idiom of the convoluted Viennese language, I asked her permission to introduce myself. "My name is Stella Kotschnig," she replied, extending her hand.

Only the many years of my professional experience kept me from outwardly reacting to the thunderclap detonating in my mind. Stella? After an evening filled with "Quante stelle", Butterfly's appeal to the stars, the woman's first name turned out to be Stella? I had met a star! And it was she who had approached my table during intermission.

I didn't want any more synchronicity in my life. Too much pain, too much heartache had been associated with synchronous events. I wanted to walk to my hotel, away from this woman named Stella, and I almost did. Instead I wondered aloud, haltingly, if she would care to go somewhere for a late supper, or just a dessert perhaps, like an applestrudel?

Stella Kotschnig looked away, then up at the sky, as if waiting for a message, what to say to this doctor. What kind of a doctor was he, she asked, as if her decision might depend on his answer. I explained that I was a psychoanalyst, born in Vienna, but living in New York; that I was now back in Vienna for a few weeks of opera and theater. "But this is the last week of June," said Stella, "and everything shuts down at the end of the month."

"I know", I replied, "but I've been here for two weeks already. Tonight was my fourth opera." She still had not reacted to my invitation.

We walked slowly alongside the opera house, crossing the street past the Hotel Sacher, home of the world-famous torte, and stopped in front of the Cafe Mozart. I pointed to the tables on the sidewalk and cocked my head. Stella nodded. Lowering herself on a metal chair, she winced, one hand involuntarily touching her abdomen. "I've had an operation," she murmured.

In the obsequious manner practiced for generations by Viennese waiters, a true specimen of these worthies stood by our table, notepad at the ready. Stella ordered a dessert called Palatschinken, thin crepes filled with apricot jam. I was hungry. Scanning the menu I noticed a dish I hadn't tasted in ages: Krautfleckerln, square noodles married to bits of spicy cabbage. Stella smiled at my choice. "I know you can't get these in New York," she said. "I've been there three times."

She volunteered that she was a vice-president at Bank Austria, dealing in international accounts, and currently on medical leave. I waited for her to go on, but she returned to the subject of opera. In the course of the next hour, we discovered each other's expertise in the field, and quotations ranging from Wagner and Verdi to Puccini and Richard Strauss started to fly between us. It made for an unexpectedly curious intimacy until I unwittingly quoted from *The Fledermaus* (The Bat) – "Happy he who forgets what cannot be changed".

Stella Kotschnig reacted with a flood of tears, excused herself and stayed away for a good twenty minutes. I was about to ask someone to check in the ladies room when she returned, apologizing profusely for what she called an unseemly outburst in front of a stranger. It took some time to convince her that emotions were familiar and acceptable to me, and to please not be concerned about having exposed herself in an inappropriate fashion.

"You must be pretty good at what you do," Stella said. "I don't feel I need to be so apologetic." I thought it was time to gently probe. Why had *The Fledermaus* triggered those tears? Did it have to do with her operation?

"May I call you Stella? I know people who have just met don't call each other by their first name in Vienna, but since you've been to New York…" I let the phrase hang.

Stella gave me a shy smile and said it was okay for me to do so, but she was not ready to reciprocate. "You are so much older than I am, and we are taught to be respectful to our elders." I said I understood, yet part of me didn't want to be labeled her elder. Would my youthful feelings never surrender to the reality of my age? Was I destined to remain a "puer aeternus", as the great Swiss psychiatrist Carl Jung had labeled men who refused to grow old?

Stella broke into my thoughts. "Yes," she said, "you touched my tears with that silly quotation." She waved to the waiter and ordered a glass of peppermint tea. "I'm thirty-seven years old, and I had cancer. They took it all out, so I can never have children." The tears started to flow again. I looked away, at the Albertina across the square where the great Duerer collection was housed. Why was this happening? What role was I meant to play in this young woman's life? The professional analyst was wrestling with the man. I ruffled my hair and polished my glasses, trying to intuit what to say next.

The peppermint tea arrived. Stella sipped and seemed to relax. "I was engaged to be married, but after the surgery he broke the engagement. He wanted a family. That was just six weeks ago." She looked at me.. "I feel like apologizing again telling this to someone I just met. I haven't even told my mother that Hans left me."

My feelings got the better of me. I touched Stella's hand, conveying genuine empathy. They sat in silence. It was close to midnight. Stella lived nearby on Anna gasse and I walked her home. At the heavy door of the ancient building Stella said, "Thank you, Dr. Stone… Michael." And in the darkness he imagined her blushing ever so slightly.

"I'm staying at the Astoria hotel," I said, "a stone's throw away." I tripped over the pun, unsure if she'd caught it.

Stella surprised me. “Two stones in one evening – quite extraordinary.”

I grinned. “Could I take you to lunch tomorrow?”

“I would like that very much,” said Stella. “I’m on indefinite leave from the bank, not ready to get back to work. Tomorrow night is the last opera performance of the season, *The Tales of Hoffmann.* I have a ticket.” I said I would try to get one as well. Gently touching her hand I waited until she had turned the heavy key and let herself in.

I walked to my hotel trying very hard to get a reading on the events: Butterfly’s cry to the heavens, “Quante stelle”, and the woman named Stella who’d had a hysterectomy and been dumped by a man to whom she was now an empty vessel, cured of her cancer but barren. Did Hans love her? Whose sacrifice was the greater one?

Emerging on the bustling Kaertnerstrasse, an elegantly dressed hooker winked at me. It jostled me back into the pulse of the city. I walked over to the hooker. “What’s your name?” I demanded. She was very young, small breasts straining against a tight yellow dress.

“Lisa,” she said. “Three thousand for the night. I can come to your hotel room.”

It was all too much. What cruel games was fate playing with him? I thanked her for the offer and gave her a thousand Schilling note. Perplexed, Lisa said something that sounded nice and inviting, but I strode away, immune to Circe’s song.

Twenty minutes later I was fast asleep, but not before asking the concierge, that mighty procurer of the impossible feat to get me a ticket to tomorrow night's opera, *The Tales of Hoffmann.*

Two

A lone space-suited astronaut had landed on the moon. He sat down in a very small crater and unpacked a bundle of dry twigs and a frying pan. He then opened a can of stew, poured the contents into the pan and placed it on the branches. Lighting a match, he gently heated his stew over a merry little fire.

I awoke from this dream, recorded it in my dreambook, and wondered about the incongruity of the image. The moon's atmosphere – itself a misnomer – contained no oxygen, and without oxygen there could be no fire. What kind of stew was I trying to warm in the realm of the moon, ubiquitous symbol of the Feminine, over a fire that could not be ignited? Yet in the dream there was no doubt that the astronaut's stew was heating up nicely.

Stella? A foolish attempt to start a process without the necessary element? Was the dream mocking me, pushing the star-bound traveler into another May-December affair, proving myself fit for an adventure in space? But wait: the spacesuit made it impossible, did it not, for the astronaut to eat the stew, even if he succeeded in warming it up with the help of an impossible magical fire!

I dismissed the whole thing as a bad joke my unconscious was teasing me with, and went to have breakfast at the Cafe Oberlaa on Neuer Markt, several stone-throws away from my hotel. Walking past the Capuchin Tombs where the Hapsburg emperors and their consorts rested in ornately sculpted sarcophagi, I recalled last night's pun and smiled. How sharp of Stella to have caught it! It had brought a little lightness to her story: to be saved from a fatal malignancy only to lose her nurturing womb and the man she wanted to marry! I felt unreasonably angry at the guy; but would I have reacted differently given this particular deck of cards? Didn't it all depend on that undefinable emotion, love, the uniquely individual way a person would experience it and then act on? Of course, the Viennese would never think of adoption: "If it's not my flesh and blood, I don't want it," the Emperor Maximilian was reputed to have said when a scandal-embroiled Countess had challenged his paternity. And the hypocritical Viennese gleefully adopted their liege's posturing rather than someone else's baby.

After a sunny repast of coffee, eggs and the buttery crescent-shaped rolls called Kipferln, I went to the opposite end of the emotional spectrum. St. Stephen's, a dark mystical cathedral of diverse architectural styles but overpoweringly gothic, was the place where I'd been confirmed at age fifteen. It was also the time when I had first discovered, shocked and bewildered, the beauty of the female body with its breath-catching allure. The incident occurred in my home parish, St. Rochus, where a boy of Jewish ancestry was attending Sunday mass as part of his Catholic upbringing and required by his school's curriculum. Sunday mass meant communion, and communion meant prior confession. Every impure thought – and that meant any fantasy a boy had about a girl – was to be confessed (and repented!), for without absolution damnation was assured. If you were lucky, it was to be purgatory, a waystation where the final destination would be decided.

On the Sunday, which marked my radical departure from the church, I had just received the wafer symbolizing the body of Christ; returning to my pew, I tried without much success to swallow the host. To take my mind off the hard wafer, which I knew mustn't be chewed, I looked across the aisle which separated the boys from the girls. Several rows ahead knelt a girl with whom I had never talked. She was a couple of years older, in a higher grade, blond and long-legged. She was also the object of the impure thoughts I confessed to Monsignor Scheffel with embarrassing regularity. As the wafer finally slid down my throat, my eyes took in a sight which started the whole impurity business again: because of her kneeling position, the girl's skirt began to ride up, revealing ever more of her legs and the seamed silk stockings which were central to my fantasy.

At this point an epiphany burst in my mind, blindingly clear, as if a great veil had been lifted. What I beheld was nothing impure, nothing that could be called a sin, oh no! I was face to face with God's creation of beauty so sublime, so beatific and enchanting, even spiritual – here was the true transsubstantiation: the wafer, finally swallowed, had miraculously turned dark repressed lust into the golden image of a shrine where worship was not merely appropriate but demanded as a holy pilgrimage. Now blissfully illuminated, I resolved to be true to the goddess who had displayed herself in the mundane shape of a girl's legs, clad in seamed stockings.

The next day I sought out Monsignor Scheffel, stating my resolve to no longer confess something that was so clearly the face of beauty itself. Predictably, the Monsignor called up visions of purgatory, tortured souls screaming for mercy, but I stood my ground. I tried several times to approach the girl, Erika, to share my epiphany, but Erika smoked cigarettes and wore lipstick and would probably think that an epiphany was some kind of disease, like maybe epilepsy.

Now in the gloomy nave of the immense church I watched a funeral mass in progress. The deceased was evidently a person of some renown since the Cardinal Archbishop himself officiated. Mozart's requiem streamed softly through the hallowed space, and a throng of mourners all but obscured the High Altar in front of which stood an open coffin. I thought of how the Viennese were often unable to separate reality from legend and truth from make-believe: grotesque and theatrical in their sentimentality, they loved a "schoene Leich" (a beautiful corpse); it was all part of their infatuation with drama and music, and behind it lay a callous and mean streak; the joy when misfortune befell someone, especially a Jew. "It served him right," they would say, inventing some fable of why the hapless person deserved to be struck down by a cruel fate. A few hundred feet from where I stood, Mozart's

weaving a woman's face, flame-red hair cascading, into the distant background of the temple.

I was searching for words that would give coherent expression to my astonishment. When I kept stumbling, Stella laughed out loud. "l haven't had fun in a long time and I hope you're not offended, but I seem to have reduced a famous psychoanalyst to wordless wonder." She was becoming animated, and her eyes, I now realized, glinted like emeralds. Just as the chimes announced the beginning of the third act, I found my voice.

"I'm very grateful for having met you, Stella." The simple affirmation summed it all up.

Returning to the Cafe Mozart after the conclusion of the opera, we discussed the epilogue.

"It is the muse, after all, who remains faithful to the poet; so is she his true anima?" Stella wondered.

"Yes, the three other women are phantoms, ungraspable and unreal creations of his mind that make him want to unite with these feverish fantasies, trying to defeat the devil who walks off with them. But he's doing Hoffmann the great service of recognizing that the muse will never leave him. I don't suppose I have to tell you the muse's name."

Stella blushed. "Don't get too personal, please, Michael," she said, hiding unsuccessfully behind the small mirror of her makeup kit.

Like the night before, I looked away at the Albertina. I nodded, wanting to respect Stella's plea, but could not escape the fact that the woman I was sitting with bore the same name as the drunk poet's muse. In spite of the mild breeze which carried the scent of lilac being hawked a few feet away by an old woman who could have stepped out of a Breughel painting, I shivered.

Four

Il awoke to one of those golden days when Vienna's pedestrian zone, bathed in the sunshine of early summer, was a riot of flowers, the scent of lilac everywhere. I telephoned Stella, wondering if she felt like an excursion to the Prater, the city's huge park, part of which contained the amusement section with the giant Ferris wheel on which Orson Welles and Joseph Cotten had feuded about *The Third Man's* nefarious doings. While still in my pre-teens, my father had taught his son how to drive on the wide lanes of the Prater where in imperial days the aristocracy used to ride the Spanish horses alongside the carriages of the courtly ladies, offering intimate suppers and nocturnal trysts.

Now riding the modern subway to the amusement park, I related these early memories to Stella. She wore an embroidered blouse, a long blue cotton skirt and a wide-brimmed straw hat from which strands of her mahagony hair kept escaping. Her hair sparkled. Stella said she was feeling rested, and was happy to have accepted his suggestion. It was a weekday and school vacations had not yet begun, so the Prater was uncharacteristically uncrowded. We rode the Liliput railway and the Ferris wheel, and then indulged in Vienna's archetypal lunch: franks with mustard and fresh horseradish, washed down with ice cold beer. For cash, I had persuaded the driver of a horse-drawn carriage to lend us a blanket, and we relaxed on the grass in the shade of a great oak tree.

"I'm feeling quite peaceful and content," said Stella. "It surprises me. I think of myself as somewhat conservative, and here I am with someone I barely know, yet it's a very comfortable feeling of warmth and security."... "Last night," Stella went on, "it was difficult for me to get up to my apartment. I felt peculiarly alone in the ancient building where I live. I climbed up to the third floor on those indented stone steps thinking of how many nailed boots had tramped up during the two centuries since those stones were first laid by an unknown mason. When I finally reached my door, I dropped the key. And bending down to retrieve it made my scar act up; it just throbbed and throbbed." She paused for a while, then said, "Am I boring you, Michael?" I shook my head gently. Stella smiled. "I don't want this to be like one of your professional sessions, but I need to share some of my background with you. It'll make things a little clearer for me." My eyes told her I understood..

"So anyway," Stella resumed, "all I could manage was to get into bed. I felt drained. But," her voice was becoming more animated," my mind was very much alive. It was searching and probing, images kept arising and disappearing, connections were formed and broken. I was making a strong-willed attempt to understand what was happening in my life. Our talk about my name seemed so important, the coincidence with the opera, but I couldn't find a focus for my emotions." There was a long pause.

"This is getting very personal, Michael. I liked you from the moment we met, but this business about being your muse just because of the way the opera ended was somehow inappropriate and disquieting. But I was fascinated when we talked about projection."

"Please tell me more about your background," I urged her. "I'm just as eager to know what meeting the way we did may mean to both of us. And believe me, my interest is not professional. We're just two people trying to find out a little more about one another."

Stella patted my hand. "That was nice the way you put it. All right, it's confession time." I heard the false jocular tone and squeezed her hand reassuringly.

"There were three men I've been in love with. Hans Hartmann was the last one. My first lover was my high school sweetheart, Fritz Lehmann. He was killed on his motorcycle at age twenty-two. Then came Walter Hollwitz, a medical student with whom I lived through his graduation and residency in orthopedic surgery. In the end we decided that our careers took precedence over getting married. I had already started at Bank Austria, was very quickly promoted to an executive position in charge of attending international monetary conferences. When I turned thirty, I was made a vice-president of the bank. By that time I had found and decorated my present apartment. That made me feel settled and happy. After a couple of brief affairs I met Johann Hartmann. Guess where?" She released a quick giggle. "At the opera, of course. He was an engineer, a member of the opera's technical staff, mildly fond of music, but totally committed to the complex machinery, which moved sections of the stage, some of which he'd helped design. That was two years ago when I was thirty-five. My father had just died after long suffering a paralyzing stroke. My mother now lives alone in a small house in the spa town of Baden, half an hour south of Vienna. She's an old-fashioned disciplinarian. She had wanted me to marry years ago to just about anyone whom she considered suitable. I know she was impressed with my accomplishments in the world of international finance. But she never said so."

Stella got up, stretching herself and looked at me intently… "I need a little more encouragement that I'm really not boring you."

"Just look at my face," I said. "Can you see a bored expression? I'm not a very good actor, Stella. My feelings are what we call right on my sleeve." I made weaving movements with my shirtsleeve.

Stella laughed. "I hadn't heard that one before, but your blue shirt has convinced me. Okay, on with my story. It gets more interesting anyhow.

"Johann Hartmann, the man I mentioned first, began to court me. Not with great passion but with a solid no-nonsense attitude about wanting to marry and have a family. So I started to sleep with him. It was comfortable but less romantic than what I would have hoped for, not operatic enough" – a lovely quick smile – "and so I said yes to his proposal. My mother was overjoyed. I guess what made me say yes was the unusual engagement ring he gave me. I thought it was a good omen for our future. He had acquired the ring at an auction of operatic memorabilia; it had belonged to Selma Kurz, arguably the greatest coloratura of all time. How the ring had gotten to the auction was unknown, but since it was engraved with the same initials as my name, and its authenticity unquestioned, Hans had bought the unique jewel and I was just delighted. Given the ring's age, part of the engraving had paled a little, not the S.K., but the small letters beneath, which were barely legible as J.H. Hans was bowled over by the double coincidence of our common initials, and now I just had to marry him.

"Then everything collapsed. I was told that what looked like a harmless fibroma in my uterus was in fact an aggressive malignant tumor. Nothing short of a prompt hysterectomy could prevent the rapid spread of the cancer. The surgeon said I would be dead within a year. When I told Hans about it, it was the beginning of the end. There was pain, fury, and finally resignation. Hans wanted children, surely I could understand that, and when I tentatively raised the issue of adoption, Hans thought I was crazy. If it's not my own flesh and blood, he said, I don't want it. Funny, now when I think back, I was less devastated than I would have expected. So that was the end. You know, Michael, what kept me reasonably balanced were my operatic friends. They provided tickets, and I dragged myself to the opera house. You know that I live only a few blocks away, but I was in great physical discomfort; still, I managed to cheer Placido Domingo's *Otello,* and to weep over Kiri te Kanawa's *Manon Lescaut.* At the Bank they were enormously solicitous, and urged me to stay away until I was fully recovered. On full pay, of course. God, I seem to be talking non-stop!"

I was pleased with the easy flow of Stella's story. "Isn't it astonishing what love of music can do for us? And opera is such a curious art form – I think only in Vienna and in Italy where opera was born can you find people like us who get carried away by great voices. I'm sure your painful trips were the best medicine."

Stella nodded. "You know, that brings me back to last night. I was hoping to get to sleep quickly, but I kept seeing the character of Stella, the diva, when she turns away from the drunken poet, and how Stella, the muse, then appears in her place; how the muse consoles Hoffmann and promises to be forever faithful to him. In my mind I heard that sweet B-flat theme with which Hoffmann serenades the muse. That put me to sleep, finally." She hesitated to go on. "I'm sending you my encouragement look again," I quipped. "It's my special laser that cuts through all wavering."

"I've felt it before," said Stella. "And it worked. You know, it's a funny thing but I rarely dream. But last night, or rather early in the morning I had a very strange dream. Would you like to hear it? Or am I imposing on you?"

I had expected it. But here, on the sunny meadow of the Prater, lying on a blanket, which smelled of horses and stables, I wasn't at all sure I wanted to hear Stella's dream. And it wasn't just the buzzing of insects, the light blue sky, and nature's soft promise of a drowsy summer day that filled me with anticipation; yes, I loved all that, wanted it to happen, in the carefree joyous ways of long ago, when I was with other women on other meadows. It was rather the anxiety, a premonition perhaps, that getting into Stella's unconscious was connected with the astronaut in his impossible situation; would he be heating the stew over an unrealistic fire?

But the call had to be heeded. The reluctant hero who would not go on the journey was inviting penalties I'd prefer not to speculate about.

"Sure," I said. And Stella told me..

"Well, I saw myself outside a small house, more like a hut. I was highly pregnant. There was a starlit sky, and three men in outlandish garb were waiting some distance away. They were carrying gifts. Then a fourth man, wearing a Cardinal's hat – is mitre the correct word? – gave me a twig on which white blossoms had sprouted. It was such a vivid image."

I saw the colorful strokes with which Stella was painting her dream. She sounded excited and curious, not unlike a child who'd been given finger paints when crayons were no longer sufficient to express feelings. I remained prone, the lids over my closed eyes fluttering slightly. The multi-layered meaning of her dream lay before my inner vision with the clarity of an illumined folio. It held out several promises, all dangerous, all scaring me. I felt like the moment after the *Butterfly* performance when I wanted to run back to my hotel having heard Stella's name. Now once more the urge to flee was in my body. "Go before it's too late," said a voice. "No, let him live it," countered another. "It will close the circle."

Abruptly I sat up. "Let's do this right. An analyst never reveals a dream's meaning, even if he has an inkling what it might be. Only soothsayers, painted palmreading women in circus tents do that. No, he asks for associations: recollections, feelings which will enlarge the coded message. These are clues in a puzzle, so that with patience the dreamer comes to an understanding by herself, perhaps with a few intuitive hints from the analyst."

Stella became instantly serious. I had noticed these rapid mood changes before; it was as if feeling was being replaced by a switch which activated facts stored in her intelligent mind. Indeed, an associative chain started to click, providing relevant background information. "I'm reminded of Mary and the three wise men from the Orient. But they didn't show up until after Jesus was born, so that does not make much sense. And for me to be pregnant is a cruel joke." She got up and walked around the oak tree. She astounded me by what came next. "And, of course, the twig with the blossoms reminds me of Tannhaeuser. But what all this has to do with me, I haven't any idea."

Il heard the challenge in her voice: it was now up to me to weave things together and offer some kind of interpretation. Tannhaeuser! It had been my association as well. Once again I was taken with how accurately she picked up interior clues. Surely this wasn't just a sharp intelligent mind: there had to be plenty of intuition which she trusted without equivocation.

Tannhaeuser, the twelfth-century minnesinger, had spent time in the realm of the love goddess, Venus. Tiring of sensuality's surfeit, he left, and courted the virtuous Elisabeth who was to award laurels to the singer who could best define love. Annoyed over the courtly piety of his fellow contestants, Tannhaeuser delivered an ardent paeon to erotic passion. Shocked, Elisabeth demanded that he join pilgrims journeying to Rome to seek absolution from the Pope. But the Pope refused: Just like his dry staff would never green again, said his Holiness, so Tannhaeuser's soul would remain condemned. Furiously turning his back on Rome, the singer re-entered the pagan world of Venus who welcomed him, arms and loins orgiastically open. But the returning pilgrims announced a miracle: the Pope's staff had sprouted new leaves, disavowing the Pontiff's prediction. Tannhaeuser was redeemed. But the news came too late for Elisabeth: her prayer for Tannhaeuser's salvation had been heard, but she died, leaving him bereft of both animas, the virgin, and her shadowy counterpart, the goddess of carnal love.

My mind went back many years to when my supervisor, the renowned Esther Harding, had issued a stern warning: never interpret a dream to someone who is not emotionally equipped to absorb it. Unless there is sufficient consciousness to integrate archetypal, non-personal material, said Dr. Harding, better to keep your mouth shut and resist the temptation to show off. There was no way at this moment, with the tinny sounds of merry-go-rounds nearby, that I could lay out the different paths revealed by Stella's dream. Obviously, she was pregnant with the Savior; the Magi's gifts were waiting; the detour into carnal, possibly incestuous love was forgiven – but the outcome of it all was not part of the prediction. Elisabeth had died for love of the minnesinger's soul, but he had lost all access to his anima! Wasn't that just like the astronaut who thought he was going to nourish himself on the moon, yet had no way to eat his stew, for if he removed his space helmet, he would promptly suffocate.

While these thoughts percolated through my mind, Stella was growing impatient. Tauntingly, she said, "If you won't tell me, I'll find a painted lady with a crystal ball." She pointed in the general direction of the amusement park. The child required an answer even if she wasn't grown up enough to hear the truth. "You're right on the mark," I said, returning the horseblanket to the driver. "The three symbols hang together: your pregnancy, the wise men, and the Cardinal with the blooming branch. But carrying Jesus and connecting this with poor Tannhaeuser is a very complex story. It requires a lot of discussion."

Stella was mollified, but like a child wanting her candy, she stuck to the story. "Remember how quickly I understood the mechanics of projection," she complained. "Surely you can tell me more than just repeating what I already told you!"

"Dream interpretation is a serious business, Stella," I said gently. "This is my field of expertise and I ask for your trust. I promise you we'll unravel it together."

A streetcar took us back to the city. I had wanted to drop her off at the house on Annagasse, but Stella was feeling both exhausted and reluctant to be by herself. "Please come up for a while, perhaps we can talk more about my dream?" Unsure of myself, I decided to let her take the initiative.

In contrast to the ancient house, Stella's living room was a showcase of modern furniture with deep plump cushions covering a multi-sectional sofa. Her color scheme was rose and gold, oozing comfort and warmth.

"I'm so impatient to get my strength back," Stella sighed as she relaxed in a large armchair. I pulled up a footstool. 'I'm quite good at massaging feet," I said, trying for a lighter touch. "Would you like that?"

Stella leaned back and closed her eyes. "Very much," she whispered. Five minutes later she had dozed off.

We had gotten uncannily close in a very short time. As I watched the sleeping woman, I examined my feelings. There was no doubt that I liked Stella. Besides the opera, about which topic we bantered constantly, we also communicated easily. Stella's wit had a self-deprecating ironic tinge, and she caught every pun, joke, and double-entendre I had uttered, both in English and the Viennese dialect which had come back to me with surprising fluency. On the serious side, her dream had now deepened matters, and the compass heading was undecipherable.

I stood by the window which faced the elegant hotel "Zum Roemischen Kaiser" (At the Roman Emperor's) and recalled staying there in the depth of winter, many years ago, when I was still living with the only woman I had ever been married to. I still had enormous fondness for Agnes, but we had been so different temperamentally that it had been better to separate. She had become a well-known pianist, was in fact scheduled for a recital in Vienna some days from now. We had remained friends and Agnes had married a philosopher who knew nothing about music but was her spiritual guide and mentor. How distant it all was! And what of the present? A few feet behind me slept Stella whom I'd met less than a week ago and who evidently was meant to be a part of my immediate future.

Stella had awakened and stood next to me. I told her about my connection with the hotel across the street and she put a tentative arm around my shoulder. It was a first expression of intimacy, a thank-you gesture for the foot massage, quite asexual, yet oddly warm and comforting. "Would you like to go to Agnes' recital?" she asked softly. "I don't much care for solo piano, but…"

I interrupted her. "Neither do I. And you know what? I think we should go away, someplace to the country; it'll do you good, speed your recovery – I'll rent a car and we'll just go for it. Anywhere, south, west, but out of the city!" I had no idea where this burst of energy came from, but I felt charged, as though it were suddenly a foregone conclusion that we would indeed do it.

"Let me sleep on it, Michael," Stella said. "I'm amazed at myself. Normally, I would think it very strange to go on a trip with a man I've met a couple of days ago. But the idea doesn't surprise me. Perhaps it has to do with regaining my strength."

Five

The next morning Stella phoned with a suggestion which Il found quaint and endearing. "Let's go visit my mother," Stella proposed. "I'm a little old-fashioned, which might surprise you coming from a vice-president in international banking; but I'd like to introduce you to her."

"Are you asking for Mom's approval of me? If she likes me, we'll go on a trip?" I meant it to sound ironic, but it came out just as old-fashioned and surprisingly caring.

Stella laughed. "No, I've already made up my mind about that. I'd like to go away with you, but I don't want her to worry, so meeting you will make her feel I'm in safe hands."

We took the Blue Train which runs from the Opera through the vineyards of Gumpoldskirchen to the ancient spa town of Baden. The sulfur springs had been known to the Romans and were pitched as wondrously healing today as when Marcus Aurelius, the Roman emperor who loved Vienna and died there, praised the thermal baths two thousand years ago. Stella's mother lived in Helen's Valley, west of the city, on the road to Mayerling, the scene of the double suicide, which presaged the end of the Hapsburg empire. The area abounded in nineteenth century villas, and the valley itself was bordered on both sides by the ruins of stone castles that clung to the hills high above the road which led to Margaret Kotschnig's house.

Finding myself in Baden opened a floodgate. Memories of Christina, my first love, tumbled through my mind as I and Stella walked by the house where she had torn her stockings climbing a fence, finding herself locked out because her stepfather had forbidden her to date Michael. It had been a wintry night, in a snowy park, when Christina had finally consented to make love with him. They had kissed forever, drunk with love and the bubbly local wine they had consumed too much of.

Pausing on a bench close to their destination, I told Stella the story of Christina. When I came to the operatic ending of our first night together, Arabella's smashing the glass of water as token of their betrothal, Stella burst into tears. She continued crying softly as I related the discovery of my Jewish roots and my flight to Italy, never to kiss Christina again.

"I wouldn't have suggested coming here had I known what pain this would cause you," she said between small sobs. I reassured her. "It's bittersweet, Stella, but only because of the passage of time – how it's all coming full circle." I looked up at the familiar hills where the old castle still stood in ruins as if the stones had been cemented again to make the memory accurate, then added, "But being here with you is both an end and a beginning – which is how it should be."

"The Cardinal who offered me the blooming staff just came to my mind, Michael," Stella said. "I'm beginning to feel quite relaxed about our trip. Maybe we shouldn't discuss my dream any more."

Mrs. Kotschnig offered tea and cookies. A short stocky woman with crystalline green eyes and yellow hair (the coiffeuse, Frau Amalie – "You remember her, Stella?" – didn't get the blond right, she explained), proved a relaxed and welcoming presence. She apologized to Stella for a remark she had made that the cancer had been god's punishment. "I was so upset," she said, addressing me. "I went to my parish priest and he put the idea in my mind, but then I thought about it and I decided it was cruel to say that to my only child. I went back to the priest, and he said he didn't mean to judge Stella whom he doesn't know, so he was sort of taking it all back. But I changed churches anyway," she concluded, wiping her slate clean.

"Mother, Dr. Stone knows Baden from his youth; his first love used to live near your house." With one thing leading to another, I learned that Christina had married an American when Vienna was occupied by the Allies after World War II, and that she and her husband had returned to Baden some years ago.

"Are they still living here?" I asked, intuitively anticipating unwanted emotions.

"They're both dead, I'm afraid," Margaret Kotschnig replied. I rose and went to a window from which I could see the house Christina had lived in, an eternity ago. Stella followed me. "You seem to be looking out of windows which open up into your past," she said softly.

I was tempted to put my head on her shoulder, wishing I were back in New York where the present consisted of work and patients, away from this place which threatened to open scars, which I'd believed untouchable. But the astronaut was on the moon, wasn't he? So this, too, was the present, and the woman standing next to me was the current resident of this lunar landscape, and there was no getting away from it.

Animated and relaxed, Stella recounted to her mother how she and I had met. Without touching on dreams, she spoke of our mutual love of opera, how she'd never met anyone who had so many scores in his head, and, oh yes, I had proposed a trip to the country to speed her recovery. She had come to think of that as a really wonderful idea; we were planning to stay away for a couple of weeks, driving to the lake country near Salzburg.

Mrs. Kotschnig excused herself and went to the kitchen. She returned with a cake she'd forgotten to serve. "Oh, mother," Stella exclaimed. "Don't look so worried. Dr. Stone will take good care of me." She and I were still standing by the window, framed against the soft summer evening. A breeze of serenity was gently moving through Mrs. Kotschnig's living room. She smiled. "I know he will, Stella,' she said, stroking her daughter's hair.

Six

Two days later, Stella and I were driving in a small Fiat heading west along the Danube through the area known as the Wachau. We passed the great abbey of Goettweig, then the town of Duernstein in whose castle Richard the Lionheart was imprisoned for thirteen months. Legend had it that his servant, the faithful

Blondel, was playing the lute nightly beneath the battlements and was rewarded by hearing Richard's answering voice. We stopped at Melk, grandest of baroque abbeys, wandering through its immense library, and emerging, looked across the river at the little town of St. Michael, perched upon a thousand foot cliff.

"The town of your namesake has quite a commanding position," said Stella. "Are you the lord of all that one surveys from up there? Fortifying yourself against your enemies?" Her eyes canvassed the lush landscape surrounding them. The Danube, looking remarkably blue, flowed in fast swells through the narrow valley below, and on either bank the steeply arranged vineyards glistened dewy and green. Stella's face had lost its pallor, her cheeks sported a healthy color, and the sun was painting her chestnut hair with a vermilion tinge.

"You're looking so much better," I said, casually putting my arm around her shoulder. "I'm still confused about us," she replied, searching for a relaxed tone. "Your arm feels protective but also vibrant, as if gentle tremors were coursing between us. They're coming from you, but I know the echo is mine."

"There is no place I would call a hometown, not even if it bears my name," I said, referring to her earlier question. To myself, I sounded wistful and forlorn. "I'm just a traveler through time. Fortified, you say? Well, yes, maybe – certainly not against enemies, but perhaps watchful about unexpected turns in the road." Or missing a sign spelling "one way only", I was on the verge of saying.

Stella's intuition tuned in quickly. "We're on this trip together," she said, giving me a warm smile. "And we can both watch out for unexpected turns."

Late in the afternoon we followed a sign reading, "Schloss Ernegg. Guests welcome." We drove through a crumbling archway into a courtyard surrounded by three mighty towers. Beyond, we glimpsed a garden and heard loud British accents. A woman who introduced herself as Countess Auersperg, one of the oldest aristocratic names, gushed at our good fortune: a suite was available, would we care to see it? She led the way upstairs into a tower, then through a halbard-filled corridor into an enormous room. Against one wall stood three single beds, facing another room, a vast distance of open space away, with yet another bed, next to which a door led into a bathroom featuring the largest tub either of us had ever seen. A million ants were frolicking on its marble surface. The entire place smelled moldy. The Countess opened two great windows beneath which a small river gurgled pleasantly. "That's the Erlauf," said the Countess, as if the name was as well-known as her own. Dismissing the ants and the stale odor, she departed, announcing that her presence was needed to coach a group of boisterous British tourists who wanted to learn a simple Austrian folktune. Dinner would be at eight o'clock sharp.

Stella started to giggle. "The three beds look like the fairytale of Grumpy, Schlumpy – and who was the third?"

I was less amused. "You're thinking of Snow White, but there were seven dwarfs. What about Papa Bear, Mama Bear and Baby Bear?"

Stella giggled some more, though the phrase "Mama Bear" made her swallow momentarily.

"But you're right," I said. "This place isn't out of a fairytale, I'd say, but it surely dates back to the days of the Holy Roman Empire when the Countess' forebears tore into boar steak in the courtyard – and that smell! Do you think you can take it?"

Stella approached one of the three beds. "It'll be okay once the air gets in." She selected the middle bed, and I moved to the opposite end of the chamber, putting my things on the bed that faced the three bears a football field away.

We were introduced to the noisy Brits, but excused ourselves right after dinner. Strolling in the bug-infested garden, we heard the Countess yodeling, "And so you can *sprecben Sie Deutscb!"* The tourists joyously repeated the stupid line. "It's been a long day," Stella sighed. "I've exhausted my energy." While I inspected the Eriauf, she excused herself to go to bed. By the time I walked in, she was asleep.

In my bed, I looked across the great space at the woman with whom I was on a journey. It was the second time I had seen her asleep. It was calm and reassuring.

When I awoke, pale daylight was creeping in through the open windows. Momentarily disoriented, I suddenly realized that Stella was lying next to me. She looked very sick. "I've been throwing up for hours," she said, reacting to my puzzled expression. "I feel so bad, I had to snuggle up to you."

"The food last night… but we ate the same thing?"

"No, Michael, I had a different dessert, a kind of eggcream." The word made her gag. I got up, took a quick shower, and went in search of some tea.

Stella sipped slowly, gratefully. "You don't mind my getting into bed with you?" The question was tentative, shy, but her eyes were firmly locked on mine. "It's all so very peculiar. Lying next to you I felt so many contradictory emotions: there was warmth and security, but there was also discomfort – it made me wonder if our age difference has something to do with it. I mean," she halted and looked away, over my shoulder, "after all, you could almost be my grandfather. I'm trying to be honest with myself and with you. A woman doesn't acknowledge that she might be attracted to her grandfather." In spite of the intense blush, which rose from her neck and went past the bridge of her nose, Stella's eyes remained locked on mine..

I felt her gaze as a soft languid caress, and was immediately back on the moon. How many women had taken me there, though never under such peculiar circumstances when nourishment seemed inaccessible. But it had always been a fantasy feeding my blood.

"It's not a very good beginning of a trip, is it?" Stella murmured, hoping the tea would stay down. "Those ants were so horrible, I saw them all over me."

I felt buoyant and optimistic. "You'll be up in no time," I pronounced. Indeed, Stella recovered within a day, eager to leave the creaky castle with its moldy beds. We continued west, exchanging the local roads for the autobahn and made good time reaching the outskirts of Salzburg.

"Coffee at Tomaselli's?" I asked. "And then plan our second night?"

"Anywhere, just no molds or ants." Stella allowed how she loved Salzburg passionately and I shared her feelings. She hadn't missed a festival in twenty years, and though that annual time was two months in the future, the baroque charm of this magical city embraced us as we sat on the high terrace of the famous coffeehouse where the ghosts of Toscanini and Reinhardt were still a living presence.

"There is a favorite place of mine on lake Wolfgang," I said, putting a sharply etched image into words.. "Like Baden, it's full of memories, but I believe going there with you might put a light present on a nostalgic past." I had a sudden insight. Could it be that the meaning of this trip, at least for him, was the transformation of a painful and distant past into a present so different and new as to be a rebirth, a fresh start, and yet a consenting to the closing of the circle, a readiness for wherever the next plane of the soul's existence turned out to be?

But what about Stella? My inner eye did a frantic search: what was he meant to do for this woman whose dream had forecast a birth and a forgiveness… for what? What was the Pope's blooming staff forgiving her for?

A sudden rainsquall, expelled from a single angry-looking cloud directly overhead, cascaded into the square. Water from the sky was needed to make the earth fertile, the Sky God impregnating Mother Earth. It was the process of the ever renewing life cycle, the most profound of nature's secrets. And Stella, barren though she was, needed to become once more a guardian of that secret way by which she could rejoin the eternal cycle. And I began to wonder if that was perhaps the task fate had assigned to him.

Seven

In mid-afternoon they arrived in the town of St. Gilgen and stopped at the Hotel Billroth named after a nineteenth century Viennese surgeon who had made medical history. After the retirement of the owners whom I had known well, it had changed hands and appearance. Gone from the lobby were the overstuffed chairs; the new interior had sofas in a soft grey fabric, chrome and silver everywhere. But the large terrace from which the view took in the Wolfgang lake, framed in the background by the snowy peaks of the Dachstein range, was as spectacular a place as ever.

Catching her breath, Stella gripped my arm. "I have never seen anything as beautiful," she managed to say after gazing silently at the scenery. The white paddle-wheeled steamer named like nearly everything else in Austria after the revered emperor Franz Joseph, was crossing from St. Gilgen, the town at the head of the lake, to the next village, Fuerberg. Tiny boats, electrically powered, shared the deep blue water with a flotilla of colorful sailboats. It all smelled of sun and summer, the meadow below the terrace was a riot of flowers, nature's bounty a dazzling display of the assertiveness of life.

There was only a double room available: two queen-size beds, separated by a nightstand. A picture window opened onto a covered balcony. Perfect for breakfast, I thought. Below, the expanse of the lake shimmered cerulean. I looked at Stella while the bellboy hovered discreetly by the door, balancing their bags. She turned away from me, entranced by the view. "This is the true fairytale," she whispered, nodding slowly.

Il tipped the bellboy and said, "Why don't you get settled? I'll take a stroll, and then I'll be on the terrace, having coffee."

Which is what he did. While on my second cup, I was joined by a young couple and a small boy wearing *lederhosen.* We chatted animatedly for some time until I happened to glance up at the balcony of our room. There stood Stella, wearing a white tank top and a skirt of the same color. Colorful spring flowers danced over its wide pleats. I waved, urging her to come down. She walked onto the terrace just as the couple and their young son were leaving. Her lips had a glossy sheen and on her ears were small round earrings, gold with a tiny gem in the center. "He is the son of the former owners," I explained. "I've known Peter since he was a boy; they now have a small restaurant in the area."

Stella ordered strawberries. "And lots of whipped cream," she called after the departing waitress.

"You look rested," I observed. "And very pretty." It was the first time I had complimented her on her appearance. "Don't embarrass me, Michael, please. I have enough trouble figuring out the nature of our relationship. Its all so irregular and unexpected, not that I mind, you know, but I'm not used to adventures. I'm still surprised at myself that I said yes to the whole idea."

The strawberries arrived, accompanied by a cloud of whipped cream in a silver bowl. The fragrance of the luscious ripe fruit was heady.

"And strange things keep happening to me." She took a deep breath. "I was taking a nap just now, but before I dozed off, I discovered that my scar has changed dramatically: the raised welt-like red has become a thin, flesh-toned line, practically indistinguishable from the adjacent skin. Almost as if time has speeded up the healing process – time spent with you. You know, since the morning at the moldy castle when I couldn't help but snuggle up against you, feeling sick and forlorn, my feelings have changed. I thought I was seeking protection, but my feelings now have a kind of erotic quality, not sexual, you understand, but it scares me, Michael." She rushed on, obviously anxious to get it out.. "I feel like touching your hair, tracing, your face, stroking your fingers one at a time. Those are feelings I haven't known with any man I've been intimate with. And now I want to do this with you – you who are twice my age! I think the grandfather thing is spooking me again. Also, what about my dream where I was pregnant, and the three wise men, and the blossoming staff? We never talked about that again. And now I don't want to talk about it any more," she finished lamely. But the steam rose again quickly and she kept shaking her head, looking frustrated and bewildered. A breeze swept over the terrace carrying the scent of honeysuckle. Il didn't know what to say. Stella's words kept tumbling out. "Then I had this incredible dream."

"Wait, Stella, please not now. I can't seem to sort out my own feelings. I've never been with a woman where things were so completely... open, and undefined. Part of me knows why we're doing this – to get you away from Vienna, help with your convalescence; all this makes sense on a very rational level, but there are other vibrations. And dreams, which confuse me, too. And now, looking at you, as one of your elders – remember you called me that when we first met – it doesn't seem to fit at all. I see a very pretty woman with whom I'm sucking strawberries on an early summer evening. And it looks positively romantic!" Il threw up my hands. "Contradict me if you can."

"I have no intention of doing so," Stella said. She held a strawberry to his lips. "Shush," she said. "I told you I took a nap and had the strangest dream." The cream-coated berries made for a two-toned swirl around her mouth.

Il recalled the meadow in the Prater. There, like now, I didn't want to hear her dream, and the ever watchful analyst knew the reason. Getting deeper into Stella's unconscious was bound to increase the feelings I had for her, however undifferentiated they still were. Moreover, the astronaut was becoming acutely aware of his predicament: his stew was almost ready to eat, but he couldn't risk taking off his space helmet. Could the dilemma be resolved?

"You have a choice, Michael," Stella said, splitting the last strawberry with me. "If not now, then after dinner. But I must share this dream with you. I really need your help making sense of it."

"I'm a coward," I said smiling.. "I'll take the delay."

As it turned out, Stella was unable to keep her eyes open when dinner was over. With their juicy lamb shank they'd shared a half-bottle of Burgundy, and the wine had made her groggy. She went up to our room while I took a walk into the town of St. Gilgen. I went into the cemetery where years ago I had suffered agonies over Lisa's betrayal; at the time, I had hammered a single red rose into a crumbling wooden Christ erected over an old grave. Il searched for the grave, and was strangely relieved when I couldn't find it. "That part of the past is truly buried," I thought to myself, as I stepped into the small church adjoining the cemetery. On impulse, I dipped a finger into the holy water font, made the sign of the cross, and thought, "Now let me deal with the living present."

As I slipped into my bed, Stella woke up briefly. Drowsily, she reached over and held my hand. She stroked each of my fingers, softly and tenderly, then withdrew her hand and went back to sleep.

Eight

In the morning, we drove to the village of St. Wolfgang on the far end of the lake. We made fun of the White Horse Inn, the setting of many movies and a famous operetta, then went into the sixteenth century parish church to admire Michael Pacher's Winged Altar, arguably the finest example of Gothic wood carving in the world. Since it was Sunday, the wings were open, and the crowning of the Virgin was on view, with its workmanship so minute that even the stitches on her clothing were clearly discernible. Familiar as she was with the Salzburg lake country, Stella revealed that she had never seen Pacher's masterpiece. She knelt in front of the numinous image and prayed. Il who stood next to her wanted to move away to respect the privacy of the moment, but Stella reached for my hand and tugged on it. This unexpected invitation to join her in a sacred time was terrifyingly intimate, and though I did kneel, my eyes were caught by a painting to the far left of the altar: Satan tempting St. Florian, the hermit in whose honor Bruckner had composed his cataclysmic "Te Deum". The painting showed the fallen angel pushing a bare-breasted woman toward the praying saint.

My heart was suddenly in my throat. Gently disengaging myself from Stella's hand, I rose and walked out of the church. Outside, the sun-washed streets, the two shades of blue of sky and lake, brought me down to reality. Still, kneeling at Stella's side, ceding to her wordless demand, had shaken me. Obviously, what was flowing from her to me was a spiritual communion. But the crowning of the Virgin was, if not offset, certainly disturbed by Satan's presence and the temptation of the flesh.

Stella emerged from the church, the flared blue skirt swinging around her bare legs. Her hair came down over her forehead, brushing the large sunglasses. Complementing the skirt was a sleeveless crocheted blouse in soft ivory. Through the open spaces in the material the outlines of her white bra were clearly visible. My head spun. Feelings were sweeping over me, which made this woman who was pausing on the church steps looking for me, immensely desirable. The Devil and the Virgin were fighting for my heart. I had to shield my eyes to regain some composure.

Briskly, Stella walked towards me. She took off her sunglasses, threw her arms around me, and kissed me on the mouth. "The Virgin commanded me to do so," she said, releasing. me. "I have just given birth to you, not as the Saviour, that would be blasphemy, but as someone who is bringing the Magi's gifts into my life. And if that means a journey to Venus, so be it, because I know that whatever happens between us I will be redeemed. My dreams predict this," she concluded. "I can feel it."

I could not respond. Stella took my arm, and we walked to the cog-wheel railroad, which was still being pulled by an ancient steam locomotive up the steep incline to the summit of the Schafberg – sheep mountain. We rode in silence, too many emotions scrambling for expression.

It was high noon, and on the top of the mountain the view of four different lakes lay before us, awesomely beautiful. "All this is ours to enjoy," said Stella, her arms arching over the grand aerial view. "Do you think we will?"

I looked at her doubtfully. I had not recovered my speech. My lips brushed Stella's shoulder. On a slope covered with mountain gentians and cyclamen, we sat down on a rock, looking at the Mondsee – moon lake far below. Stella quickly identified the lake, which separates the province of Salzburg from Upper Austria. "My whole life seems to have revolved around the moon," said I, tracing the lines in her left palm. Her eyes coaxed me to go on.

Now that I could speak of symbols, I felt more comfortable. I gave Stella a short review of my past. "The moon has always meant the feminine to me, and the women in my life were the personifications of the moon's symbolic characteristics; from the benevolent full moon to the terrible Hecate, the goddess who reigns over moondark. And now once again, I find myself with you in the realm of the moon, happy and scared at the same time." I wondered if Stella was ready to hear about the astronaut, but decided against it. There was too much energy around already, especially since that remarkable epiphany a scant hour ago.

Stella listened attentively. "You must open yourself to my dream now, it may help us find the right way." Taking my hand, she proceeded to tell it.

"I was watching a woman in labor. A white-coated man with dark eyes and a great beard kept looking at his gold watch, timing the woman's contractions. The watch was on a gold chain and he kept moving it at regular intervals from his vest pocket to his hand. Then the woman gave birth to a boy. It was very easy. The doctor handed her the baby. Then he looked again at his watch and said, "I'm very sorry, but if I stay longer I'll miss the bell song. You have a beautiful boy, and he will marry you some day. And then he went to the opera!"

Stella's voice expressed curiosity and exasperation. "Of all these dreams I've been having, this one is really puzzling. Maybe because of this mix of opera and the baby marrying his mother. But I thought about it in the church just before, and it gave me the courage to say to you what I did. What is going on, Michael?"

She could not have anticipated my reaction. I started to laugh, unable to stop until tears made me choke. The man who seemed to have both feet on the ground was simply beside himself. Opposing emotions were criss-crossing his features, and his arms kept making flailing circles in the air.

Stella grabbed my hands and held them fast. Her grip calmed me down. "Oh, Stella!' It was a half-moan, but the words that followed were clear and coherent. "Where is your engagement ring, the one Hans got you at the auction?" The question took Stella aback. "I haven't worn it since we broke up; why do you ask? And what is this all about?"

I was still wiping the tears from my face. "Please forget my crazy behavior… just give me the ring if you still carry it with you." Fishing in her purse, Stella produced the ring. I pointed to the faint set of the second initials on the ring. "J.H. stands for Joseph

Halban, the husband of Selma Kurz. He was the obstetrician who delivered me."

Stella stared at me. "This is magic or madness," she managed after a few tense moments. "If I were the hysterical type, I might fling myself over the precipice, straight down into the distant moon lake. But the vice-president of Bank Austria, in charge of international monetary matters, isn't going to let this happen." She swallowed hard. And a light dawned. "My god, the bell song! Of course! How could I have missed it? It's the famous coloratura aria from Lakme, a part that Selma Kurz must have sung many times! But how in god's name can I dream about your birth, Michael? And that you, as a baby, were going to marry your mother… Me?"

I was stunned at her instant grasp of the dream figure's subjective meaning. Stella had intuitively realized that the woman in labor was an aspect of her own unconscious psyche, her own pregnancy coming to fruition. But that didn't help with the Oedipal implication: the boy, Michael, was going to marry his mother, any mother, perhaps Stella who could not be a mother but would become one if the incest were carried out.

Unthinkable? Wasn't this the precise counterpart to my astronaut who couldn't eat his stew without risking suffocation? Yet if she accepted the Magi's gifts – which she had consented to in front of the church in St. Wolfgang at the command of the Virgin, had even spoken of a journey to Venus – she would rejoin the fertility cycle, and the Pope's blooming staff had already predicted her redemption.

Slowly, gradually, with no words being exchanged, I realized that Stella understood what was happening. More than ever it became clear to me that she was not only a natural in assimilating unconscious imagery, but some sort of a seeress as well. It relieved some of my anxiety, which had erupted earlier when I'd been at a loss how I could ever tell her what it all meant.

Stella was calm. We were about to speak at the same time when Stella prevailed. "We don't have to act on any of this stuff, Michael," she said with quiet assurance. "Certainly not yet." She got up from the rock and went into the crowded restaurant nearby returning with an iced orange drink and two sandwiches.

I was overwhelmed with gratitude. I wanted to say so, but Stella put a finger on my lips, and said, "Eat your sandwich."

"Yes, mother," I said and we exploded into fits of laughter which released the tension these stupefying insights had imposed.

At dinner on the terrace of their hotel in St. Gilgen, Stella asked me about Selma Kurz's life. She had changed into a green silk dress with a high-neck raffled collar. At the end of a long pendant, a polished black stone rested on her chest. I recognized it as an obsidian, the glassy end-product of hot volcanic lava. On her left hand she wore Selma Kurz's ring.

"My recollection is vague. I know she came from one of the eastern provinces of the empire, studied in Paris and Vienna where she was discovered by Gustav Mahler. Richard Strauss was so taken with her voice that he rewrote the part of Zerbinetta in his *Ariadne auf*

Naxos, creating what is probably the most difficult coloratura aria in the repertory. Her ability to trill was supposed to be without peer. In addition to her fame as a singer, she became socially prominent by marrying Professor Halban. His reputation as a gynaecologist extended to America, but in Vienna the couple were known for their lavish parties where Selma would spontaneously sing, but only when her husband permitted it. The story goes that his watch was their secret code: as long as he toyed with it, she could sing, but when the watch went back to his vest pocket… *'finita la cantata.'* Selma was said to have worshipped him, and they had a daughter, Desi, who had a brief career as a soprano."

"How did it happen that he delivered you?" Stella asked.

"My father and Professor Halban belonged to the same club, and I believe it was Halban who warned my father that my mother's heart was not likely to withstand the strain of labor. He was right. But as you see, her son is hale and healthy, even though he's now your elder!"

"Please don't tease me, Michael," Stella pleaded. "The term has become meaningless." She spooned some apricot mousse into a meringue cup. The terrace was tastefully lit, and the moths of summer were dancing around the small table lamps, drawn to and repelled by a hostile energy which disturbed their nocturnal flights. A waxing crescent moon hung over the lake, throwing its pale reflection over some rowboats moored at the hotel's small wharf.

There was a commotion at the door, which opened onto the terrace. Several guests had risen, surrounding a plumpish white-haired woman. She shook hands with them, but moved nimbly toward the table where I and Stella were sitting.

"Frau Murli!" I was on my feet, hugging the woman who returned my exuberance by kissing me on both cheeks. *"Mein lieber Herr Doktor!"* she said. "Peter told me you were here and I couldn't wait to see you!" A waitress had pulled up a chair and was rewarded. *"Bist schon wieder da?* – You here again, Mariandel?" The girl blushed over being recognized by her former employer and nearly curtsied before fleeing toward the kitchen.

Michael introduced Stella. Murli, the former *grande dame* of the hotel sat down heavily. She made small talk with Stella, but her eyes were checking out the daughter going out for a date: was the dress appropriate? The hair in place? "M*ein liebes Fraeulein Kotschnig,"* said Murli. "You have no idea how pleased I am to meet you. You see, this man, my dear Herr Doktor, has not just been a favorite guest for many summers, but he's a dear friend as well." She looked at me for permission to elaborate. I gazed at her with affection and nodded. "He has suffered a great loss some years ago, but if I'm not mistaken – and my husband says I never am, but that's just to avoid an argument!" Murli winked, "he's been very fortunate in meeting you. You are a very beautiful woman."

Like a little girl caught in some forbidden activity, the vice-president of Bank Austria blushed crimson. Acting as if she hadn't noticed, Murli turned to me.

"You must tell me how you and Fraeulein Kotschnig met and how long you're staying here." Following an old routine, Mariandel, the waitress, served Murli some hot chocolate. The plump lady patted her hand. "Trained you well, didn't I?' Mariandel fled again.

Stella had regained her persona. She told the story of the accidental meeting at the opera, their mutual love of this art form, and how Michael had suggested this trip to speed her convalescence from major surgery. "I hope you're not too upset about your condition," said Murli. "There are many other ways to have children."

Stella put her hand to her mouth. Her face, barely restored to relaxed serenity, became flushed again. She gulped down her espresso. "Words fail me, Frau Murli. You know, the strangest things have been happening to me, actually to both of us. We dream about events in each other's lives that we have no conscious knowledge of; and now, you have said something that refers to my condition even though I didn't speak of it. It makes me feel I've entered into another life, like'Stella in Wonderland', and it's pretty scary."

Murli took hold of Stella's hand, and like a blind woman traced the Selma Kurz ring on her finger. "Some of us are connected by non-verbal means," she said confidently. "It could be this ring that is the bond between you and Dr. Michael. When I looked at you I knew that you too had suffered a great loss, and that surely is a tie to this man."

I had the familiar sense that there was too much unconscious energy circulating and wanted to bring the conversation back to concrete reality. Murli talked about family and her grandson, and how much she missed running the hotel.

Stella excused herself. Murli looked after the slender figure in the shimmering silk dress walking the length of the terrace, weaving in and out between the softly lit tables. Then she saw the curiosity in my face.

"*Lieber* Herr Doktor, we've been friends for many years, but I have never dared take your face in my hands… may I?" The question was rhetorical. She held my face and stroked it gently. "We're not too far apart in years," Murli said, "though I wish I looked as young as you do." There was a long pause. "I think you know that I'm a pious woman who believes in prayer. I've prayed for you many times, asking God to help you get over the loss of your Lisa, the Frau Doktor, and I remember telling you that she is not replaceable because she was the great love, the only true love in your life. And I don't think Fraulein Kotschnig is a replacement. But she is something else. The two of you need each other for something special, something very unusual that you can give to each other." Murli paused again. "Besides," she said, making it sound like a casual afterthought, "she's a very beautiful woman aching to redeem her unlived life."

I knew Murli was speaking true. I bent over her hand and kissed it, as the years with Lisa rushed by my inner eye, the tape doing a fast backward. When I looked up, Stella was coming toward us.The past vanished. And Stella did look beautiful.

Murli rose and said goodbye. "You two go well together," were her parting words. We took her to her car, then walked around the garden. Stella kissed me. It was a tender kiss, as full of feelings as the sky above us was decked out in stars. With one voice we said, *"Quante stelle!"* Of such comings together, love can grow and fear put to rest.

"Let's leave tomorrow," she said, and I agreed. Our sleep was deep and dreamless.

Nine

At breakfast, Stella said, "I've been thinking of a place I heard about, a hunting lodge, somewhere in the Pinzgau. Do you want to explore it?" The girl at the reception was helpful in locating our destination. The "penthouse" suite awaited them, said the woman at the other end of the line. It was Stella's turn to pay the bill; expenses, they had agreed, were to be shared equally. I left instructions for a bouquet of roses to be delivered to Frau Murli, and we signed the card, "With love."

Stella was driving. I marveled at the many outfits she managed to extract from her valise. She wore a pair of sleek grey pants and a red V-neck sweater over a simple white blouse. The Selma Kurz ring was firmly in place, a symbolic celebration of Michael's birth to whom she was now bound more meaningfully than to the man who had given it to her.

The lodge called "Hubertushof" was secreted away in an alpine hollow ringed by majestic firs. Named after the patron saint of hunters, it had been in the family of Count Recksdorf for over two hundred years. It was a two-story wooden structure with two tower-like features on either side. Tower East was the penthouse suite: a cozily furnished living room connected by an open archway to a bedroom with two comfortable looking beds and mountainous down comforters. An ultramodern green-marbled bathroom offered two sinks, a large tub, toilet and bidet. From the living room, one entered a wide terrace on which dwarf spruce was growing in deep rocky planters. The view encompassed the meadow in front of the lodge and, in the distance, the mountain range of the Corinthian border. To someone with animal hearing, the rumble of the Krimml waterfalls, the highest in Europe, would have been discernible.

Count Recksdorf offered a cheery welcome. The season didn't start until July, he explained, which accounted for the small number of guests currently present. Stella and I were enchanted with the place.

"The penthouse is really delightful," said Stella. "I love the privacy, and if the food measures up, this place is worth the long drive." They had been on the road for over three hours, driving past the mighty fortress of Werfen and the bustling town of Zell am See. The Count sent up drinks and tiny brioches filled with chopped spicy sausage. Relaxing on the terrace, we took in our new surroundings. Stella decided to take a bath while I dozed in a deckchair, a spruce tree shading me from the late afternoon sun.

I didn't know how much time had elapsed, but when I opened my eyes, I saw something I hadn't even toyed with as fantasy but which now presented itself as stark reality. "I felt I should reveal myself to you, Michael," said Stella, standing nude before me. In the soft twilight of the approaching sunset, her appearance was neither sexual nor even mildly erotic. She looked to me like a breathtakingly beautiful statue come to life, a naked Hermione stepping before a startled but grateful Leontes. I looked at her face, purposely avoiding the loveliness of her body. I remained silent, but Stella saw love for her in my eyes and she bent down, lightly brushing my lips with hers. "Time to get dressed," she said and disappeared.

I showered and when I came out of the bathroom Stella was sitting on the terrace wearing still another dress I hadn't seen before. It was a tight-fitting sheath of metallic blue with a deep plunging neckline. A choker of what looked like diamonds and sapphires was around her neck, and her hair fell in soft waves to her shoulders. Stella laughed at my gaping expression. "It's all fake, Michael, but it did fool some people. You're seeing me in my professional persona at fancy banking parties."

The dining room faced another open-air terrace, beyond which a few far-away lights testified to the presence of distant neighbors. Our table stood next to a gaudily glazed porcelain stove, and on the walls hung antlers of various sizes. The stuffed head of a giant moose graced the far wall where two waitresses in folkloric costumes were handling plates from the kitchen beyond.

Stella's entrance stopped the conversation at the two occupied tables. The Count, a jaunty man with a nervous twitch over his left eye, made the introductions. A physician from Vienna with his wife, and a Swiss businessman whose female companion left no doubt that she'd been supplied by a high-class escort agency. I shook my head disapprovingly. "Be tolerant, Michael," Stella warned. "Harried businessmen need relief from stressful deals." She gave me a dazzling smile. "Not everyone has mysterious dreams to guide them."

Her light mood was infectious. She chatted amiably with the doctor's wife at the next table, while the Swiss businessman was making obvious attempts to attract her attention. I felt remarkably comfortable. The image of the naked Stella had left a soothing impression which I didn't comprehend. The absence of an erotic response puzzled me; yet I trusted that our emotional compass would eventually provide a true heading.

The waitress, Margit, turned out to be Hungarian with scant command of German. Stella surprised me once again as she discussed the menu in halting Hungarian. "My father came from there, he taught me when I was little, and I recently brushed up on the language when the Bank assigned me to Budapest for a few weeks." She took a sip of the light Rosé the Count had recommended. "I have some more surprises in store, Michael!" Stella was openly flirting with me, but there was nothing seductive in either her tone or her body language. The feelings she transmitted were something so natural as if she and I were already one flesh and one spirit, hermaphroditic or androgynous, with no sexual tension between them. I had never experienced anything like it in a woman's presence, but I surrendered to it, absorbing it with a sense of wonder and curiosity.

The menu discussion over, Stella informed me about our choices. Against my habit to make my own selections, I let Stella choose. My attention was not on food, but on the radiant presence emanating from the woman who only two weeks ago was recuperating from the double trauma she had suffered. "Your mother should see you now," I said. "She'd be very happy."

"She'd be grateful to you, Michael, for suggesting it. As am I. From the bottom of my heart."

A couple of hours later, we took possession of our bedroom. And a new note was introduced in the complex orchestral score fate was creating for us: we went to sleep in one another's arms, two travelers entwined on the narrow and crooked path to dreamland which can suddenly become a broad cosmic highway to the stars.

Ten

"Are we behaving like brother and sister?" I asked her the next morning as we munched hot buttery rolls lathered with strawberry marmalade. "I have never spent a night like the last one, with a beautiful woman in my arms, and me in hers, and yet sleeping as deeply as a new-born baby."

"The same is true for me, Michael. My sleep was so peaceful and you – you were simply a part of me."

I shook my head and wanted to continue the conversation when the Count stopped by our table.

"I'm organizing a small outing, well, not too small; have you ever been on the Grossglockner road?"

"Oh, yes," I said, but it's been many years." Stella chimed in. "l was there as a child… is that where you're planning to go?"

"The day is brilliantly clear," said Count Recksdorf, the twitching eye much in evidence, "and my other four guests don't know this awesome mountain, so I thought we might all go and my station wagon is big enough. Would you care to join us?" His bubbling enthusiasm was interrupted by two people walking into the dining room. "This is my nephew, Paul Scheibling, the son of my late sister. And this is Julia, his daughter, called Mausi." Everyone shook hands. Mausi was perhaps five or six, a genuine goldilocks girl wearing a pink dirndl. Paul too had blond hair. He wore a traditional Austrian hunting suit of dark grey with green stripes along the side of his trousers, the color repeated on the lapels and elbows of his jacket. He had a friendly open face with a stubble nose and deepset brown eyes which reminded me of a fawn. I guessed Paul's age to be in the mid-forties.

"Paul is an architect in Vienna," Count Recksdorf added. "He and Mausi are eager to go up the Grossglockner," he gushed on," so if you two don't come along, you'll be here all by your lonesome selves." Lonesome selves? Hardly, Stella and I thought in unison, smiling at each other. We decided to join the party. Sweaters and blankets were provided, and the trunk of the station wagon, which was actually a minibus, swallowed two large picnic hampers. With the Count at the wheel, the little group set off to make the ascent to Austria's most spectacular mountain road, the Grossglockner High Alpine Highway.

Relishing his role as a guide, the Count delved into local lore as they rode toward the village of Bruck, an hour away, the starting point of the vaunted road. "There's a mystery about the road. Before it was built, there was no passage way through these mountains for a hundred miles east or west. Yet when the engineers started blasting, they found deep in the bowels of the mountain a Roman statue; it proved the legend of the impossible tasks performed by one mythic man, Hercules!"

Soon we were above the timberline. Grass became sparse, then disappeared altogether. "Moss is the only vegetation at this altitude," said the Count. "We're at seven thousand feet, and this gully," he pointed to the right where great boulders were lying about as if dropped by a giant's hand, "is called the witches' kitchen." A little house was sitting precariously between two enormous rocks. "This inn has been here for five hundred years, centuries before there was any passage through these impenetrable mountains. I know the people who run it: they're stubborn folk, staying here most of the year, serving the mountaineers who do the ascent the hard way."

The road was sweeping around a curve and suddenly the Grossglockner burst into view. The sight of the glittering snow covered peak, thirteen thousand feet high, drew involuntary gasps. Mausi cried out, "Look at the black ants crawling out there!" The distant specks were climbers struggling across Europe's oldest and biggest glacier, the Pasterze.

We pulled into a huge parking area. Paul got out first, helping Mausi, and close behind her Stella, to dismount from the minibus. Mausi grabbed Stella's hand. "Aunt Stella, can we go up the ice, please?" From the glacier, sparks flashed and scintillated, and even with protective sunglasses it was hard to look at the twinkling eruptions. The glacier seemed alive, leaping, dancing pinpoints of colored light streaming ceaselessly from its icy surface. The group sat down at wooden tables, breathing the thin sharp air, as they watched the Count unloading the hampers. Paul and I went inside the crowded restaurant and returned with hot coffee, tea and lemonade. The three women, Stella, the doctor's wife whose name was Steffi, and Verena, the Swiss lady who seemed relieved to have company other than the dour man she was with, busied themselves with the traditional task of setting out sandwiches and cakes.

Paul who had been rather silent during the trip, now opened up like a lightbulb programmed to be switched on at a pre-set time. "I wish I could design a tall structure, maybe an obelisk, to be erected up here, something that would transmit a beacon to the universe. At night, it would be our own star, a star from earth, reaching out to other stars! And just think what the stars must look like from this altitude!"

Mausi chuckled. "Daddy has a telescope at home in Vienna; he likes to look at the sky at night. Sometimes he stays up all night, and once he showed me the planet Jupiter – but that was before my bedtime."

Paul looked at the child affectionately. "Ever since her mother went away, she's been daddy's helper; after she's done her homework, she likes to help our cook in the kitchen, sometimes she even sets the table before I get home." He caressed Mausi's hair.

"Don't mess with my hair, daddy," the girl admonished him, sounding very grown-up, "remember how long it took to do it this morning!"

Stella, guessing the truth, addressed the child. "Where did your mother go, Mausi?" she asked gently.

"To the stars," came the serious reply. "That's why daddy looks at the stars all the time, because some day she'll come back from there."

Count Recksdorf seemed uncomfortable with this turn of the conversation. He launched into the details of Paul's career. "He's designed concert halls in France and the Netherlands, also one in America, in Pittsburgh. He specializes in acoustics. And his dream is to design a modern opera house."

This caught Stella's and my attention. The talk turned to matters operatic which interested the doctor and his wife as well. Only the Swiss couple looked bored. The man excused himself. "We'll take a walk toward the glacier," he mumbled, gripping Verena's arm. Her bored expression changed to a puppet grin: her master was calling. Mausi asked permission to come along which brightened Verena instantly, and the three vanished into the blinding sunlight.

"We're both opera lovers," I said, stroking Stella's hand. She related the *Butterfly* meeting and how her name had become the crucial link between the love duet of the first act and getting to know me.

"And now we're back with stars, Paul," said Stella. "Mausi's explanation was very moving to me; what a beautiful, poetic way to make a mother's absence acceptable."

"My wife died in a boating accident when Mausi was two. Somehow the star story is still real to her. Probably not much longer," he added wistfully. "But I'm quite a romantic myself, so I guess a part of me believes the story too. Symbolically, of course." He shielded his eyes, searching for the little girl among the gawking, chattering crowd. "Is your name really Stella?"

"It is," I answered quickly. "And she has become my morning and evening star."

Paul reddened. "I did not mean to put my foot in, please forgive me." Genuinely embarrassed, he looked away.

Stella reached for his hand. "Never mind, Paul. No harm done." Then she turned to me. "Are you playing jealous and possessive?"

The tone was light, even joking, but I felt rebuked. "The old triangle," I said. "Put a beautiful woman at a table with two men, and the green-eyed monster stirs in the background. Especially when both men are into stars, and the woman's name is Stella. I apologize, Paul."

Relief appeared in the person of Mausi who came tripping back, carrying a small shiny rock. "Look, everybody, I got a piece of the glacier!" A bluish vein streaked across the rock she held in her tiny hand. No one knew anything about geology, but I hazarded a guess. "The blue part may be Lapis, that's a very lucky stone."

"Like the one on your pinkie?" She'd eyed my ring earlier.

"Yes," said Stella. "Uncle Michael has been a very lucky man all his life."

"Let it hold out just a little longer," I murmured. Stella heard me and put her arm around my neck,. her lips seeking mine.

"Gee," said Mausi, looking up at her father. "They sure like to kiss!"

"Show me where you found the glacier stone," said Paul, his eyes on Stella's hair. A lambent glow shone from the thick mahogany strands as if the sun might set it afire. He averted his stare and walked away.

Mausi ran after him. "What's the matter, daddy? Don't you like auntie Stella?"

Eleven

In the crook of my arm, Stella was peacefully sleeping. The dinner had been convivial, with everyone reminiscing about the mountain's grandeur. Even the Swiss businessman had relaxed, coaxing the group to call him Seppli. Steffi and Verena had found a guitar and were singing Austrian and Swiss folksongs. Mausi had kissed them all goodnight, and told her father that she was too tired for a bedtime story.

"I'm very grown up tonight," she announced. "I'll put myself to bed. But tomorrow it'll be different!" She shook a mischievous finger at her father and went upstairs. Only Paul had remained quiet. He excused himself early, claiming it was a good night for comet watching. In our bedroom, I had kept one nightlight on. Sleep eluded me. My position was cramped, but as the guardian of Stella's sleep, I didn't want to dislodge her. In the semi-darkness I kept looking down at her, immense tenderness in my heart. The top of her lacy white nightgown was open, one ivory breast half exposed. For the umpteenth time I wondered about the absence of an erotic impulse. Yet wasn't my tender affection part of Eros as well? My mind tried different projections: were my feelings those of a son for a mother? A father's for a daughter? It was clear that I was reunited, through her, with something exquisitely feminine in myself – but where did that leave Michael, the man?

Stella moved, and the left breast slid out completely. I looked at the nipple with a sudden yearning that frightened me. That small pink bud, flat and fragile, was the secret door to every temple I had ever been to; the access to every shrine I had ever worshipped at; it was the channel to eternal life, providing the pilgrim with the password that would gain him admission if he was pure of heart and spirit. I thought I qualified. And I bent down and put my lips on that round pink spot. A sweet scent, like a gentle narcotic, rose from her skin. My eyes closed, and I fell asleep on Stella's breast.

The dream I recorded in the morning was as sharply etched as Michael Pacher's woodcarving of the Virgin's mantle in the great winged altar of St. Wolfgang.

The astronaut was taking off his space helmet. I held my breath, terrified that the man would suffocate.

But he was okay. Shielding him in a great big bubble were the three goddesses of the moon, for once united in a single purpose. There was fresh air in the bubble, air from a piney forest on earth, and the astronaut spooned down his stew. When he was done, the scene changed to my office in New York. In a child's large scrawl a sign said, "The doctor is in."

Twelve

In the morning, Stella wasn't feeling well. Her forehead felt feverish, and I asked the Viennese doctor to take a look at her. Egon Nussbaum was a general practitioner who checked her pulse, pressure and temperature, and thought she had a touch of the "summer flu", a harmless twenty-four-hour bug. "Fluids and bedrest," said Dr. Nussbaum. He reassured the Count that Stella was in no danger.

Paul shyly asked me to please give her his good wishes, and little Mausi was upset when Dr. Nussbaum forbade a visit to Stella's room.

"But sick people like to hear stories," she complained.

Steffi Nussbaum asked Paul's permission to take the child shopping to the next village, Neukirchen. She'd seen a charming blue dress, and it would give her great pleasure to give it to Mausi as a present. The Swiss couple decided to stay put. The pool looked inviting, and Verena wanted to model a barely decent looking bikini.

My dream kept revolving in my mind. I wasn't sure what to make of it; even my intuition remained silent. On impulse, I suggested to Paul a walk to some nearby ruins – a shady path would take them there in less than an hour. At first, Paul hesitated, but I was persuasive; feeling like making amends for yesterday's uncalled for rebuff. The path wound in serpentine turns past several haylofts and then entered a forest so dense that sunlight was splintered into thin shafts, bouncing back into dappled patches of green. We walked in silence, each reluctant to broach the issue, which had lodged itself between us.

"I have great respect for your profession, Michael, and I know we're not in your consulting room, and perhaps you don't want to hear about my private life…" Paul waited for a reaction. I gave him an encouraging nod, though the gesture was costing me dearly. Without warning, my third eye had opened, revealing both parts of my dream's meaning and where Paul was heading as well. I felt faint. The need to lean against a tree was overwhelming. Fighting for control, I put my hand on Paul's arm.

"I know what's on your mind, Paul. But I don't know if I want to answer you." As sometimes happened to me, an operatic quotation raced through my mind, wanting to be recognized. I fought against it, but Wotan's voice was not to be stilled. "You want to talk about Stella. Go on."

"I'm not a brash person, Michael; I'm sure you've marked me as a rather shy introvert, a romantic who likes to look to the stars for hope, for comfort and reassurance in his loneliness." He paused, sitting down on a stump, the decaying remnant of a once living tree. "You said yesterday that Stella was your morning and evening star. The phrase struck me, it rang like a gong." Paul stumbled, hesitated, then forced himself go on. "A gong, a sound which covered the entire scale the human hear can receive – as if you were her father, lover, son, spiritual healer, I don't know what else. She chided you, lightly, yes, for being possessive – but I know she was right, not in the jealous way of the green monster, but as if you were her saviour, holding her very lifeline in your hands… I'm sounding awfully melodramatic to myself." I raised my hand. "If you were a patient of mine, I'd be awed by your connection with what's behind the word; by your symbiotic relationship with the unconscious, and if that patient were interested, I might recommend him for training as an analyst. You, Paul, do more than awe me: your reading of my mind terrifies me! You haven't a clue how straight on the target you are!"

I was shouting. From somewhere an echo came back, like thunder that was still miles away announcing itself by sheet lightning, invisible since we were under the canopy of the shielding forest.

"I'm all you say for Stella, and she is the universe in which I'm contained. We're still contained in each other; she and I are what you look for in the heavens, we're a galactic mass, spinning around each other, until a cataclysm will throw one of us off, to form a new solar system, no longer dependent on the mother who spawned us." I tried to breathe more quietly.

Paul appeared shaken by this powerful outburst. He groped for words. "If I'm out of bounds, I apologize,

Michael. But I think I heard a confession. Maybe like a defiant sinner who dared some priest to deny him absolution." Both men were silent. A forest bird warbled near by. Finally, Paul risked the question, which pounded away in his mind. "And Stella? Does she affirm what you just told me?"

Like a man desperately trying to throw off the stranglehold an adversary had wound around his neck threatening to break his windpipe, my fury was getting the better of me. I felt infused with vast powers, with a voice drumming in my ear, "Kill him, kill him." With a twisting effort I turned away from Paul, and dug my finger into a decaying tree, clawing at the bark which came loose in moldy chunks. Red ants were swarming inside.

"Part of me knows you're the new man in her life. She can't have children, and you have little Mausi whom she will love. You're the right age for her too, and you like the stars… Stella!" I began to sob. Great muffled wracking cries escaped from my throat; between swallowing and heaving, my air threatened to be cut off and I choked convulsively.

Reflexively, Paul drummed on my back to restore normal breathing. Gradually I calmed down. Then I gripped Paul's shoulder.

"I know I just blasted you into space. But there is an archetypal precedent here. In the third opera of the 'Ring' cycle, Wotan, whose reign is ending, makes a last futile attempt to bar the hero's, Siegfried's way to Bruennhilde's rock where the world's Anima is sleeping. He extends his spear on which all his previous deeds and misdeeds are recorded. But young

Siegfried shatters the spear with the sword, which Wotan had originally bequeathed to him. The way to awaken Bruennhilde is open, and Siegfried begins his ascent. Wotan, compelled to accept his fate, says, *'Zieh hin, ich kann dich nicht halten!* – Go forth, I cannot prevent you.' I may not look it and don't feel it, but I'm getting close to the end of my life, Paul. Stella is my final link to the Eternal Feminine, the last star on my firmament, and we've met under circumstances which command us to explore what it is all about, for both of us. For the moment, her star shines like Venus in the evening and morning sky. But my voyage to her may be about to end. But make no mistake, Paul, what I'm saying to you, is my story. Stella is as sensitive to unconscious happenings as you seem to be, so I would not be surprised if she picked up what's going on between you and me. But the decisive, the conscious step, must come from her, in her own good time. And because of this, I want to swear you to secrecy about my confession." Paul bowed his head. "Thank you, Michael, for your trust. Of course, all you've said is safe with me." It was barely a murmur.

My impassioned speech had silenced the warbling bird. Now the winged minstrel was heard again, joined by another trilling voice. "A mating call," I said, shivering.

Paul raised his eyes, wrestling with himself to shape another question. "How can you speak so knowingly about the future? I haven't dared to think Stella might be interested in me. I don't even know my own feelings yet."

Walking slowly, we resumed our trek to what was left of an ancient castle. Its rocky tower was crumbling, a shapeless heap of boulders. I felt as if I had suddenly aged, not in my body, but that my outpouring to Paul had sapped a reserve of emotional energy I had protected for a very long time.

A different path led back to the Count's lodge. We came by a small shrine. A wooden cross over a stone altar on which three cupped candles were throwing a feeble light on a simple painting of the Madonna, was leaning crookedly against a tree. "I'm not much into prescribed rituals," Paul said. "But I'd like to stay here for a moment, if it's all right with you."

I knelt down, wrapping my hands around one of the candles. My mind went back to the church in St. Wolfgang where Stella had wanted me to kneel with her, and I had glimpsed the painting of Satan, the seducer. Now I was praying, not to the Virgin, but to the Goddess whose loving protection I had been granted all my life. I didn't know what to ask for, but it was a vague plea for an appropriate exit ritual – to be released from her arms, with boundless gratitude, and permitted to continue my pilgrimage until my time was up. Paul remained standing, one hand over his heart, his own silent wish too unformed to be expressed in prayer. When we arrived at the lodge, I sensed a new bond was alive in both men; how long it would keep the faith was uncertain.

Stella had evidently recovered from the touch of the "summer flu." She was sitting by the pool, chatting with the Swiss couple who had become astonishingly companionable. Il had never seen her in a bathing suit, and was immediately yanked back to the moon. The force of the transition amazed me: a short time ago, I'd been praying for an exit; and now, looking at Stella in a form-fitting white swimsuit my anima soared high like a bird of the wild being suddenly released from enforced captivity. For his part, Paul saw the stars dancing in my eyes, but he no longer concealed his own starry look at the woman in the dazzling white outfit. "Let it be a fair contest," he said to himself.

Count Recksdorf ambled over, trailed by Steffi and Mausi. The child was wearing a blue summer frock, and everybody around the pool applauded. "You look enchanting, Mausi," said Stella, opening her arms to hug the little girl. Paul saw his daughter being embraced by Stella and his prayer found a sharply defined focus. "I'm going to court this woman," he said to himself. "And some day I will marry her.'

"We have fresh crayfish for dinner," the Count announced. "I caught them myself in a swift brook coming from the Krimml falls. You must go see the falls soon as long as this great weather continues. Maybe tomorrow?"

The gathering by the pool broke up. Stella and I went to our room for a rest before dinner. "How was your walk with Paul?" she inquired as she slipped out of her swimsuit, replacing it with a silk robe the color of her hair. The nude intimacy between us had become routine, but I looked away as she was changing.

"What do you think of him?" I parried her question. "You know, I'm really not sure, but I'm developing quite a crush on Mausi. She's the child I've always wanted, a little dreamy but self-assured and lovely looking."

"But what about her father?" I persisted. Stella looked at me curiously.

"You know, we never got back to our talk about the brother and sister stuff; maybe we should resume it. Perhaps after dinner?"

She disappeared into the bathroom. I heard the water running, and knocked on the door. Hearing no reply, I walked in. The window and the mirrors over the double sink were steamed up. Stella liked her bath very hot. Groping my way to the tub, I sat down on its rim. Her body was submerged beneath a froth of scented bubbles; her head, with eyes closed, rested against the porcelain end of the tub. She sensed my presence and extended a wet hand, seeking mine.

"About brother and sister," I said. "I'm still confused." I told her about the astronaut eating his stew under the protection of the lunar goddesses.

For a long time Stella didn't say anything. "Will you wash my back, please?" She sat up, her breasts floating above the bubbles. Soaping her back, I gently massaged the skin.

"I like Paul," she said unexpectedly. "But that's all. You, on the other hand, are as mysterious to me as ever. I think the brother sister thing is just surface because we're both afraid. So we make believe there's nothing else. And last night I woke up briefly, and found you asleep on my breast. It excited me, Michael. Now go away." She withdrew her hand and submerged herself, preparing to wash her hair.

I left the steamy bathroom, perspiring, and upset about Stella's revelation.

The opposing stimuli assaulting me were almost too much to assimilate: first the soul-baring with Paul; then, at the pool being yanked back to the moon; and now hearing from Stella's mouth something that swept away their placidly comfortable brother-sister behavior. What next?, I wondered, looking for balance. Although I rarely drank hard liquor, I deliberately went down to the bar. The Swiss couple was having pre-dinner drinks and I joined them, downing two double scotches in rapid succession. Verena was wearing a red dress whose cleverly designed neckline plunged almost to her navel. Seppli had a possessive arm around her waist, and the Count was telling the story of the stuffed moosehead. It irritated me, and carrying my third scotch, I walked onto the outdoor terrace where Dr. Nussbaum and his wife were enjoying their gentle Camparis. I sat down at their table.

"How long have the two of you been married?" I asked. The Nussbaums beamed. "Nearly thirty years," said Egon.

"And has either of you ever been unfaithful?" I demanded, uncharacteristically blunt. Egon was shocked. Steffi blushed.

"What a question, Dr. Stone!" she parried. I intuited a secret in Steffi's past of which Egon was not aware. "Before Egon and I became engaged, there was a young man who courted me. He was a romantic dreamer, and maybe if I hadn't known Egon already, I might have fallen for him. When I turned him down, he pursued my best friend, Tina. They had a stormy affair, and when she refused to marry him, he killed himself."

Now Egon remembered the long-forgotten saga. I knew a half-truth when I heard one. There was no doubt that Steffi had acted out a brief fling with the romantic dreamer and then settled for the solid Egon. Her next sentence confirmed my hunch.

"I loved Egon's stable character, and he's been the best husband and father I could have wished for. You dear, dear man!" She pinched his cheek affectionately. Egon bloomed.

"Why did you ask, Michael? Have you ever been married?"

I didn't want to talk about Agnes or any other woman in my past life. My whole being was filled with Stella. "Do you think I'm too old to marry Stella?" The question was out of my mouth before I consciously registered it. The Nussbaums looked at each other.

"You look very youthful," said Egon, "though I think you're probably past sixty. But in my opinion an age gap should not be an obstacle in marrying someone, unless of course one wants to raise children."

"And Stella has talked to us about her surgery," Steffi added. "So my answer is no, you're not too old if you two are really in love." Both Nussbaums were beaming at him like benevolent parents-in-law. I shook Egon's hand solemnly and gave Steffi a peck on the cheek. I went back to the bar.

Stella was sitting with Seppli and Verena, sipping a Dubonnet. She wore the green silk dress I remembered from the evening with Murli in St. Gilgen, and her hair was freshly blown dry, burnished mahogany against the creamy skin of her face. My pulse raced. I didn't know if the three scotches were responsible or if it was the woman casually sitting on a high bar stool, long legs crossed, waiting for me. The Count's voice boomed from the kitchen, giving instructions to the cook. Before I could cross the space to where Stella was sitting, Paul, Mausi and the Nussbaums entered the cozy paneled room. Mausi immediately ran up to Stella and showed her a drawing.

"I've sketched everybody from memory this afternoon," she announced proudly. "I just sat down, but I had to count on my fingers if I left anybody out." She produced the colored sheet. Alongside a table, eight stick figures were leaning against it. Realistically enough, Mausi had placed the Count in the center, herself between Paul and Stella; then came Doctor Nussbaum with a little black bag, Steffi, and finally the Swiss couple. Michael was absent.

"You forgot Uncle Michael," said Stella casually.

Mausi looked puzzled, counting slowly on her fingers. Then, brightly, "I'll just put him next to Aunt Verena now." She proceeded to correct the drawing.

Much later in the evening, I blamed the unaccustomed liquor for my extreme reaction. "You should have taught her how to count, Paul," I yelled. "You're an architect, aren't you? So teach your child about numbers!" I stormed out. There was an embarrassed silence. The Count who had missed the scene, came in, happily rubbing his hands over the fresh crayfish which were simmering in his special broth. "They only take a few minutes," he said, urging everyone into the dining room.

Of the whole group only Mausi was not upset. "Grownups are like that sometimes," she said gravely. "I know how to count, daddy. But I do make mistakes." Impulsively, Stella hugged the child. Paul tried to smile at his daughter without much success. Mausi looked at Stella beseechingly. "If Uncle Michael is still angry, you could sit at our table."

"I will, Mausi, if your father has no objections." Paul nodded lamely, still too shaken to speak freely. Along with the Nussbaums, they walked into the dining room. "You're so composed, Stella,' Steffi murmured. "Poor Paul, his feelings are so transparent."

"Sometimes it helps to be a professional banker," Stella whispered back.

Thirteen

I missed the crayfish dinner. I returned to the lodge about three hours later, finding that everybody had retired. In their room, Stella was relaxing in an easy chair, reading about the Count's family history. "The crayfish were really delicious; and we had Mango icecream for dessert." There wasn't a trace of recrimination in either her voice or demeanor. "Where were you?"

"Nowhere and anywhere, really. Mostly on a bench in the village, beating my breast and too ashamed to face you and the others. But especially you."

"It's as if some big event is hovering nearby," mused Stella. "Not necessarily something catastrophic, but a great sea change. I can feel it, but I don't fear it."

"Maybe we're in the eye of the storm, and things will overtake us when we leave it," I said, anxious and remorseful. Stella looked at me, emerald eyes caressing. "What set you off tonight? Just because Mausi forgot to draw you?" I was resisting her, but she kept probing. "Are you worried you'll be wiped off the map? Or did the child hit upon the truth, that you're going to wipe yourself off?"

I felt the anger rising again and fought hard to contain it. "Yes," I said, sensing tears behind the anger and wanting to keep them at bay. "Yes, I'm afraid that I'll get wiped off, vanish, and all of a sudden I'll be back in my New York office, having lost you."

It was no use. The sobs could not be suppressed and I surrendered to them. Stella held me. "Four weeks ago I didn't know you. And now you've become the most important person in my life. I don't want to lose you, but I think we're still too blind to see what we're doing, what roles have been assigned to us – we haven't found each other's proper place. Give us time, Michael."

They remained embraced for a long time. I calmed down and decided to go to sleep. Drowsily, I watched Stella walk into the bathroom. Through the half-open door my eyes, heavy with impending sleep, transmitted an image of Stella carefully inspecting her face. She appeared satisfied with what she saw. "How healthy she looks," I formed the unfocused thought. Stella lowered her nightgown to expose her breasts. The view of their full ripeness, not yet subject to gravity's pull, became my final send-off into sleep.

As the first peach light filtered through our open bedroom window, I stirred. I became aware of Stella's body spooned against my back, her hand resting on my stomach. For a while I lay still, luxuriating in the sultry heat our bodies generated. Like a leaf dropping from a tree, a single sheet of paper floated from their night table onto the bed. In the pale dawn, I read the dream Stella must have recorded earlier.

"I was in my apartment on Annagasse. The ceiling of my bedroom was open to the sky. It was night, and I was thinking, "Quante stelle!', when a small spaceship came out of the heavens and circled over Vienna. A lone woman was piloting the craft. I couldn't see her face, but the ship's logo was a black ring with the letters S K and J H. Then the J H disappeared, and was replaced by a P and an M just as the ship landed in front of the opera house. The pilot emerged, wearing the dark green dress I had worn when I met Michael, and walked into the opera house. The first act of *Madam Butterfly* was in progress, and Michael, wearing the uniform of an American naval officer, was singing the part of Lt. Pinkerton. The woman walked past the full orchestra section, then jumped across the pit. From the stage, she motioned to the conductor, who looked somewhat like Egon Nussbaum, to stop. She then announced in a loud voice, 'Due to the recall of the battleship *Lincoln,* this performance is cancelled.'"

As I put the paper down, Stella moved. Enfolding her in my arms, a wave of bittersweet longing washed over me. I tried not to make a hasty judgement of what I had read, but the recall of Pinkerton's ship fueled the anxiety that I was being pulled out of Stella's unconscious. I got out of bed and went to the window. Though some fresh snow glistened on the mountains, a dark cloudbank hovered over the valley. As I watched, it began to discharge thickly coiled strands of rain, shielding me from the outside world.

"Michael, come back to bed. I'm cold." I slipped in next to Stella. 'I've read your dream," I said softly.

"I know you did. Your ship was recalled just after you'd been singing the *'Amore o grillo'* phrase when Pinkerton describes his mixed feelings for Butterfly, you know, when he doesn't know whether it's love or a game, like a girl in every port. In the story, it is he who abandons her." Stella was hugging me tightly. "Are you going to abandon me, Michael?"

"I'm the grandfather who's been spooking you from the beginning," I said. "The dream's theme is abandonment. It's a question of who will abandon whom, isn't it? And the message is coming from outer space, like my astronaut on the moon. It's a cosmic issue."

Stella closed her eyes again. She lay back, wrapped in the downy featherbed squeezing my hand. "Last night I looked at myself. I'm a healthy woman again, thanks to the magic this trip has woven. No, that's not right. It's the magic our dreams have woven, and without you I'd still be in Vienna, feeling sorry for myself."

She paused. I stroked her face, inhaling the lush scent coming from the commingling of our bodies.

"But there was this other thing. I became aroused again thinking how you'd fallen asleep on my breast a few nights ago." It was her turn to walk to the window. With her back to me, Stella spoke into the rain.

"I think that's why I had the dream. I'm not supposed to go in that direction. That way lies the sin."

I was no longer surprised by the uncanny self-perception of this remarkable woman. "But the blooming staff? You've been forgiven, remember?" I heard the pitying pleading in my voice, how I wanted it to be different, and felt suddenly ashamed.

"I know," Stella said. "Let's have breakfast."

Fourteen

For the next three days it rained steadily. Seppli and Verena suffered it for two, but departed on the third, heading for Switzerland. "In the Engadin the sun shines all the time," Seppli proclaimed. The weather report confirmed this and they decided to go there.

With no new guests arriving, the lodge took on a slightly forlorn face. Everyone was reading or playing games. Paul revealed that he had played tournament Scrabble, and proved it by defeating one and all. Though I hadn't played in years, I polished up my bridge game. Partnered with Steffi against Stella and Egon, I endured Steffi's good-natured ribbing with a grin-and-bear it countenance.

"Why didn't you finesse the Queen of Hearts?" Steffi demanded in exasperation.

"I'm sorry," I replied, "but I have a lot of trouble these days with the Queen of Hearts."

"No innuendoes, please," said Stella. "Paul could misinterpret them." I realized that she was trying to draw Paul more openly into the triangle of which she was the center. For the sake of uncovering more clearly definable feelings. I knew, too, of Paul's attraction to Stella. The tragic irony of this constellation wasn't lost on me. Stella and myself, each immersed in a whirlpool of criss-crossing emotions and each under a mandate to find the true path.

Egon's bid of Three No Trumps pulled Stella back to the present. She looked at her own hand, and when Steffi passed, she raised the bid to six, a Small Slam. I who held the Ace and King of Spades doubled her bid. Stella spread her hand on the table and walked over to watch Egon play the bid. She realized immediately that he could not possibly fulfil the contract.

Disappointed, she went to the table where the Count, Paul and Mausi were playing Scrabble. In his shy way, Paul had not picked up on Stella's taunt. She hunched down next to Mausi. The child was really sharp, Stella concluded, as Mausi filled in some spaces with the word "honeymoon".

"Do you know what a honeymoon is?" Stella asked her.

"Of course I do." Mausi was piqued. "After two people get married, they go away to some nice place and love each other all the time. Have you ever been on a honeymoon, Aunt Stella?"

"I've not found a man I wanted to marry, Mausi. But I know I will some day, and then I'll go with him on a honeymoon."

"You must go to a sweet place where there's lots of honey, and the moon is full and bright," said Mausi dreamily. "When I was real little, I always wanted to marry daddy, especially after mummy left. But now, I'm not so sure."

"You're so much of a woman already, you're giving me the chills," she murmured outside of Mausi's hearing. At the bridge table Egon, surprising the others, had fulfilled the bid, but only because I had blundered badly. "Next time you play with Stella," said Steffi, really annoyed. I apologized and went out for some fresh air. My mind couldn't let go of the abandonment issue. There was also the matter of the initials. The men in their earlier lives, Johann Hartmann and Joseph Halban, had been replaced by the two men who now dominated Stella's: Paul and Michael. And Michael had been ordered to stop singing. Frustration over time's curved ball kept spitting up hot lava from his underground volcano. What a pointless duel was I still fighting?

The Count was called to the kitchen, and Mausi decided she'd enough of big words. Taking her crayola set, she sunk into an easy chair and began to sketch.

It was five o'clock and the rain had stopped. I overheard Stella inviting Paul to accompany her to the village's general store: she had a craving for mint chocolate candy. Surprised, Paul accepted and got raincoats and umbrellas. I went outside to smoke a cigarette.

Stella threw me an astonished look. “Another vice? Scotch wasn’t enough?” she asked testily. I waved them off and went back inside.

A feeling of despair, insubstantial but pervasive, was gripping me again. Just seeing Stella and Paul walking away together made me furious. I went looking for Steffi. The Nussbaums were having coffee and cake, and Il wondered if I could have some words with Steffi alone. Not trusting my own reactions, I needed an older woman’s take on the crosscurrents which seemed to be everywhere.

“I’ll go for a walk with you, Michael, after we’ve finished this delicious cranberry pie.” Outside, the clouds were breaking up. It promised to be a clear evening. I took Steffi’s arm and we walked past the Count’s well-tended little graveyard in the general direction of the village.

“Look, Michael, I have eyes in my head, and I see you’re eating your heart out because Paul is young and taken with Stella; he obviously hopes to marry again and provide a mother for Mausi. Paul is a serious man. Stella, however, is attached to you in a way I’ve never seen a woman act. It’s as if the two of you were under some kind of spell.” Steffi was bewildered.

“We have an unconscious bond that keeps the two of us tethered to one another with a dream cord.” I was trying hard to express myself sensibly. “My mind is ready to give her up, it even knows that she and Paul would go well together, but I can’t let her go. It is Stella who must leave me, on her own free decision; and this can happen only if Paul goes seriously after her. When he does, my heart will break, but I’ll consent to it because I have no other choice. I'm telling you all this, Steffi, with great dread in my heart, but I'm fond of you, and because I believe you can help this birth-and-death process along."

Steffi heard my pain and deep sincerity, but her feelings rebelled against playing matchmaker in this delicate situation so fraught with explosive emotions. She liked them all so much! If she encouraged Paul to be bolder in courting Stella, could Michael bear to watch it without losing his temper again?

"I'll think about it," she promised. "And I'll talk with Egon too; he's very sensitive in such matters."

I couldn't resist a tease. "You did have a fling with the romantic guy before you married Egon, didn't you?"

"Oh you," said Steffi, poking me in the ribs. "Of course I did. Never open your mouth in front of a psychoanalyst, people always say. But, yes, it was a lovely brief affair, and I was heartbroken when he killed himself." The exchange of confidences was like a comfortable warm blanket Michael and Steffi were wrapping around each other. When we turned back to the lodge, Steffi told me that she was going to intervene somehow. But events overtook her decision with surprising swiftness.

Fifteen

It was the kind of summer morning when the air, not yet warmed by the sun, is so crisp that inhaling it deeply is almost uncomfortable, as if a sharp draft is rushing down your windpipe and you wait for a return flow of what is still warm deep inside your body. You sense the sun coming up behind the crest of the mountain the penthouse was facing, and the inner eye anticipates the appearance of the first rays before the inexorable celestial event actually occurs.

Stella and I were having breakfast on our little terrace. Dewdrops still shimmered on the dwarf spruce in their rocky planters. “Let’s see the Krimml falls today,” Stella said. “The weather could not be more glorious.” Under her maroon silk robe Stella was naked. She had only splashed water on her face and brushed her teeth when breakfast arrived, and the fragrance of her body, still warm from long hours of downy sleep, clung sweetly to her skin.

“Your body overpowers the aroma of the coffee,” I said. “That must say something about pheromones.” I had not intended such a deliberate come-on. Was this a genuine erotic response or yet another try to forestall Stella’s moving away from me?

“Oh, Michael,” Stella said with great affection. “Let’s just put the heavy stuff aside and enjoy this great day! We love each other in a most peculiar way – and things won’t get any clearer today, okay?” My uncertain mood surrendered to her serene appeal. This morning, I decided, she was still there, in full bloom for me, and I wanted to make the most of it. We got dressed and consulted with the Count about the best approach to the famous falls.

“You have a choice to climb on either side of the falls, but I suggest you pick the left bank; the climb is steeper, but at the midpoint between the first and second cascade you have the best view of this tremendous spectacle. Also, there's a place for snacks nearby. Be sure to take your sunglasses; plastic raincoats can be rented at the box office." We were about to drive off when the Count called us back. "Tonight the falls are illuminated, which is truly magical, so you may want to go back after dinner. In fact, I'll try to arrange a little party; there's a spot, halfway up the Gerlos pass road from which we can see the floodlights go on!"

It was ten o'clock when we reached the vast parking area in the town of Krimml. Following the Count's advice, we started up on the left bank. For the first fifteen minutes, the well-marked path led in a gentle rise through meadows and woods. Then the gradient became steep. After half an hour Stella demurred. She lay down in the grass. "Neither of us is in the kind of shape this climb requires, so let's do this *andante molto e con sordino.*" Though still invisible, the roaring of the falls was constant.

I was feeling good, even as my breath was coming in short shallow drafts. I was surprised how well I was adjusting to an exercise which recalled my Army days, nearly fifty years ago, when I would do a forced march of twenty miles in the broiling Texas heat with a forty-pound pack on my shoulders. I stretched out next to Stella.

"We have all the time," I said, raising myself on an elbow and looking in her eyes. "I would have liked to say, 'all the time in the world', but I've got to stop fooling myself. I know we will eventually re-enact the third act of *Boheme,* when Mimi and Rodolfo agree to part, not for someone else, but because they can't bear staying together. You will leave me, Stella, because…' He stopped.

I sounded to myself not just like a broken record, but like a man unable to accept reality, wanting to stop time, to rewind it, so he could have a new life with this unique woman whom some benevolent goddess had sent his way, only to have her spirited away again by some mocking satanic being, laughing derisively, as if it had all been a mirage. Resuming our ascent, we came to a clearing where a first view of the falls struck us with elemental force. Leaning against a concrete railing, we looked at the roaring water as it tumbled, rushed, wave over spraying wave, on its final twelve hundred feet descent into the valley. Straining to see upward where the next level was hidden, by both distance and the blinding water coming towards them, we wondered silently if the energy required by continuing the ascent would be matched by a more stupendous view still. Over the ceaseless noise, Stella shouted, "Let's go on!" and I nodded approvingly. Strewn with small rocks, the path got steeper. We rested about every ten minutes, and after nearly an hour of strenuous effort, we did reach the plateau the Count had been praising.

We were at three thousand feet. No superlative could do justice to describe what lay before us. The falls were narrower and far more turbulent than on the first level. It was as if the water was trying to expand, breaking over the ledge on which we stood, engulfing and crushing us into the atoms we once were and would again be some day. The spray hit us, and in seconds our clothes were soaked. The plastic raincoats were forgotten and would have been useless anyway. The water was icy, but the midday sun immediately turned the soaking spray into steam, a wet but not altogether unpleasant feeling, as if standing in one's bathroom, switching the shower from cold to hot in rapid succession.

Suddenly, on the opposite bank and barely discernible through the glistening mist, Stella thought she spotted two familiar figures. She made a frantic effort to get me to look where she was pointing, but my fogged-up glasses rendered me sightless. Stella pulled me back to where my face was clear of the spray. "It's Paul and Mausi," she shouted, "on the other side!" Excitedly, she moved back and forth in search of a spot where she might signal to them.

In the midst of this unceasing roar, among mist and sprays and the gigantic power of the thundering falls, time arrested itself. It was but a fraction of a second, but enough for the four of them, two on either side of the raging waters, to recognize each other and to point upward. A thousand feet from where we stood, seen from a steep angle, a bridge had been built to enable tourists to look up and down into the foaming whirlpools. Few people were crossing over, for the closeness of the elemental energy beneath the bridge was not for timid souls. A local legend told of an adulterous tryst taking place on the bridge, and how a giant wave had swept the sinful couple into the falls, with nothing left of them to attest they had ever lived. On windy days, guards were posted at either end of the bridge, preventing anyone from crossing. But the day was soft and calm, and shortly Stella, Michael, Paul and Mausi stood together on the connecting span. The noise made it impossible to talk, so they attempted through signs to decide on which side to descend jointly. Mausi was clearly scared, holding on to both men. I looked into the madness below and thought of Sherlock Holmes and Doctor Moriarty, when justice and the criminal mind were wrestling over ultimate verities at the Reichenbach falls in Switzerland. Which of the titans had been victorious was never revealed.

Stella was raising her arm, pointing at something far downstream. The flash of a sunbeam lit up the Selma Kurz ring on her finger. Arrested by the sudden spark, Paul reached for her hand and Stella gripped his own, hard. Her face turned to me, willing me to look at what she was doing. With a fluid motion, Stella pulled the ring off her finger and threw it in a wide arc into the screaming life force below.

I understood. For the briefest moment my heart stopped. Then the gold curtain of Vienna's opera house came down for the last time. I pried Mausi loose from her father's hand, and walked with her to the right bank of the falls. There we sat down on a rock and waited for Stella and Paul to join us.

Sixteen

Inspired by the prospect of the illuminated falls (which happened only once in every summer month), the Count had ordered a champagne dinner. In addition to his six guests, he had invited several local friends who enriched the meal with tall tales. Baron Max, another hunter of moose from an adjoining valley, and his dowager mother, the Baroness Elsa who wore a dress of considerable vintage, were the liveliest of the group. The legend of the adulterous tryst on the bridge was recounted in greater detail. *"Pas devant les enfants,"* the Baroness had said, but she was overruled, and Mausi was too tired anyway to pay attention to an immoral story; she was waiting for dinner to be over so they could get going and see the lit-up falls.

"It was the old triangle, you see," said Max. "The miller, one Johann Sebastian Mahlkopf, was getting on in years, but was still in robust health and very much in love with his younger wife, Katharina. She loved him, but was secretly grieving over being barren." I was about to interrupt, but Stella threw me a glance of such warmth that I thought better of it. They were sitting opposite each other, she being flanked by the Count and Paul, while I was seated between Steffi Nussbaum and the dowager Baroness.

"Well, miller Mahlkopf had a nephew by the name of Franz Krimml."

"The Krimmls, you see," the Baroness Elsa interrupted her son, "were and still are a local family since it was customary for people moving into the valley from someplace else, to eventually adopt an already existing name."

"So Franz apparently had an inborn affinity for the falls and the brook which bore his name," Max resumed. "He fell in love with Katharina, and though she resisted his advances, she granted him one wish: he could kiss her one time, and one time only, in a place of his choice. Beside himself over the promised kiss, he chose the bridge across the falls as a place where nature's force and abundance might become his ally in seducing Katharina beyond what she had granted him. In those days, of course, it was not the bridge we have today, but several wide hardwood planks nailed together, tethered by strong hempen ropes to two sturdy trees on opposite sides of the falls.

"Too pious to renege on a sworn promise, Katharina tried to talk Franz out of his chosen location, but to no avail. At high noon, the story goes, the two exchanged a kiss on the planks. And then the wave came."

I cleared my throat. "There is another way to look at this story, not as punishment for a transgression, but as an ordained transformation where two souls destined for each other are united on a plane beyond physical reality." I paused. "We mustn't always let the devil grin, as the priests would have it. Who is to tell whether these two were not fated to merge with one another in the very element which has given life to our planet? And thereby assure perpetual renewal?"

The group around the Count's table was silent. Looking at Stella, I thought I'd never seen so much love in a woman's face. Stella's cheeks were flushed and her eyes sent out sparks of happiness. She raised her glass.

"Here's a toast to the psychoanalyst in our midst who has just turned a sordid story into a beautiful myth!" Glasses clinked as everyone was pondering this very new angle in a very old story. However, before the angle could be discussed further, the Count announced that it was high time to drive up the Gerlos road if they wanted to see the floodlit falls. Along with the Count, the locals chose to remain and open several more bottles of the bubbly spirits.

Thus the six lodgers drove through the summer night to the spot designated by the Count. There they watched in silent awe how out of the forest huge beams of light erupted, illuminating in gradual stages all three visible sections of the tremendous waterfall.

"How beautiful that is," Mausi murmured as she fell asleep on Stella's lap.

Seventeen

On our small terrace, surrounded by the dwarf spruce planters, Stella threw her arms around me and kissed me deeply. A thousand stars blazed in the sky. The moon was full.

"Our journey is ending, Michael," she whispered. "You and our dreams have brought the light of the future into my life. I owe you, and myself, the fulfillment of what brought us together that night at the opera. These four short weeks, a full lunar cycle, have contracted into the new center from which I can go forward. I've been opened up to an inner life which would have kept me barren had your own unconscious not helped me to reach beyond… I didn't know the way, nor that there was a way at all. But tonight there is total clarity, the way is marked by the light from the heavens.

"I want our bodies to unite, for I must commit the sin I'm charged with. We will possess each other, merge with one another, as our dreams have foretold. It will be our epiphany. Our lovechild will be born and it will die on the cross. For in the morning, Michael, I shall leave you forever, but in the flesh only, and give myself to another man with whom I will have a long and serene marriage, with Mausi as our guardian angel. But Stella, the muse, will be with you always, and our bond will outlast our lifetimes."

Stella didn't know herself. She had never spoken such words before. It was as if a larger than life Stella had taken over her mind, making sacred pronouncements that must be honored. We undressed each other, and I carried her to bed.

All my senses were alive, throbbing in different frequencies. My heart filled my entire chest, pulsing in hammer blows. And below, in Stella's hand, my maleness was rising, large and firm, and I kissed the woman who had united me with myself, kissed her ferociously, and they both tasted blood. There were no caresses, no titillations of fondling and stroking, but a rough entry, as if each wanted to claim the other's territory, fast and furiously, an animalistic duel for supremacy. It was a mating of polar opposites, the two sexes fighting for their respective gender, yet knowing that they would lose their uniqueness as they pushed their bodies to consume the yearning they had borne for so long, and to delay the yearning that was still waiting for the ultimate merging of their souls.

Almost immediately, Stella's orgasms broke forth, roaring beasts locked in a cage whose door was now being ripped open. With each thrust, another convulsing wave was wracking her body, as her juices flooded my testicles.

"Hilf mir, hilf mir," she moaned. "Help me," gasping for breath, as another wave made her legs thrash uncontrollably. She was sobbing against my chest, now and then grabbing my face, licking, kissing and biting, a mindless female in heat. "Oh, help me, please," she screamed, "I'm there, I'm there!"

I came, drowning her scream with a deep rumbling groan, double basses furiously moving their bows, then suddenly dying.

Stella couldn't stop shaking. I held her, now tenderly kissing the dew which covered her face. As I slipped out of her body, Stella opened her eyes. "We will be one flesh and one spirit forever," she breathed, as the tears started to flow again. "Because through you, by giving birth to you, I've become the mother I thought I could never be. I have sinned, but I'm already forgiven."

"Ich *liebe Dich,* Michael."

With love on their lips and in their hearts we slept in one another's arms for the last time.

Eighteen

In December of that same year, at Xmas, Paul and Stella were married in the church of the Nine Angelic Choirs in Vienna's imperial Courtyard. On the arm of the man she'd met eons ago at a performance of *Madam Butterfly,* Stella walked up the aisle to the high altar. She had insisted that I give her away and I had agreed.

"If you want to be true to our story," she had written me in New York, "you must come to Vienna for my wedding." Steffi Nussbaum and Mausi were the unequal bridesmaids. Also on Stella's insistence, the humdrum "Lohengrin' wedding march had been replaced by a medley of tunes from *The Tales of Hoffmann,* transcribed for organ. All these irregular doings were fine with Paul whose happiness over marrying Stella knew no bounds. Dispensing with a best man, he waited at the altar as Stella and I walked slowly toward him. Her wedding dress was all lace, layers of white tulle, and the antique veil a present from an anonymous person, signed "The Poet." This, too, Paul had accepted; he'd learned about trust.

In the first pew sat Stella's mother who kept shaking her head over the strange music the organist was playing. "Stella has always been an unusual child," she whispered to Count Recksdorf and Dr. Nussbaum. "But they're such a handsome couple." Egon Nussbaum and the Count exchanged glances.

"You may now kiss the bride," said Monsignor Sachs to Paul.

I had slipped into a pew next to Mausi. "Will you come home with us, Uncle Michael?" she asked. "For the reception?"

"No, Mausi. I have a plane to catch. But I'll come back to see all of you very soon." I left by a side door. The circle was closed and I could go home. The doctor would be in again. And dream no more.

EPILOGUE

A while ago the dream series ended. It had presented me with memories of eight different women whom I had collided with over the years; from the first incandescent passion of my youth to what felt like the final manifestation of that undefinable yet uniquely human condition we call love.

But, dear reader, don't be misled by Michael's prediction that he wasn't going to dream any more. As it happened, the dream of Stella came to me soon after I had in fact returned from her wedding in Vienna. I resumed my practice in New York, wondering if my journey with Stella was indeed the end of my connection to the eternal Feminine. It was a depressing thought. In joy and in pain, the connection had flowed irresistibly for a lifetime.

To challenge this unsettling feeling which kept clanging about in a minor key, I invoked Stella's prophetic vision that the Muse would never forsake me. Up to now, the result of this appeal were the eight stories which my dreams compelled me to record. For your delectation, I hope.

Having done so, I should like to present you with a dream which arose from deep levels of the collective unconscious after I delivered the manuscript to my publishers. Happily, it put the lie to Michael's concern that the juices have stopped running for good. Whether this dream speaks of my remaining in the continued good graces of the Muse, or if it holds the dubious promise of yet another encounter with the goddess, I should like to leave to your speculative intuition.

But the intensity of the dream was shocking.

In my dream the moon had caught fire. It was an incredibly awesome sight as orange and blue flames were criss-crossing the moon's surface. Every now and then I seemed to be viewing a close-up of craters from which giant flares were erupting. Then a cosmic event happened, so terrifying that I struggled to wake up, but couldn't.

With a feeling of utter helplessness I watched the burning moon traverse the sky in a vast arc, and fall into the ocean.

And from the sea arose a new moon, cool and golden, and it, vent back up into the sky and took its place among the stars.

The sense of relief was indescribable.

In the next scene, I was strolling through what seemed to be a country fair. It was harvest time, and farmers were exhibiting their produce. Masses of red apples were everywhere. I stopped by one stand behind which a woman was sorting out different vegetables. Suddenly she faced me, holding an object in her outstretched hand. "You need this," she said.

I woke up, knowing that she had offered me a jar of pale yellow honey.

Does this image tug on your memory? And elicit tiny tinkling bells in your mind?

If it doesn't, you might do well to turn back some pages – for if Michael has learned one thing in his journeys, it's that no one should be without the food the love goddess requires, if she's to bless your life with yearning and fulfillment.

THE END.

ABOUT THE AUTHOR

Peter Lynn was born in Vienna, Austria. Fleeing Hider, he arrived in the United States in time to join the army. Being multi-lingual, he served with military intelligence in Europe, ending this phase as U.S. Public Safety Officer in occupied Berlin. Returning to the United States, he obtained his Bachelor of Science degree in psychology from Columbia University, New York, and his Ph.D. from the University of Zurich, Switzerland. While there, he also studied with the famous psychiatrist, C. G. Jung, and received his Analyst's Diploma at the latter's training institute in Zurich. Back in New York, he went into private practice as a psychoanalyst, then became co-founder of the New York Training Institute for Analytical Psychology, serving as its Dean of Training for 20 years. Currently again in private practice, he is married.

Printed in the United States
217007BV00005B/3/A

9 781410 714756

Експрес до Галіції

Богдан Коломійчук

Експрес до Галіції

Львів
Видавництво Старого Лева
2022

УДК 821.161.2-312.6
К61

Богдан Коломійчук

К61 Експрес до Ґаліції [Текст] : роман / Богдан Коломійчук. — Львів : Видавництво Старого Лева, 2022. — 352 с.

ISBN 978-617-679-776-0

«Експрес до Ґаліції» — новий детективний роман Богдана Коломійчука, в якому на читача чекають заплутані справи та небезпечні розслідування. Весна 1906 року. Під час відпустки у Швейцарії комісар львівської поліції Адам Вістович несподівано втягується у небезпечну шпигунську гру, в якій на карту поставлено не лише людські життя, але й долі імперій. Розшифрувавши секретний документ, Вістович дізнається занадто багато, як на звичайного детектива з далекого австрійського Львова.

У цей же час з клініки в курортному Бадені зникає дивний російський пацієнт, якого розшукують розвідки одразу кількох країн, а у Венеції стається вбивство непримітного перекладача з німецької. Вістовичу доведеться з'ясувати, як пов'язані ці події і чому сліди, здавалося б, непов'язаних справ ведуть до Львова.

УДК 821.161.2-312.6

ISBN 978-617-679-776-0

Der Mensch ist Etwas, das überwunden soll

Friedrich Nietzsche,

«Also sprach Zarathustra»

Людина — це те, що слід подолати

Фрідріх Ніцше,

«Так казав Заратустра»

I

Венеція
2 квітня 1906 року

Є міста, які ненавидиш з першого погляду...

Зазвичай не тому, що їм бракує привабливості. Аж ніяк... Будь-хто мав би закохатися в них. Замальовувати в блокнот старовинні храми й перспективу тісних середньовічних вуличок. Перечитувати поетів, народжених тут, і надсилати додому прегарні листівки. А проте, щойно черевик торкається вокзального перону, як глибоко в душі народжується бажання купити зворотний квиток і забратися геть під три чорти.

Антон Піллер, 42-річний позаштатний кореспондент бернського тижневика «*Die neue Post*», крім того, вільний редактор видавництва «*Alle Sterne*», прибув сьогодні до Венеції обіднім поїздом з Цюриха. Подорож важко було назвати приємною чи бодай стерпною. Піллер понад добу змушений був трястися в незручному купе другого класу. Справи в редакції та видавництві йшли паскудно, тож місце в першому класі він собі дозволити не міг. Ба більше, прибулий не мав грошей на зворотну дорогу. Усього, що залишилось у гаманці, вистачило на дешевий готель і скромну вечерю.

Втім, чоловік був певен, що всі поневіряння перетерпів недарма. Вже завтра відбудеться зустріч, після якої його фінансовим труднощам настане кінець. Можливо, він навіть подивиться на це місто іншими очима. А поки що, докурюючи п'яту за останню годину цигарку і видихаючи дим у невелике готельне вікно, за яким чаїлася волога передранішня темрява, Антон Піллер ненавидів Венецію...

Готель, в якому зупинився швейцарець, знаходився неподалік площі святого Марка, в одному з численних провулків, де, щоб розминутися, двоє перехожих були змушені втискатися в стіну. Ці проклятущі венеційські провулки виявилися схожими один на одного, як дірки в носі, тому готельну адресу Піллер шукав більше години. При цьому чоловік ані на мить не відпускав з рук валізу, що завдавало йому додаткових страждань. І тільки опинившись перед кривими дверима «*Hotel del sole*», він опустив свій тягар на бруківку й зі страждeнною гримасою на обличчі розім'яв побілілі пальці. Після цього звів погляд угору. Під вузькою смужкою неба виднілися гострі кути прочинених віконниць. Очевидно, десь там, на третьому або четвертому поверсі, для нього приготовано кімнату...

— *Attenzione*! — раптом почулося за спиною, і хтось грубо штовхнув його в плечі.

Піллер боляче вперіщився обличчям просто в готельні двері, але втримався на ногах і одразу повернувся до свого кривдника. Втім, низький широкоплечий торговець, навіть не озирнувшись, вже поволікся далі провулком, тягнучи за собою на двоколісній тачці плетений короб, наповнений усіляким мотлохом.

— Сучий виродок!.. — сердито вигукнув йому вслід швейцарець і дістав хустинку, щоб витерти з-під носа кров.

Коли перестало юшити, сховав закривавлену шматку знову в кишеню й поправив капелюха. Потім підняв з бруківки валізу й зайшов до готелю.

Сонний рецепціоніст ліниво звів голову й подивився на гостя. На пухлій щоці лишився відбиток долоні, якою той щойно підпирав обличчя. Чорні скуйовджені вусики підстрибнули догори, а червоні, як у дівчини, губки сотворили щось подібне до привітної усмішки.

На стійці поруч з ним стояв телефонний апарат, облізлий бронзовий дзвоник і нерівна стопка паперів. На стіні висів годинник, розмірено відбиваючи тутешній час. Була четверта по полудні.

— Добридень, сеньйоре, — хриплим від дрімоти голосом привітався адміністратор.

Піллер придивився до його обличчя з червоною плямою на щоці й чомусь подумав, що такий самий слід лишився би й від ляпаса. Він навіть уявив, як щосили б'є ні в чому не винного італійця по мармизі, а той німує від болю й здивування і тільки вибалушує на нього свої чорні, як ґудзики, очі. Одночасно пригадався торговець у провулку, що так брутально його штовхнув. Швейцарця знову охопила злість.

— Добридень, — кинув він адміністратору, сам стрепенувшись від свого сердитого голосу.

— У вас заброньовано кімнату? — запитав італієць вже без усмішки.

Прибулий кивнув і простягнув йому папірець з номером резервації.

— Хвилинку... — сказав адміністратор, розгортаючи готельний журнал.

Після недовгого пошуку він озвався знову:

— Ваше прізвище Пілло?

— Піллер, — виправив його гість.

— О, даруйте... Антоніо Піллер?

— Антон Піллер, чорт забирай!

— Пробачте, сеньйоре, — зніяковів рецепціоніст. — Ви так добре говорите італійською, що я мимохіть помилився... Дозвольте ваш паспорт... О, ви швейцарець...

— Моя матір була італійкою, — примирливо сказав гість, зумівши себе нарешті опанувати.

Адміністратор швидко занотував щось у зошит.

— З вас п'ять лір, — повідомив він і повернув йому документ.

Швейцарець витягнув з нагрудної кишені гаманець.

— Сніданок завтра о пів на восьму, — додав адміністратор.

— Я можу відмовитися від сніданку?

— Можете. Але він усе одно входить у вартість.

— Дідько...

— Провести вас до кімнати?

— Ні, спасибі, я відшукаю сам.

— Третій поверх, другі двері від сходів. Номер 32...

Італієць поклав перед ним ключ з масивним грушоподібним дармовисом. Піллер мовчки взяв його й, підхопивши валізу, рушив до сходів.

— Гарного перебування у Венеції, — побажав йому вслід італієць.

Відповідати не хотілось.

Номер виявився тіснуватим, зі старезними трухлявими меблями, але постіль на ліжку була свіжою. Зрештою, нічого іншого, як виспатись після важкої дороги, постояльцеві не хотілося. Трохи пізніше він спуститься донизу й подбає собі про вечерю. Чоловік роздягнувся й пішов до ванної. Повернувся за кілька хвилин, витираючи обличчя й шию готельним рушником з вицвілим візерунком.

Перш ніж вмоститися на ліжку, Піллер відкрив валізу. Зверху було напхано змінний одяг, кілька газет, пуделко зубного порошку та інші дорожні дрібниці. Усе це швейцарець одним рухом переклав на підлогу, а тоді витягнув чималий німецько-італійський словник. Саме під ним лежало найдорожче: грубий стос паперу, загорнений у шкіряну палітурку. Швейцарець лагідно провів по ній рукою.

— Завтра, — видихнув Піллер і знову накрив свій скарб книжкою, а потім — фланелевим піджаком. Доволі непоганим і ще зовсім не зношеним. Швейцарець подумав, що вдягне його на зустріч. Під ним добре сидітиме улюблена камізелька, а до неї пасуватимуть зручні дорожні штани. А ще в цього піджака великі місткі кишені, отже, буде куди заховати револьвер.

Піллер стрепенувся при згадці про зброю. Його шестизарядний «Шмідт»* також лежав у валізі. За підкладкою, в таємній кишеньці, куди подорожні зазвичай ховають гроші або цінні папери.

---

* Ідеться про цивільну модель швейцарського револьвера *Schmidt M1882* виробництва «*Waffenfabrik Bern*».

Цього «Шмідта» подарував йому колись ще в студентські роки університетський приятель. Сталося це після того, як худорлявого й невисокого на зріст Антона ледь не до смерті побили й пограбували в передмісті Цюриха. Коли Піллер оклигав, вони з другом подалися на стрільбище. Тоді Антон вперше у своєму житті натиснув на гачок і відчув, з якою диявольською силою та гучним звуком з люфи виривається смертоносна куля. Щойно вгомонилося серцебиття, спровоковане першим у житті пострілом, він подумав, що волів би ніколи не повторювати такого досвіду. Усі ці вправи зі зброєю та іскристий азарт в очах інших стрільців були не для нього.

Втім, збираючись у подорож до Венеції, він вирішив прихопити зброю. По-перше, дорога була неблизька й часом небезпечна, а по-друге, надто вже цінний рукопис мав у валізі... Та й хто його знає, як складеться завтрашня зустріч і що за тип цей Доменіко Салтіні, який вранці, о десятій, чекатиме його в ресторації неподалік мосту Ріалто.

Швейцарець не мав певності, чи ресторани у Венеції відчиняються так рано. Хоча, з іншого боку, десь же мусять снідати всі ці натовпи американських та британських туристів, які прокидаються вдосвіта, попри те, що насолоджувались *Venice by night** і потрапили до раніших газетних повідомлень через жахливий галас, який зчиняли під вікнами городян. Одна з цих газет навіть саркастично зауважила, що венеційці тепер можуть вчити англійську не виходячи з дому, а просто відчинивши вікно в будь-який час доби.

* *Venice by night* (*англ.*) — Венеція вночі.

О сьомій постоялець спустився донизу, де, проминувши адміністратора, що знову дрімав, вийшов на вулицю. У найближчій пекарні чоловік купив паперовий пакуночок з теплими *grissini** й рушив назад до готелю. Цей хліб, що мав стати йому вечерею, приємно грів руку, й навіть через пакунок відчувався його божественний аромат, від чого рот Піллера безперервно наповнювався слиною. Врешті, не витримавши, швейцарець вирішив з'їсти частину вечері на ходу. Чоловік дістав хлібець і з апетитом відкусив одразу половину. Прожовуючи, навіть сповільнив крок, а далі й зупинився. Врешті Антон помітив, що стоїть просто навпроти собору святого Марка. Химерні гострі форми будівлі врізалися в перші міські сутінки і густо-сіре венеційське небо. Споруда видалася йому величною, і чоловік готовий був назвати її навіть гарною, але про себе знову нагадав шлунок. Різким голодним спазмом він попросив ще хліба, й Антон йому не відмовив. Запхавши до рота наступний шматок, швейцарець зауважив, як низько кружляють над ним чайки. Найпевніше, їх привабила їжа, яку вони, набравшись нахабності, готові були б видерти з його рук. Швейцарець завбачливо згорнув пакунок і, втиснувши голову в плечі, майже побіг до готелю, так і не давши собі шансу бодай трохи полюбити Венецію.

У своїй кімнаті він найперше знову розгорнув валізу й перевірив, чи на місці рукопис... Ніхто його не чіпав. Ніхто не рухав фланелевого піджака, призначеного на завтрашню зустріч, ніхто не переклав у інше місце німецько-італійський словник, якого Піллер насправді не

* *Grissini* (*італ.*) — італійські хлібці невеликого розміру.

потребував, настільки досконало він знав обидві мови, ніхто не заходив у номер за його відсутності. Антон полегшено зітхнув, доїв решту хліба й закурив.

О дев'ятій його почало хилити на сон. Не зачиняючи вікна, постоялець вклався в ліжко. З приємністю відчув, як сонливість лагідно розливається по його тілу. Проникає в кожну кінцівку, знерухомлюючи її і наповнюючи приємною терпкістю. Після цього нарешті спинився скажений маховик думок у голові, й чоловік заснув.

Піллер снив рідним Цюрихом, набережною Женевського озера і прогулянкою з сином. Після розлучення з дружиною він бачився з ним тільки раз. Поміж звичних теревенів про все на світі Антон намагався пояснити йому, що матір не у всьому права. Так, він справді почав занадто часто зазирати в чарку й втратив добру роботу викладача в університеті, але хіба це причина руйнувати сім'ю? Тепер у своєму сні чоловік тлумачив йому інше:

— От побачиш, малий, усе налагодиться. Я продам той рукопис і матиму купу грошей. Ти чуєш, малий?.. Твоя мати до мене повернеться, і все буде як раніше...

Хлопець кивав і мовчки доїдав яблуко, ніби йому було байдуже, як складеться подальша їхня доля.

— Ти чуєш мене? — повторив Піллер, трохи ображений такою байдужістю. — Чуєш, я питаю?..

Несподівано для себе Антон заговорив низьким чужим голосом, якого добряче перелякався сам. Той голос народжувався не в ньому, а десь ззовні. Так, наче й мовцем був не він, а хтось сторонній. Піллер навіть роззирнувся довкола в пошуках того незнайомця, проте вони з сином були одні на всій набережній.

— *Attenzione!* — раптом вигукнув малий.

Антон здивовано подивився на сина. Йому хотілося запитати в чому річ, але чоловік досі боявся власного голосу.

— *Attenzione!!!* — малий перейшов на вереск, і обличчя його перетворилося на страшну потворну гримасу.

— *Attenzione!!!*

Піллер підхопився на ліжку й вирячився у темряву. Хтось кричав за вікном, тягнучи за собою щось важке. Можливо, навіть той самий торговець, що штовхнув його вдень. Оговтавшись від кошмару, постоялець намацав сірники й годинника. Присвітивши вогнем циферблат, з подивом побачив, що була тільки третя ночі. Це кляте місто вже прокидалося!..

— Бісова Венеція... — упівголоса промовив швейцарець і знову черкнув сірником об стіну, цього разу — щоб знайти цигарки. — Ненавиджу.

Сон як рукою зняло. До самого світанку лишалося тільки курити й думати. На зміну нічному кошмару приходив ранішній.

Дочекавшись сьомої, Антон поплівся до ванної і з насолодою вмився. Після майже безсонної ночі голова здавалася набитою ганчір'ям, як в опудала. Зрештою, глянувши на себе в дзеркало, швейцарець зауважив, що й вигляд він мав не кращий. Скуйовджене волосся стирчало в різні боки, очі підпухли, впалі щоки набули якогось мертвотноблідого кольору. Ні, він радше людина-примара з циркової кімнати жаху.

Колись мандрівний цирк зупинився в Цюриху, й вони з сином вирішили відвідати їхню виставу. Спершу були силачі й клоуни, а далі малий потягнув батька до шатра з написом «Заходь, якщо наважишся». Всередині панувала темрява, і тільки коли хтось заходив слідом за ними, її розтинав промінь світла ззовні. За хвилину-другу, коли відчувалася присутність щонайменше десяти осіб дорослих і малих, десь у глибині яскраво-червоним світлом спалахнув електричний ліхтар, підсвітивши мерзенну пику за сталевими ґратами. Наступної миті мармиза широко роззявила рота, загорланивши так, що в присутніх позакладало у вухах. Діти з вереском кинулися геть із шатра. І навіть серед дорослих почалося сум'яття. Хтось, не стримуючи себе, вилаявся, хтось зареготав, хтось подався уперед до цієї з'яви, проте світло згасло й вона зникла так само раптово, як і виникла.

Антон разом з іншими вийшов з намету і найперше відшукав поглядом сина. Той стояв неподалік, якось по-дорослому схрестивши руки на грудях.

— Злякався? — підійшовши, запитав він у сина.

— Анітрохи, — той заперечливо хитнув головою. — Було добре видно, що той циркач просто кривляється. У житті буває страшніше.

— Ти про що? — запитав Піллер, хоча насправді добре все зрозумів.

— Ну-у-у, ти коли напиваєшся, то, буває, значно страшніше кричиш, — пояснив малий. — Ось там морозиво! Купиш мені?..

І, не чекаючи на відповідь, хлопець побіг до торговця, обліпленого дітьми, як мухами.

Антон удруге зачерпнув долонями води й плеснув собі в обличчя. Тутешня навіть питна вода смерділа гнилизною. Залишалося тільки здогадуватись, скільки хвороб дарувала вона венеційцям. Особливо влітку, з настанням перших по-справжньому спекотних днів. Ще один привід не любити це місто.

А щодо пиятики... Так, малий мав рацію. Алкоголь позбавляв його розуму. Напиваючись, Піллер не ставав агресивним, але людську подобу втрачав. Міг волати, кривлятися або повзати по підлозі. Добре, що при цьому не залишав межі їхнього дому, інакше неодмінно збирав би довкола себе купу роззяв, як у цирку, а тоді син і дружина вмерли би від сорому.

При згадці про спиртне Антон з огидою відчув, як у животі запекло. Це відчуття не сплутати ні з чим — настав ранок, і йому захотілося випити.

— Паскудство, — сердито видихнув постоялець і ковтнув слину. Точніше, спробував ковтнути. Від надмірного куріння горло було сухе, мов пісок. Сплюнувши на підлогу, чоловік опустив голову просто в миску з водою. Примусив себе стояти так з пів хвилини, а потім випрямився, судомно хапаючи ротом повітря. Повторивши цю процедуру тричі, Піллер відчув, що тепер почувається краще й може йти донизу на сніданок.

Їжа була препаскудною. З ніжністю пригадуючи свіжий хліб, який був у нього на вечерю, Піллер запхнув до рота черствий бутерброд і, прикликавши на поміч усю свою силу волі, змусив себе прожувати. Потім запив його ледве теплою кавою і вийшов з ресторації.

До зустрічі залишалося більше двох годин, та швейцарець не хотів стирчати в готелі. Ранок був прохолодний, але днина заповідалася погожа: небо над містом простягалося блакитним чистим куполом, і перші червонуваті снопи сонячних променів важко осідали на старому камінні. Піллер загорнувся в пальто і глибоко насадив капелюха. Тоді взяв під пахву згорток з рукописом і швидким впевненим кроком, наче й справді достеменно знав, куди йти, вийшов з готелю. Найголовніше зараз — рухатися, бо від хвилювання і думок, що, мов павутина, тягнуться за ним ще з ночі, можна було збожеволіти. Дивлячись збоку, кожен би сказав, що бачить перед собою якогось тутешнього клерка або чиновника, що поспішає до своєї контори, аби без запізнення взятися до роботи. Але Піллер і гадки не мав, куди йшов. Минаючи провулок за провулком, площу за площею, переходячи один міст за іншим, він невдовзі опинився перед Головним двірцем, звідки почалися його вчорашні поневіряння. Це був край міста. Далі виднілася безкрая затока, яку стрілою розтинала штучна земляна коса, насипана, вочевидь, спеціально, аби до цього острівного міста протягти залізничну колію, що сполучила б його з материком. Материк звідси не проглядався, тому здавалося, що коса тягнеться в нікуди. І так само в нікуди з острівного перону, чахкаючи, хмикаючи й видихаючи гігантські клуби диму й пари, відправляється вранішній експрес. Піллер зупинився, спостерігаючи за тим, як поїзд неквапно набирає хід і як від несподіваних гудків над дахами вагонів злякано затріпотіли зграї птахів. Це були чайки і голуби, два пташині клани, що населяли Венецію.

Провівши очима поїзд і навіть дочекавшись, поки той зникне за обрієм, Піллер повернувся й уже неквапом подався назад до міста. Йому подумалося, що насправді це міг бути поїзд до Цюриха. Можливо, навіть той самий, яким він прибув сюди учора. І ось він рушає в зворотньому керунку вже без нього. Спершу до Мілана, а звідти — в його рідні Альпи. Від цієї думки на душі стало ще мерзенніше, ніж було.

Швейцарець міцніше притиснув до себе рукопис, і в ту ж мить його зап'ясток відчув руків'я револьвера, що лежав у кишені піджака. Чоловік стрепенувся всім тілом, наче це хтось інший, а не він поклав туди зброю, менш ніж пів години тому. Він притишено вилаявся й спробував пригадати, чи його «Шмідт» на запобіжнику. Дідько! А якщо ні?.. Швейцарець раптом уявив, як револьвер випадково вистрілює просто у піджаку. Здається, він поклав його так, що той націлений йому в геніталії. Чудово! Ось він передає рукопис і, перш ніж узяти гроші, тієї ж миті гучним пострілом відбиває собі яйця. Дурнуватішої ситуації годі й уявити. Швейцарець зупинився і ще раз торкнувся револьвера, цього разу навмисне. Кортіло просто дістати його з кишені й перевірити, але Піллер стояв посеред вулиці. Можна, звісно, сховатися десь у закутку, але й тоді не буде певності, що він не потрапить на очі містянам або ще гірше — поліції.

Чоловік глибоко вдихнув, намагаючись заспокоїтись, і спробував пригадати ту частину ранку, коли збирався виходити з готелю. Ось він одягнувся, обережно, мов порцелянову вазу, поклав на стіл рукопис... Згадав про «Шмідта». Дістав набої, зарядив... Поклав револьвера до кишені, а рукопис узяв під пахву. Та чи клацнув він запобіжником? Піллер не пам'ятав!..

Хоча... Хоча, здається, так. Перш ніж покласти зброю до кишені він подбав, щоб не сталося випадкового пострілу. Хвала небесам!

Полегшення виявилось таким же несподіваним, як і ця нова гризота. Від серця відлягло, й гумор миттю поліпшився.

З подивом швейцарець помітив, що у Венеції трапляються й тихі куточки. Вчергове звернувши навмання,

Піллер навіть завмер від несподіванки. Типовий, але дещо облущений аркоподібний міст, перекинутий через невеликий безіменний канал, сполучав між собою два стрімкі квартали, що складалися з високих п'ятиповерхових будівель, оповитих плющем темно-іржавого кольору та квітами. Квіти цієї ранньої весни ще мали б бути несміливими й слабкими, а проте вони рішуче виривалися назовні зі старих балконів, пробивалися крізь балюстраду, як в'язні-смертники крізь ґрати, з надією вдихнути чи вхопити якомога більше повітря й сонця. І вся ця квітково-кам'яна тиша раптом здалася неприродною, ба навіть болючою та нестерпною для вуха. Тому коли її розітнула пісня гондольєра, десь так, як гостра шабля розтинає шовк, Піллеру полегшало. За мить він побачив, як з-за рогу виринув високий загнутий ніс гондоли, в якій стриміла постать чоловіка в традиційному *канотьє**, білій сорочці, чорних штанах і червоному поясі довкола стану. Він тримав у руках довжелезне весло, проте, здавалося, майже ним не орудував. Так, ніби човном керував думкою або тією самою дещо непристойною *баркаролою***, що злітала з його губ:

La biondina in gondoleta
L'altra sera g'ho menà:
Dal piacer la povereta,
La s'ha in bota indormenzà.
La dormiva su sto brazzo,
Mi ogni tanto la svegliava,

* Канотьє — солом'яний капелюх.

** Баркарола — традиційна пісня гондольєрів.

Ma la barca che ninava
*La tornava a indormenzar...**

Провівши його поглядом, чоловік вирушив далі. Перейшов міст, за яким починалися нерівні сходи і провадили вниз, до чергового провулку. Той виявився темним і сирим, мов кротяча нора, тому Піллер прискорив крок, аби якнайшвидше його пройти. Ще бракувало наштовхнутися на якихось грабіжників чи просто тутешніх бевзів, котрі не від того, аби нам'яти боки випадковому перехожому. Байдуже, з якого приводу.

Провулок вивів до загородженого саду. Кілька тендітних, майже безлистих дерев визирало з-за кам'яної стіни, здавалося, самі дивувалися, як могли опинитися тут, серед міських будівель на цьому острові. Йти уздовж загорожі довелося довго. Піллер навіть з тривогою почав поглядати на годинник, всерйоз побоюючись запізнитись на таку важливу для нього зустріч. Найстрашнішим було те, що він гадки не мав, де перебуває і в який бік від домовленого місця прямує.

Врешті, коли вже, мабуть, вдесяте прокляв себе за цю ідіотичну ідею прогулятися містом, стіна закінчилася. Перед Піллером знову був канал і місток, до дрібних деталей схожий на попередній, біля якого він слухав пісню гондольєра. Швейцарець встиг подумати, що й справді

---

* Білявку минулого вечора
Привів я в гондолу свою,
Та заснула вона з насолоди
В обіймах моїх.
Я будив її без упину, та човен
Її заколисував знов... — (*з італ.*)

якимось дивом опинився на попередньому місці, проте зауважив, що тут було значно людніше. Все через плавучий ринок, точніше велетенський човен, навантажений зерном, борошном, свіжою зеленню, сушеною рибою та спеціями у дерев'яних пуделках. Двоє жвавих торговців у засмальцьованих жакетах вправно передавали товар на берег, у той самий час швидко перераховуючи гроші і — що найдивніше — не перестаючи при цьому торгуватись зі своїми покупцями. Складалося враження, що в човні працювало не дві пари рук, а значно більше. Так само на березі, де зібралося заледве півтора десятка містян з порожніми кошиками в руках, панував такий галас, наче насправді сюди збіглося пів Венеції. Стоячи в безладній черзі, люди користалися з нагоди привітатися, похвалитися, поскаржитись і навіть посваритись. Очевидно, в тутешньому кварталі це був усталений і довгожданий час. Час на закупи, хоча ті — як було видно — відігравали далеко не головну роль у цій сповненій життя, емоцій та жестів виставі.

Піллер подумав, що добре було б запитати в цих людей, де знаходиться ресторація «Марко Поло». Бо саме там він має бути вже за сорок хвилин. Чоловік сягнув рукою до нагрудної кишені, звідки дістав блокнот, куди ще в Швейцарії занотував цю назву. Щоб зробити це, йому довелося дужче затиснути під пахвою рукопис. Це виявилося некомфортно й трохи лячно. Піллер боявся, що може впустити його на землю. Так ніби той був із кришталю або фарфору й міг розбитися на друзки. Розгорнувши блокнот, він побачив їхню з сином і дружиною сімейну світлину (насправді єдину, як він за мить згадав). Молода пара, всього рік після одруження. Синові два чи три місяці. Дитина, дбайливо загорнута в пелюшки, на руках у матері. Антон поруч, ніжно тримає її за лікоть. Фотограф тоді мордував їх майже сорок хвилин. Малий час від часу прокидався і плакав... Знимка коштувала *два франки*.

Рукопис таки вислизнув з-під пахви й упав прямісінько у витоптане болото.

— Трясця! — розпачливо вилаявся Піллер і швидко заховав блокнот назад до кишені.

Сталося найгірше, мабуть, що могло статися в цій ситуації: пакунок розгорнувся й сторінки рукопису розсипалися на долівці. Швейцарець заходився збирати їх, проте з жахом помітив, що мокрий бруд встиг безжалісно вчепитися до країв паперу, а часом і відбитися гидкими плямами посередині тексту. За лічені хвилини цей рукопис увібрав у себе все, чим дихало ближнє торговисько: грязюку, гнилизну, риб'ячі рештки й цигарковий попіл.

— Ох, ви бідолаха, сеньйоре! — поспівчувала Піллеру якась жінка. Вона стояла за кілька кроків від нього й скрушно хитала головою.

— Шановна пані... — звернувся до неї швейцарець. Він стояв, притиснувши підібрані сторінки до грудей, і відчував, що готовий заплакати, як скривджений хлопчак. — Скажіть, заради Бога, де знаходиться «Марко Поло»?..

— Даруйте, сеньйоре, я не знаю, де таке продають, — відповіла жінка.

— Це не товар, — пояснив Піллер, — це ресторація.

Венеційка раптом спохмурніла й окинула його зневажливим поглядом.

— Звідки мені знати? — буркнула вона. — Я не вештаюся по рестораціях.

І, відвернувшись від нього, рушила у бік ринку.

— Йдіть далі цією вуличкою, сеньйоре, — порадив юнацький голос позаду Піллера.

Швейцарець озирнувся. Перед ним стояв молодий чоловік у затертому одязі й дивився на Піллера крізь дим від своєї цигарки. Погляд мав примружений, як у карткового шулера за гральним столом.

— І як довго йти? — перепитав Антон.

— Зо чверть години. Минете три провулки праворуч від себе, перейдете схожий на цей місток і побачите яскраву вивіску з написом «Ресторан "Марко Поло"», — пояснив юнак. — Головне — йдіть увесь час прямо.

— Щиро дякую, — кивнув йому Піллер, все намагаючись подолати внутрішній розпач.

Як, у біса, тепер віддати тому Салтіні рукопис? Що він подумає? Що Піллер діставався до Венеції в баржі зі свиньми? Чи у вагоні з нечистотами? І це ж треба стільки часу його леліяти, щоб отак безглуздо й випадково загидити!

— Пасувало б узяти з вас копійчину, — продовжив молодик, — бо ж я таки допоміг, але...

Юнак махнув рукою й подався кудись геть. Вочевидь, Піллер мав настільки жалюгідний вигляд, що молодий пройдисвіт утратив будь-який азарт.

Зрештою, Антон вирішив себе опанувати й не гаяти більше часу. Почувався він кепсько, але й добре розумів, що спізнення на таку важливу зустріч не покращить його становища. Мов у тумані, подався за вказаним напрямком, дивлячись перед собою невидючими очима. Зупинився тільки тоді, коли просто перед носом виник напис «Готель та ресторація «"Марко Поло"».

Заклад був типовим для Венеції: низькі продовгуваті вікна, стіни, прикрашені копіями Тінторетто* й вицвілими карнавальними масками, та невеликі акуратні столики під білими скатертинами. З вулиці виднілася дерев'яна тераса, де на парапетах тіснилися горщики з квітами.

Запах яєчні з тунцем вітав перших гостей, мов невидимий метрдотель на вході, і швейцарець вкотре з ненавистю згадав свій жебрацький сніданок, від якого відчував тепер неприємні спазми в шлунку. Хоч, може, були вони в нього радше від хвилювання.

З відвідувачів усередині сиділа тільки пара літніх американців чи англійців. Крім яєчні, ці двоє мали перед собою велику тарілку підсмажених бобів і корзинку зі свіжим хлібом. Усе це вони запивали чаєм з великих керамічних горнят. Пара неспішно перемовлялася між собою, час від часу голосно сміючись і закашлюючись. Загалом же вони досить гармонійно вписувались у тутешній заспокійливий інтер'єр. Напроти швейцарця непомітно з'явився лисуватий усміхнений кельнер.

— Бажаєте поснідати, сеньйоре? — привітно запитав він у Піллера, трохи спантеличено глянувши на розтріпаний рукопис, що той досі притискав до грудей.

Піллер стрепенувся, наче поява тут кельнера була якоюсь несподіванкою.

— Ні, дякую, — відповів гість, — я маю тут зустріч...

На цих словах він роззирнувся довкола, втім, нікого, крім тієї самої англо-американської пари, не побачив.

---

* Тінторетто (справжнє ім'я — Якопо Робусті; 1518–1594) — венеційський художник, представник високого Відродження.

— Зустріч? — перепитав офіціант. — То, можливо, це на вас чекає сеньйор Салтіні?

Ім'я він вимовив притишено, ніби говорив щось непристойне або надто сакральне. Втім, попри стишеність, воно вкололо Піллера розпеченою голкою. Щоб якось приховати чи виправдати хвилювання, швейцарець зиркнув на годинник. Насправді до зустрічі ще лишалося приблизно вісім хвилин.

— Так, на мене... — відповів Піллер. — Але...

— Сеньйор Салтіні просив, щоб ви піднялися нагору, до готелю. Він чекатиме на вас у кімнаті 77.

«Отже, Салтіні вирішив, що внизу занадто багато вух», — майнула в Антона думка.

Він мовчки кивнув у відповідь і попрямував до сходів, глянувши чомусь наостанок на чи то англійців, чи то американців, що й далі балакали про своє і не звертали на них із кельнером жодної уваги. Здавалося, Піллеру було цікаво, скільки бобів, яєчні й хліба лишилось у них на столі. Не надто багато. Найпевніше, ці двоє, попри вік, не скаржилися на поганий апетит.

Потрібні двері у напівтемному коридорі вдалося відшукати не відразу. Швейцарець зауважив подумки з неабиякою прикрістю, що пошуки зайняли в нього не менше десяти хвилин. Отже, на зустріч він запізниться приблизно хвилин на п'ять.

Чоловік постукав, і з того боку грубуватий голос запросив його увійти. Номер 77 виявився чимось на кшталт тутешнього люксу, де в просторому передпокої спиною до балконних дверей на нього чекав Доменіко Салтіні. Між ним і Піллером стояв журнальний столик, на якому в попільниці диміли залишки двох сигарет.

Мабуть, саме стільки встиг викурити італієць, доки Піллер ішов сюди з ресторану. Біля столика стояли два широкі крісла. Швейцарець уперше відчув, що добряче находився за цей ранок, тому вони видалися йому навіть привабливими.

Салтіні був чоловіком високого зросту і кремезної, як у борця, статури. Мав коротку міцну шию, на якій трималася цілковито лиса голова. Піллер спробував розгледіти обличчя, проте зробити це було важко — заважало вранішнє світло, що пробивалося в того з-за спини. Втім, чоловік із дещо несподіваною люб'язністю зробив кілька кроків назустріч гостю й простягнув руку для привітання. Коли обличчя його опинилося ближче, швейцарець з подивом побачив, що воно не позбавлене приємних рис. І навіть світилося привітністю. Зіпсувати це враження міг тільки зламаний ніс. Такий, що зазвичай мають кулачні бійці або вуличні шукачі пригод.

— Радий зустрітися, пане Піллере! — широко усміхаючись, промовив Салтіні. Він говорив чомусь німецькою, причому зовсім без акценту. Антона це трохи здивувало і, відповівши на привітання, він одразу ж зауважив:

— У вас перфектна вимова, пане Салтіні.

— Вимова? — не зрозумів той. — Що ви маєте на увазі?

— Я гадав, ми говоритимемо італійською.

— Он як? Що ж, втім... Якщо ваша ласка, давайте продовжимо німецькою.

На цих словах Салтіні жестом запросив Піллера сісти. «Але ж цей рукопис я переклав для вас саме з німецької, — ледь не вирвалось у швейцарця, — на біса вам знадобилися мої послуги, якщо ви могли прочитати його і без мого посередництва?..»

— Бачу, ви принесли те, про що ми домовлялися, — вдоволено сказав Салтіні, кивнувши на папери в руках Піллера.

— Так, — відповів той, відчувши, як недоречно в нього почав хрипіти голос. — І якщо ваше видавництво й надалі зацікавлене...

— Звісно, що зацікавлене, — перебив Салтіні. — Більше того, ми одразу виплатимо вам суму, яку обіцяли.

Нарешті замість неспокою швейцарець відчув щось подібне до радості й полегшення. Італієць запропонував йому сигарету, і той з удячністю її прийняв. На кілька секунд, поки чоловіки закурювали, в передпокої панувала тиша. «Дуже непогані „*Eckstein*“, — подумав Піллер, впізнавши етикетку на пачці й з приємністю затягуючи дим глибоко в легені, — італійці, виявляється, також поціновувачі німецького тютюну...» Він поклав рукопис на столик і став чекати, доки видавець захоче його переглянути. Проте Салтіні тільки покосився на нього крізь пелену диму й критично гмикнув, зауваживши на ньому сліди венеційського болота.

— Гроші я маю при собі, — продовжив італієць, стежачи тепер, як від його слів змінюється обличчя Піллера.

— Радий це чути, — промовив швейцарець.

— Втім, є одна умова... — сказавши це, Салтіні відкинувся на спинку крісла й заклав ногу на ногу. Потім підніс до рота цигарку й стиснув її своїми тонкими акуратними губами. Ці губи не пасували до його лисого черепа і зламаного носа. Здавалося, на цьому обличчі вони опинились випадково.

«Яка ще, до дідька, умова», — швейцарець відчув, що знову нервується, проте залишив ці слова при собі.

— Насправді нічого надзвичайного, — поспішив заспокоїти його співрозмовник, і слова вилітали з його рота слідом за темно-синім цигарковим димом. — Мені потрібен оригінал цього рукопису.

— Але... але я не маю його при собі, — відповів Піллер.

— Звісно, що ні, — посміхнувся Салтіні, — я бачу, що ви прийшли сюди лише зі своїм перекладом. Оригінал, мабуть, залишився в готелі.

Швейцарець заперечливо хитнув головою.

— Оригінал залишився у Цюриху, — сказав він.

Запала мовчанка, яку зрештою порушив сам Піллер:

— Послухайте, пане Салтіні... Все це якось дивно. У жодному листі ви не згадували, що вам потрібен оригінал твору, — заговорив він, — та навіть якби й згадували, боюся, що це неможливо. Адже рукопис мені довірила сама авторка, і не пізніше, ніж за два місяці я мушу надіслати його їй назад до Ґаліції... Ми домовлялися, що я перекладу текст італійською й передам його вам у домовлений час. Себто сьогодні... Я день і ніч працював, аби встигнути! Витратив останні гроші на квиток до Венеції, аж тут виявляється...

Видавець примирливим жестом, виставивши перед собою долоню, зупинив його емоційну промову.

— Маєте рацію, пане Піллере, — сказав Салтіні, — визнаю, усіх умов я вам не повідомив. Проте, як мені здається, двоє інтеліґентних людей завжди можуть домовитись. Я, скажімо, готовий подвоїти суму вашого гонорару, аби компенсувати це непорозуміння. Що скажете?

Піллер важко ковтнув слину.

— Не знаю, чи ви почули, пане Салтіні, — промовив він, — я сказав, що авторський рукопис залишився у Швейцарії.

— У вашому помешканні?

— Ні, в надійнішому місці.

— На бога, пане Піллере! Ми живемо в прогресивні часи! — раптом вигукнув італієць. — Відправте додому телеграму, попросіть кого-небудь вислати вам цей бісів рукопис до Венеції поштою. Звісно, ви не завтра отримаєте посилку, доведеться трохи почекати, але всі витрати, пов'язані з вашим перебуванням у Венеції, я беру на себе.

— Чому вам так потрібен оригінал? — поцікавився швейцарець. — Ви не довіряєте моєму перекладу?

Загасивши недопалок, він дістав з кишені хустинку й протер спітніле чоло.

— Ну, що ви! Звісно, довіряю, — запевнив Салтіні.

— То в чому річ?

— Це професійна таємниця, пане Піллере. Дозвольте її не відкривати, — голос видавця став категоричнішим і навіть жорсткішим. — Просто зробіть те, що прошу.

— Я вже казав, я дав слово авторці...

— Хай йому біс! — Салтіні несподівано ляснув рукою по стільниці. Від його врівноваженості не залишилося і сліду.

Піллер схопився з крісла і став як укопаний, не знаючи, як йому бути далі. Італієць також звівся на ноги. Якусь мить вони просто дивилися один на одного, а тоді Салтіні рвучко подався до дверей, замкнув їх, а ключ поклав до кишені піджака.

— Ви звідси не вийдете, добродію, доки ми не домовимося, — повідомив він швейцарцю.

— Відколи це у видавців такі мафіозні методи? — запитав Піллер.

— Що вдієш, — розвів руками Салтіні, — ринок жорсткий, на полицях купа дешевих французьких романів, читачу не догодиш, влада дере податків три шкури, тож доводиться отак — перекладача до стіни.

— І що ви зробите? — злякано перепитав швейцарець.

— М'яко переконаю вас пристати на мої умови.

— А як же авторка?

— Їй ми подаруємо один друкований примірник. А рукопис — скажете, що загубили.

Не довго думаючи, Піллер кинувся до балконних дверей, де ще кілька хвилин тому стояв Салтіні.

— Зупиніться, чорт забирай! — почув він за спиною його голос, проте не зважав і щосили наліг на дверну ручку. Вона не піддалася. Він спробував відчинити двері ще раз і ще раз, проте марно. Почув, як італієць наближається до нього, а тоді раптом згадав про свій револьвер. Миттю сягнув рукою до кишені й вихопив звідти «Шмідта». Попри хвилювання, зумів зняти зброю з запобіжника, після цього наставив її на Салтіні. Італієць спинився за якихось два кроки від нього.

— Ані руш! — наказав лисому Піллер, з насолодою помітивши, як у того від подиву відвисла щелепа.

— Ви збожеволіли? — промовив той. — Брати зброю на літературні перемовини?

— Ви ж самі кажете, що справа ця небезпечна, — криво посміхнувся швейцарець, — особливо якщо маєш справу з псевдовидавцем.

— Це ви про що? — на обличчі Салтіні спалахнуло обурення.

— Годі комедій! Ви схожі радше на костолома з дешевої кнайпи, ніж на людину з книжкового світу, — кинув йому Піллер. — І звідки у вас така добра німецька?

— По-вашому, італієць не може знати німецької?

— Звісно, що може. Але навряд чи говоритиме з баварським акцентом!

Салтіні раптом зітхнув і посміхаючись кивнув головою. Мовби у дружньому товаристві хтось розгадав його хитру загадку.

— Австрійським, — уточнив він.

— Що? — не зрозумів Піллер.

— У мене радше австрійський акцент. Я родом із Зальцбурга і ніколи не був у Баварії.

Вчергове запанувала мовчанка. Піллер не опускав зброю, але гарячково намагався придумати, як найкраще вчинити в цій ситуації. Найгірше — що рукопис він лишив на столі, і щоб знову до нього дістатися, мусив би пройти повз цього здорованя.

Десь під ними хтось почав грати на фортепіано. Піллер навіть упізнав мелодію — Шуберт, «Соната ля-мажор», друга частина, «Анданте». Пригадується, його дружина вважала цей твір найдосконалішим фортепіанним твором. Він не погоджувався, хоча також любив Шуберта. Іноді в них доходило до суперечок... Це ж треба, сперечатися через музику! І чи існує в цьому світі краща причина для суперечки?

Салтіні раптом зробив різкий крок до нього, і швейцарець майже рефлекторно натиснув на спуст. Гримнув постріл, заглушивши сонату, розбивши її на друзки, мов кришталеву вазу. Італієць пригнувся, куля його не зачепила. Піллеру від цього навіть полегшало. Проте тієї ж миті він помітив, як здоровило також вихопив зброю й одразу, не вагаючись, вистрілив у нього. Це, власне, й усе, що побачив перед смертю Антон Піллер.

Його тіло, відкинуте пострілом, продавило скло балконних дверей і перехилилося через низьку балюстраду. Трохи так повисівши, зрештою сторчголов полетіло в канал, де, здійнявши купу бризок, завмерло і мирно подалося далі за течією.

Місце тут було напрочуд гарне й безлюдне.

II

Баден
9 квітня 1906 року

Нічні чергування молодий асистент Фелікс Краут ненавидів понад усе. Він знав, що всім асистентам доктора Ріцке доводиться чергувати вночі біля цих психів, знав тоді, коли випрошував для себе місце в тутешній лікарні. Ба більше, ще студіюючи медицину в Дюссельдорфі, добре усвідомлював, що спочатку доведеться виконувати найнуднішу й найбруднішу роботу, проте підготувати себе не зумів. Вдень час минав швидко. Доктор був трудоголіком, а тому з головою пірнав у роботу, змушуючи до того самого й підлеглих. Іноді Феліксові здавалося, що промайнула тільки година, а тоді з подивом помічав, що вже закінчується день. Асистент любив медицину, був удячний доктору Ріцке за можливість працювати й вчитися, але ці проклятущі нічні чергування ненавидів усією душею.

Воно, зрештою, й не дивно. Фелікс мав заледве двадцять п'ять років і ночі волів би проводити під ковдрою зі своєю Ґретою, аніж наодинці в затхлій комірчині, що гордо йменувалася його кабінетом. Спати тут було ніде, хіба що сидячи й спершись руками на стіл. П'ять разів за нічну зміну в товаристві двох санітарів йому доводилося робити обхід. Усі тридцять палат «Психіатричної клініки святого Климента», в кожну з яких слід було обережно зазирнути, аби переконатися, що з хворими все гаразд, і водночас не потривожити їхнього сну.

До першого за цю ніч огляду лишалося двадцять хвилин. Достатньо часу, аби заварити чергову каву, і замало, щоб трохи подрімати за столом. Цікаво, що робить зараз його Ґрета? В нічні зміни, окрім маруди й утоми, його ще шалено мучили ревнощі. А що коли його двадцятирічна дружина спить з іншим? Ці думки гризли його зсередини, й щоразу він ледве стримувався, аби притьмом не помчати додому.

Злі язики не втомлювалися повторювати, що вона надто гарна для нього. Надто струнка, надто пишногруда, надто соковита. Або ж він надто хирлявий, сутулий і надто ревнивий. Кохаючись із нею, Фелікс намагався вдивлятися Ґреті в обличчя. Чи достатньо їй добре? Чи достатньо вона задоволена? І кожного разу йому здавалося, що ні... Що його можливостей їй замало. Любовних і, по щирості, фінансових. Жили вони без особливої розкоші.

Кава трохи збадьорила, і коли в двері постукав санітар, Краут почувався значно краще. Він вхопив список пацієнтів і вийшов у коридор. Санітари стовбичили під стіною, мов два големи, не кажучи ані слова й дивлячись прямо перед собою. Без сумніву, їм також понад усе хотілося спати.

— Ну гаразд, панове, — ніби переконуючи їх у необхідності цієї справи, промовив асистент, — хутко пройдемося і знову по своїх норах.

Після цього рушив уздовж лікарняного коридору, ледь-ледь освітленого тьмяним електричним світлом. Більшість пацієнтів спали, дехто мовчки сидів на ліжку й розглядав стіну перед собою, ще один стиха вів монолог. Загалом, як подумав Краут, ніч мала бути спокійною.

Підходячи до палати під номером 28, асистент сповільнив крок, щоб відшукати у списку пацієнта, який утримувався там останні два місяці. Його історію хвороби доктор Ріцке тримав у своєму кабінеті, жодного разу не показавши її Феліксу, а в обхідних списках він значився тільки як «Яша, росіянин, 43 роки». У примітках вказувалося, що пацієнт спокійний і погано говорить німецькою. Як він сюди потрапив і чи довго тут пробуде, асистент також не знав.

Відхиливши металеву стулку на дверях, Краут зазирнув усередину палати. Перше, що він помітив, — там було ввімкнено світильник, хоча в цю пору хворим заборонялося ним користуватись. Режим, як стверджував доктор Ріцке, був украй важливим для пацієнтів, тож після одинадцятої їм дозволявся лише невеличкий нічник над ліжком. Сам Яша, худий змучений чоловік з підстриженою борідкою, сидів за столом, поклавши перед собою книжку. Побачивши у прорізі дверей обличчя Краута, він махнув рукою, запрошуючи того всередину.

— Відімкніть двері, — наказав Фелікс санітарові, що носив на поясі чималу в'язку з ключами. — Цьому пацієнтові щось від мене потрібно.

Голем у білому халаті неохоче підкорився. Відчинивши двері, він спершу зайшов до палати сам, а тоді впустив туди Краута. Фелікс уперше чітко й при світлі побачив цього пацієнта. Вдень доктор Ріцке відвідував його сам, а вночі Яша зазвичай слухняно спав, не створюючи черговим жодних проблем.

— Уже пізно, — лагідно заговорив до пацієнта Фелікс, — вам слід погасити світильник.

— Прошу вибачення, пане лікарю, — відповів той, — я залишив його тому, що хотів з вами порозмовляти.

Росіянин і справді говорив з акцентом, але назвати його німецьку поганою аж ніяк не випадало.

— Зі мною? — здивувався Фелікс. — Можливо, з доктором Ріцке?

— Ні, саме з вами, — наполіг Яша.

— Але ми не знайомі.

— Чому ж? У вас є моя історія хвороби, а я бачив вас кілька разів під час прогулянки. Хіба цього замало для знайомства?

Асистент уважно придивився до співрозмовника. Той відповів йому таким самим прискіпливим поглядом чорних дещо запалих очей. Над очима й різкою дугою брів височіло широке аристократичне чоло. Волосся гладко зачесане назад. Щоки акуратно виголені рівно до того місця, де починалася акуратна борідка. Губи тонкі й бліді. Міцно стиснуті, мовби зі страху сказати зайвого.

— Помиляєтесь, я не бачив вашої картки, — відповів Фелікс, — доктор Ріцке тримає її в себе й особисто займається вашим лікуванням. «Та чи хворий він? — одразу ж подумав асистент. — Якщо це так, то я не здоровіший за нього».

— І все-таки я проситиму вас про розмову, пане лікарю. Повірте, справа дуже важлива, — запевнив Яша. — Будь ласка, наодинці.

— Стосується вашого здоров'я?

— Впевнений, що так, — кивнув той.

Фелікс озирнувся на санітарів. На їхніх кам'яних обличчях читався сумнів і стійке бажання забрати звідси Краута, забратись самим, захряснути двері палати й завалитися спати до наступного обходу.

— Гаразд, — погодився Фелікс, — якщо вам потрібна допомога, то я не маю права відмовити. Почекайте за дверима, — наказав він големам.

Ті знехотя, весь час зиркаючи на Яшу недобрими очима, підкорилися.

Лишившись з асистентом сам на сам, росіянин якийсь час мовчав, мовби збираючись з думками. Краут сів на стілець навпроти нього, пильно стежачи за мімікою і найменшими рухами пацієнта. Подумки він перебирав усе можливе, що могло б хвилювати цього Яшу. Врешті той заговорив:

— Мені потрібна допомога, пане Крауте.

Слова Яша вимовляв притишено й обережно, час від часу поглядаючи на двері, за якими стояли санітари. Здавалося, йому дуже не хотілося, щоб ця розмова досягнула їхніх вух.

— Звісно, — відповів Фелікс, — для цього існує клініка...

— Облиште, — нетерпляче перебив Яша, — я зараз не про медицину. І якщо вже бути відвертим, то я хворий не більше, ніж ви й ті двоє довбнів у коридорі.

Асистент отетеріло глянув на нього й вже хотів підвестися, коли ж псевдопацієнт м'яко його притримав за руку.

— Благаю вас, не йдіть, — прошепотів він.

— Ось що, добродію, — трохи знервовано мовив асистент, — не знаю, чому ви тут і що вам потрібно, але стосується це тільки вас і доктора Ріцке. Я у це не пхатимусь.

— Заради Бога, — знову попросив той, — я віддячу...

На цих словах Яша сягнув рукою до кишені і витягнув звідти золотий перстень зі смарагдом.

— Ось. Ця річ коштує цілого статку. Вона ваша...

У Фелікса пересохло в горлянці. Він жадібно глипнув на коштовність, а тоді підійшов до дверей і сам перевірив, чи добре вони зачинені. Кілька секунд вичекав, прислухаючись до розмови санітарів на коридорі. Тоді повернувся і сів знову на свій стілець.

— Візьміть, переконайтеся, що він справжній, — сказав росіянин, тицяючи перстень тому просто в руки, — це фамільна коштовність. Ви в житті такої не бачили.

Останнє точно було правдою. Найдорожчий скарб у їхньому з Ґретою домі — це срібний кулон його дружини, який вона отримала в подарунок від хрещеної матері ще в дитинстві. Ще його годинник. Виглядав він коштовно, проте кожен ювелір з першого погляду сказав би, що позолота на ньому несправжня. А отже, й вартує він заледве обіду в посередньому ресторані.

Втім, персня Фелікс так і не взяв. Десь у глибині його єства раптом прокинулись обережність та підозрілість.

— І що ви за це хочете? — запитав він.

— Одну дріб'язкову послугу.

— Яку?

Не зводячи зі співрозмовника очей, Яша на секунду замовк, мовби тільки для того, щоб прикусити свою безкровну губу, а тоді промовив:

— Завтра в місті у готелі «Під золотим оленем» зупиниться один російський вельможа. Граф Орлов. Високий чоловік років сорока. Дещо огрядний. Ви без проблем його впізнаєте... Здебільшого він буває у двох місцях: у себе в номері або в клубі «Пігмаліон». Там він марнує час за гральним столом.

— І що потрібно від мене? — запитав Фелікс.

— Я хочу, щоб ви передали йому від мене листа. Особисто в руки.

— І все?

Яша кивнув.

— Я ж казав, що послуга дріб'язкова.

— Однак, ви готові щедро за неї заплатити, — Краут виразно глянув на перстень, що залишився в руках пацієнта. Той майже недбало тримав його двома пальцями, мовби підкреслюючи, що лікар будь-якої миті може взяти його собі.

— Мені вкрай важливо, аби граф отримав це послання.

— Що в ньому?

— Повідомлення про те, що я тут, і прохання мене відвідати.

— Невже більше нічого?

— Нічогісінько.

Асистент не поспішав з відповіддю. Було видно, як його діймають сумніви.

— Ви говорили про це доктору Ріцке?

— Говорив про що?

— Про цього графа... Орлова... Про те, що збираєтеся з ним зустрітися.

— Ні, — різко вимовив пацієнт. — І вас проситиму ані словом не прохопитися про нашу розмову доктору.

Краут стенув плечима, показуючи, що не має ані потреби, ані бажання патякати про це зі своїм начальником.

— Пообіцяйте, що мовчатимете, — не вгавав Яша.

— Обіцяю, — відмахнувся Фелікс.

Росіянин перегорнув кілька сторінок своєї книжки й дістав з-поміж них запечатаного конверта. На ньому не було жодної позначки, тільки сліди від клейкої суміші.

— То як? — перепитав він. — На вас можна покластися?

Фелікс врешті мовчки кивнув і сховав листа в кишені халата. Після цього взяв у пацієнта перстень і, затиснувши його в руці, вийшов з палати. Санітари курили просто в коридорі і, побачивши асистента, миттю загасили свої самокрути. Курити тут заборонялось, але големи знали, що асистент Краут їм не дорікатиме. Вночі правила й приписи ставали м'якшими і вже не такими обов'язковими до виконання...

Додому Фелікс повернувся, як завжди, о пів на дев'яту ранку. О восьмій до клініки приходив доктор Ріцке. Хвилин п'ятнадцять він розпитував асистента про те, як минуло чергування, а тоді відпускав його. Сьогодні доктору здалося, що Фелікс поводився дещо незвично: говорив мало і трохи плутався у словах.

— Ви не захворіли, пане Крауте? — турботливо перепитав він підлеглого.

Той відповів, що й справді почувається трохи недобре. Хоч це було брехнею, бо насправді йому з голови не йшов росіянин, лист і перстень, що, лежачи в кишені жилета, легенько тиснув під ребра. А ще Фелікса розпікав сором, оскільки він уперше робив щось за спиною свого наставника.

На щастя, доктор нічого не запідозрив і порадив асистентові випити чарку коньяку та добре виспатись. Пообіцявши, що так і зробить, Фелікс поспіхом вийшов із клініки. Дорога додому зайняла ще п'ятнадцять хвилин.

В їхній із Ґретою спальні було порожньо. Його дружина, як завжди в цей час, вже була на роботі. Вона служила гувернанткою в багатій швейцарській сім'ї, що переїхала два роки тому до Бадена. Навчала дітей французької, танців та водила їх ввечері до театру. Не роздягаючись, Фелікс ліг на ліжко й зарився обличчям в її подушку. З насолодою вдихнув знайомий щемкий запах, у якому добре знав кожну нотку: мило, олійка для шкіри й мазь для доброго сну, яку дружина намащувала собі на скроні. Ґрета завжди так пахнула, коли засинала. Цей запах пробуджував у ньому одночасно пожадання й ревнощі. А також знову витягував на поверхню сумніви й власну невпевненість.

З пів години Фелікс намагався заснути, але марно. Врешті плюнув на сон, підвівся й привів себе до ладу. Ще за кілька хвилин подався снідати до улюбленої кнайпи за рогом вулиці. Рука його щоразу тягнулася до кишені жилета, аби переконатися, що перстень, який він отримав уночі від російського пацієнта, досі на місці. Збоку можна було подумати, що в молодого чоловіка поколює десь біля селезінки.

У кнайпі, як завжди у ранішній час, вільних місць майже не було. Сніданок тут коштував недорого, тому їдців кожного ранку набивалося чимало. Були це молоді лікарі, як-от Фелікс, небагаті вчителі, дрібні торговці, а також робітники, що обслуговували тутешні лікувальні басейни та бювети з мінеральною водою. Дим від їхніх цигарок тягнувся до низької дерев'яної стелі, де збирався у прозорі хмари, створюючи цим людям власні тимчасові небеса. Вікна у кнайпі не відчиняли, бо знадвору було досить прохолодно. Отож цей вранішній світ був замкнений сам у собі. Спокійний і самодостатній. І навіть не вірилося, що за якусь годину він розчиниться у світі зовнішньому, коли ця публіка, поспішаючи, піде геть і візьметься до щоденної рутини.

Фелікс зняв плаща, капелюха й почепив їх на кострубатий вішак. Тоді вмостився за столиком під стіною. Кельнер, кругленький верткий чоловічок, підійшов одразу. Він знав і цінував постійних клієнтів, тому рідко змушував їх чекати. Його короткі вусики підстрибнули у привітній усмішці, і Фелікс міг бути певен, що вона в нього щира.

Асистент замовив підсмажений хліб, яєчню, шматочок баварського сиру і каву.

— Маєте трохи стомлений вигляд, — співчутливо зазначив кельнер.

— Була нічна зміна, а вранці заснути так і не вдалося, — сказав Краут.

Чоловік з розумінням кивнув.

— Якщо не надто сьогодні поспішаєте, то я принесу дещо. За рахунок закладу.

Кельнер підморгнув йому і зник за шинквасом. Повернувся за якусь хвилину, несучи на таці прозорий келишок, наповнений горілкою. Вдруге підморгнувши клієнтові, чоловік поставив його перед ним на стіл.

— «*Wyborowa*» з Позена. Вчора отримали. Чиста, як сльоза немовляти, — промовив кельнер притишеним змовницьким голосом. — Саме те, що потрібно після важкої ночі.

— А чи не надто рання година? — з сумнівом у голосі запитав Фелікс, хоча тієї ж миті пригадав, що випити йому радив також і доктор Ріцке.

— А хіба буває рано для ліків, пане Крауте? Людина п'є їх, коли потребує, — промовив офіціант. — Заждіть лише, принесу вам сніданок.

«А й справді, — подумав Фелікс, вкотре перевіривши, чи на місці перстень, — гірше мені точно не буде, а от впевненості трохи додасться...»

Яєчня ще шкварчала в нього на тарілці, а хліб і сир мали апетитніший, ніж зазвичай, вигляд. Асистент підніс зі столу келишок і з приємністю відчув долонею його прохолоду. Тоді вже без сумнівів перехилив горілку собі до рота. Алкоголь приємно спалахнув у горлі і розлився нутром. Одразу після цього Фелікс глибоко вдихнув — він робив так завжди, коли випивка припадала до ґусту. Тільки після цього заходився їсти сніданок. Після їжі закурив, обдумуючи, що робитиме сьогодні вдень. Найперше — слід піти до готелю «Під золотим оленем» і довідатися, чи прибув уже граф Орлов. Якщо так, тоді він одразу ж передасть йому листа від Яші... А далі — піде до ювеліра, покаже йому персня і з'ясує, за скільки може продати цю коштовність. Якщо гроші в ювеліра знайдуться одразу, купить Ґреті якийсь подарунок. При згадці про дружину Фелікса знову охопило бажання. Він купить їй подарунок і запросить до ресторації. Або принесе вино і солодощі додому. Вони вип'ють, і Ґрета кохатиметься з ним — не так, як завжди. По-іншому — як із сильним чоловіком. Пристрасно й безсоромно, мов колись. Він більше не вдивлятиметься їй в обличчя, бо й так буде певен, що їй добре. Що вона віддається йому не з жалю чи обов'язку, а тому, що по-справжньому його хоче.

Фелікс загасив цигарку й виклав на стіл *пів марки* за сніданок. Підвівся, вдячно кивнув на прощання кельнеру, одягся й вийшов на вулицю. На вулиці було похмуро й трохи вітряно, тому асистент одразу ж підняв комір плаща й глибше насадив на голову капелюха. Попри те що був уже квітень, весною в місті навіть не пахло. На узгір'ї, біля руїн Старого Замку*, лежав сніг і, судячи з погоди, пролежить там ще довго.

Вузьким брукованим провулком, що незручно звивався вгору, чоловік вийшов на залюднену Фрідріхштрассе, де, тримаючись хідника, щоб не потрапити під екіпаж або під колеса якого-небудь автомобіля, пройшов кількасот метрів до повороту на Вердерштрассе. Тут, неподалік від міського парку, височів чотириповерховий розкішний готель «Під золотим оленем», найстаріший і найдорожчий у Бадені.

Швейцар відчинив перед ним двері, проте якось недбало, вочевидь тому, що не мав жодної надії отримати від Фелікса чайові. Той зі свого боку, звісно, й не збирався давати йому ані *пфеніга*. Обмінявшись з ним холодними поглядами, Краут зайшов у вестибюль.

Інтер'єр зблиснув перед ним світлом і розкішшю, золотом і велетенськими картинами у коштовних рамах, гладким мармуром і товстезними колонами, поміж якими на підвищенні, наче вівтар в античному храмі, знаходилася стійка рецепції.

---

* Старий Замок (нім. *Altes Schloss*) — відомий також як замок Гогенбаден. Архітектурна пам'ятка поруч Баден-Бадена, датована XII ст.

Роль жертовних ягнят, схоже, дісталася двом рецепціоністам, які, завмерши й не сміючи вимовити ані слова, вислуховували істерику якоїсь мадам. Її чоловік стояв позаду, чи то підтримуючи дружину, чи то разом з адміністраторами чекаючи, коли в неї скінчаться запаси жовчі. Іноді він ніжно брав її за лікоть і лагідним голосом промовляв щось російською, проте щоразу вона жестом наказувала йому не втручатися. Кричала вона французькою, час од часу зупиняючись, щоб набрати в легені повітря і підібрати потрібне слово. Фелікс не знав французької, тому нічого не розумів. Бідолахи за стійкою, найпевніше, воліли б не знати французької, щоб також не розуміти.

Фінал цієї сцени виявився доволі яскравим і несподіваним. Дама вигукнула останню свою фразу якось надто голосно й натужно, від чого заточилася назад і впала просто на руки чоловікові.

— Дивіться, що ви зробили, негідники! — замість неї вигукнув той.

Фелікс уже хотів кинутися на допомогу, проте побачив, що дама встояла на ногах, хоч вигляд мала виснажений. Чоловік простягнув їй флакон із ароматичною сіллю, після чого, гнівно зиркаючи в бік рецепції, повів її до сходів. Щойно вони пропали з виду, як адміністратори за стійкою зітхнули з полегшенням і одночасно взялися витирати хустинками зволожені лоби. На Фелікса вони не звертали жодної уваги, аж поки той не підійшов достатньо близько. Один із них був зовсім молодим, мав не більше двадцяти років. Інший — старший, з рівною поставою і дещо манірними рухами. Обидва зміряли гостя поглядом, намагаючись, видно, одразу зрозуміти, хто він і що йому треба.

Фелікс вирішив усміхнутися.

— Ну вона й істеричка, — співчутливо сказав він.

— Це ще мадам Панфілова не надто сердита. Ви й уявити не можете, що тут відбувається, коли в неї по-справжньому поганий настрій, — відповів молодший.

Старший колега кинув на нього суворий погляд, і той замовк, винувато опустивши очі.

— Чим можемо служити, шановний пане? — звернувся він до Краута.

Голос цей чоловік мав рівний, слова вимовляв чітко, з підкресленою штучною приязню.

— Я шукаю одного російського вельможу, — сказав Фелікс, — він зупинився у цьому готелі.

Тепер навіть старший адміністратор не стримав усмішки.

— Добродію, — мовив той, — у нас майже всі номери займають російські вельможі. Чи не могли б ви назвати його ім'я?

— Звісно... — відповів Краут, сам дивуючись зі своєї недалекоглядності. — Це граф... граф Орлов.

Рецепціоніст, схоже, зрозумів, про кого йшла мова.

— Його світлість повинен був прибути на світанку. Одну секунду, я перевірю в списках.

Він рушив до прочинених дверей за стійкою, й було чути, як десь у сусідньому приміщенні чоловік перегортав невидимі сторінки.

— Чого та мадам збісилася? — пошепки запитав Фелікс у молодшого, скориставшись нагодою.

— Не подали в номер кав'яру, — так само пошепки відповів йому рецепціоніст. При цьому він скорчив таку серйозну міну, ніби йшлося про справді страхітливий злочин, за який ще сьогодні його привселюдно стратять. Фелікс розтулив рота, щоб запитати більше, але не встиг, бо тієї ж миті з журналом у руках повернувся старший.

— Так і є, — на ходу говорив він, — граф Орлов поселився сьогодні ще перед восьмою і просив за жодних обставин не турбувати його аж до вечора.

На цих словах адміністратор категоричним рухом закрив свої списки.

— Я маю для нього листа, — сказав Фелікс.

— Ви чули: «За жодних обставин», — повторив старший. — Мені шкода. Навідайтеся сюди десь після сьомої.

«Найпевніше, доведеться шукати його в клубі», — подумав Краут і, подякувавши, рушив до виходу. Там знову наштовхнувся на швейцара, який цього разу вирішив не відчиняти перед ним дверей. Фелікс прочинив їх сам, зійшов зовнішніми сходами і неквапно рушив тією самою Фрідріхштрассе, яка привела його до готелю.

Йдучи тепер у протилежний бік, асистент Краут намагався вигадати, як убити час аж до сьомої. Приємний ефект від випитої чарки потроху вивітрювався, і на зміну йому знову приходила їдка втома від безсонної ночі. Можна було повернутися до кнайпи й випити ще, проте Фелікс побоювався сп'яніти. Краще вже потім, коли віддасть тому графові листа і побуває у ювеліра...

Раптова думка, що промайнула у стомленій голові, повернула Феліксу добрий гумор: до ювеліра він може піти просто зараз! Звісно, пасувало б зробити це після виконаної роботи, але що складного в тому, щоб передати комусь листа? До того ж ввечері ювелірні крамниці вже зачинені, й доведеться чекати до наступного ранку. А в нього грандіозні плани ще на сьогодні.

Підбадьорений цими роздумами, Краут вирушив на Кайзерштрассе, де була найбільша в місті ювелірна крамниця Вайсманна. Йти було недовго, проте чоловіка раптом охопило таке хвилювання, що він мусив зупинитись і закурити. Несподівано йому здалося, що за ним стежать. Пильнують кожен його крок ще, мабуть, від кнайпи... Викуривши одну цигарку, він одразу ж запалив другу, одночасно намагаючись себе опанувати. «Ніхто не знає, що в мене в кишені. Ніхто не знає, куди я йду...» — переконував він себе, одночасно вдаючи байдужого перехожого, який просто зупинився покурити й порозглядати Кургауз* навпроти.

— Треба попросити доктора Ріцке ставити мені менше нічних чергувань, — пошепки сказав він сам до себе, — від них в мене нерви, як у параноїка...

Коли сяк-так вдалося заспокоїтись, асистент рушив далі. Докладаючи, щоправда, чимало зусиль, аби не озиратися кожної хвилини.

Крамниця Альберта Вайсманна розташовувалася поруч із міським казино в самому центрі Бадена. Розміщення це виявилося досить вигідним. Власник часто затримувався в ній до ранку, знаючи, що десь після півночі можна сподіватися візиту якого-небудь азартного невдахи, котрому негайно треба продати якусь свою коштовність, аби за отримані гроші спробувати відігратись.

Про Альберта Вайсманна ходили різні чутки. Подейкували, що свій ґешефт він розпочав понад тридцять років тому з того, що завозив дешеве золото з російського Уралу. Відстань у тисячі миль він раз або двічі на рік долав

---

* Кургауз (нім. *Kurhaus*) — будинок дозвілля. Місце, де проводяться розважальні заходи, концерти тощо.

самотужки, не покладаючись на посередників та не беручи собі спільників. Довгі роки він уникав грабіжників, підкуповував митників і терпів усі дорожні негаразди, аж поки одного разу ледь не загинув у пащі ведмедя. Звір підстеріг його і напав, коли ювелір пішки йшов до залізничної станції. Як завжди, сам, звично не довіряючи жодній людській душі в цілому світі. Врятував його мисливець, що вистрілив у тварюку з відстані ста кроків і, на щастя, не промахнувся. Розповідають, що вдячний Вайсманн віддав мисливцеві все, що мав у торбі й кишенях, залишивши собі тільки гроші на дорогу. Повернувшись до Бадена, чоловік вирішив так далеко більше не їздити. Та й узагалі не виїжджати далі рідного міста, тим більше, що золота за ці роки трохи назбирав. Якраз вистачило, щоб купити в збанкрутілого аптекаря його аптеку й облаштувати там ювелірну майстерню, а потім і крамницю.

Втім, за короткий час поповзли чутки, що Вайсманн знайшов у аптечній пивниці забуту алхімічну лабораторію і з допомогою того-таки аптекаря-банкрута навчився перетворювати бронзу на золото, а вугілля — на діаманти. Олії у вогонь підлила звістка про наглу смерть аптекаря. Він начебто вкоротив собі віку за допомогою міцної конопляної мотузки і малярської драбини, що стояла в його коморі бозна-скільки часу без діла. «Не інакше, як Вайсманн звів зі світу спільника, щоб той не вибовкав їхні секрети», — говорили підозріливі містяни. Поліція навіть завела справу й узялася до розслідування, втім, жодної таємної лабораторії у ювелірній крамниці слідчі не виявили (хоча ретельно шукали), та й версія про причетність Вайсманна до смерті аптекаря не знайшла жодного підтвердження. Зате з'ясувалося, що боргів у покійника лишилось, як у собаки бліх, і кредитори писали йому довгі листи подекуди з досить відвертими погрозами.

Розслідування закінчилось, і хоч репутацію Альберта Вайсманна було добряче зіпсовано, клієнтів йому не бракувало. Насамперед тому, що майстром він був непоганим і працював на совість.

Феліксові, звісна річ, були відомі ці чутки. Проте, як людина раціональна, вірив він тільки в те, що могло бути правдою. Зайшовши до крамниці, він зняв капелюха й привітався з господарем. Той сидів за велетенською дерев'яною рахівницею, цілковито заглиблений у розрахунки. Почувши, як рипнули двері, підвівся й рушив назустріч відвідувачу.

Вайсманн був невисокого зросту сивий чоловік з уважним, проникливим поглядом. Обличчя мав злегка жовтуватого кольору, а зморшки різкі, як лінії на контурній карті. Зовнішність його здавалася малоприємною, а проте заговорив ювелір приязно, мовби Краут був тут частим гостем.

— Вітаю, молодий чоловіче, — сказав ювелір, знімаючи зі свого гострого носа делікатні окуляри в дротяній оправі. — Чим можу допомогти?

— У мене є дещо... — почав Краут. — На продаж, якщо ваша ласка.

— Он як, — посерйознішав господар. — Що ж, показуйте. Подивимося, чи воно мене зацікавить.

Фелікс озирнувся на двері, мовби побоюючись, що за ним міг зайти ще хтось, а тоді дістав з кишені перстень. Ювелір насадив окуляри на носа й, узявши коштовність до рук, уважно до неї придивився. Розглядав кілька хвилин, а тоді перевів погляд на гостя.

— Отже, на продаж? — перепитав Вайсманн.

Клієнт ствердно кивнув.

Господар повернув йому персня, швидко підійшов до дверей і замкнув їх на ключ.

— І скільки ви хочете? — мовив ювелір, повернувшись на попереднє місце.

— Рівно стільки, скільки він коштує, — по-діловому відповів асистент.

— Він коштує чимало, молодий чоловіче. Зізнаюся, я стільки не маю. Тобто не маю тут, в крамниці... Але викупити його у вас готовий.

Він задумався на кілька хвилин, заклав руки за спину й кілька разів пройшовся вздовж крамниці. Фелікс затамував подих, стежачи за ним і дослухаючись одночасно до цокання годинника на стіні. Під годинником одна біля одної стояли книжкова шафа і засклена вітрина, де лежали прикраси. Далі було облаштовано робоче місце майстра: масивний дубовий стіл, заставлений вагами, скриньками з інструментами, кількома записниками, чималою лінзою на підставці й двома лампами. Одна була гасова, інша — швидше за все, електрична.

— Зробімо так, — зупинившись, сказав ювелір. — Частину грошей, а саме п'ять тисяч марок, я видам зараз. На решту ж суми напишу боргове зобов'язання. У ньому буде сказано, що я повинен повністю з вами розрахуватися не пізніше, ніж за два тижні. Рівно стільки часу мені знадобиться, аби отримати необхідні кошти в банку. Що скажете?

Він пильно глянув на співрозмовника, ніби оцінював вартість і його самого.

— П'ять тисяч марок, — повторив Фелікс, — а решта суми — це скільки?

Асистент нетямився від щастя, проте боявся це показати й удавав із себе прискіпливого продавця.

— Решта суми — це ще десять тисяч, — відповів Вайсманн.

Феліксу перехопило подих.

— Згода, — вимовив гість.

Мабуть, він сказав це занадто поспішно й охоче, бо ювелір посміхнувся і на якийсь час зник у себе в комірчині. Чути було, як господар відмикає важкий замок, відчиняє двері сейфу, відраховує потрібну кількість купюр і знову надійно замикає свій сховок. Коли повернувся до гостя, то обличчя мав почервоніле, ніби вся ця процедура вартувала йому значних зусиль.

— Ось, можете перерахувати, — сказав він, простягаючи Феліксові акуратний паперовий згорток.

— Немає жодної потреби... — хотів заперечити той, але Вайсманн його перебив:

— Гроші люблять порядок, тишу і добру лічбу. Крім того, я міг випадково відрахувати вам більше... Перерахуйте, а я тим часом помилуюся своїм новим надбанням. Ви дозволите? — ювелір простягнув руку.

— Звісно, — відповів Фелікс, віддаючи йому перстень, — він тепер ваш.

— Саме так... — якимось хижим голосом промовив господар, сідаючи за свій стіл. — Тепер мій.

Чоловік увімкнув електричну лампу й підніс коштовність до лінзи. Уважно роздивившись її з усіх можливих ракурсів, ювелір ствердно промовив щось сам до себе й узявся писати боргове зобов'язання. Тривало це близько чверті години, аж доки врешті Вайсманн широко розписався під текстом, а поруч з підписом поставив печатку. Потім зачекав ще зо дві хвилини, аби висох атрамент. Далі підвівся й приніс документ Феліксу. Той взяв його й перечитав текст. Усе там було так, як і говорив ювелір: решту грошей, тобто десять тисяч марок, він обіцяв віддати Крауту не пізніше полудня 23 квітня 1906 року. Залишалося тільки потиснути один одному руки і попрощатися, що вони і зробили.

Коли гість пішов, ювелір не поспішав повертатися до своєї звичної роботи. Точніше, чоловік вирішив на сьогодні про неї забути. Якусь хвилину він ще потримав перстень перед очима, а тоді швидко поклав його до кишені жилета, точнісінько як перед тим Краут, і заходився одягатись. Швидко накинув пальто, шарф, до кишені поклав пару тонких рукавиць. Спершу вирішив узяти капелюх, але передумав і насадив на голову зручного теплого кашкета. Наостанок зняв свої делікатні окуляри, замінивши їх більшими, що мали масивніші лінзи й міцніше сиділи на обличчі. Після цього Вайсманн поспіхом вийшов на вулицю й зачинив крамницю ззовні. Більше сьогодні повертатись до роботи він не збирався.

Ювелір подався до заднього двору казино, де під широким навісом стояв його «Даймлер» поруч із кількома іншими авто. Нечисленні баденські автомобілісти облаштували тут стоянку, щомісяця сплачуючи певну суму власнику закладу й прилеглої території. Той, зі свого боку, зобов'язав сторожа пильнувати автомобілі вдень і вночі. Навряд чи хтось намагався би їх вкрасти, а от розібрати й зазирнути всередину механізму — на це охочих знайшлося б чимало.

Вайсманн вмостився на водійському сидінні, вдягнув рукавці й завів двигун. «Даймлер» затрясло, а з вихлопної труби почулося знайоме чмихання. Понад усе він зараз боявся, що авто не поїде. За останній тиждень воно вже тричі виходило з ладу. Проте сьогодні йому щастило. Сторож, що ліниво виповз зі своєї будки, відкрив перед ним браму, і Вайсманн виїхав зі стоянки.

Далі слід було набратися терпіння, щоб проїхати гамірною Фрідріхштрассе, не зіткнутися при цьому з кінним фіакром і не наскочити на випадкового роззяву, якому раптово заманулося перейти вулицю. Цей відрізок дороги до виїзду з міста завжди коштував йому шалених нервів. Руки після нього ще довго тремтіли, а єдиним бажанням було зупинитися в найближчій кнайпі й перехилити чогось міцного. Проволікшись так до Страсбурзької Дороги, Вайсманн врешті зміг впевнено натиснути на газ і поїхати швидше.

За містом починалися виноградники. Безлисті лози сільванера, рислінгу і дорнфельдера в цю пору мали вигляд сірий і непривітний, як випалений ліс, і залишалося тільки домислювати, як зміниться в кольорі тутешній ландшафт вже за кілька місяців, з настанням літа. Втім, найчарівнішою порою в цих місцях була осінь, коли минають спекотні дні, а в місцевих *Weinstuben** з'являється молоде вино. Найвеселіший час для довколишніх гультяїв і найприбутковіший для виноробів.

За якийсь час Вайсманн виїхав до Райну, і його «Даймлер» помчав уздовж плину ріки, іноді обганяючи навантажену баржу або пароплав, що курсував, найпевніше,

---

* *Weinstuben* (*нім.*) — винні кнайпи.

між Страсбургом і Майнцом чи Мангаймом. Протилежний берег Райну виглядав казково: зі скелястих виступів виростали середньовічні замки й сторожові вежі. А часом і саме гігантське каміння вибудовувалося у велетенські химери, що стриміли над водою, заворожуючи туристів і погрожуючи річковим суднам.

Втім, Вайсманну, по щирості, було плювати на всю цю мальовничість. Він дивився перед собою, намагався не вскочити колесом у випадкову яму і дістатися до цілі якнайшвидше. Водій сповільнився, тільки коли побачив попереду стару портову вежу. Ніякого порту в цьому місці давно не було, і навіть берег Райну встигли перепланувати, укріпивши його схили бетоном і камінням, аби дорога, що проходила всього за кілька метрів від води, не нищилася повенями. Та попри те, вежа виглядала добре збереженою, хоч і не виконувала більше ніякої функції. Видно, річкові транспортні компанії вирішили не покидати цю споруду напризволяще й час від часу виділяли кошти на ремонт.

Портова вежа була для Вайсманна орієнтиром. Тут він збочив, об'їхав її і попрямував далі вузькою лісовою дорогою, аж доки та не закінчилася біля важких металевих воріт, за якими виднілася невелика струнка вілла з двома шпилястими вежами і кількома різьбленими балконами. Такими зазвичай були маєтки тутешніх багатих виноробів або власників судноплавних компаній.

Вайсманн заглушив двигун і вийшов з авто. Браму було зачинено зсередини, тож довелося почекати, доки його побачить сторож і прийде відчиняти.

— Автомобіль прошу залишити ззовні, пане Вайсманне, — озвався той до прибулого, — такі нові правила.

Сторож, хоч старий і сивобородий, але поставу мав рівну, як у вишколеного вояка. Зрештою, нічого дивного. Цей чоловік був військовим емеритом і ще десять чи п'ятнадцять років тому носив унтерофіцерський мундир. На гостей дивився трохи зверхньо й говорив таким тоном, ніби віддав накази новобранцям. Вайсманн його недолюблював і намагався спілкуватися з ним якомога менше. Тому й зараз не сперечався і слухняно залишив авто поза брамою, попросивши тільки, аби той, не зволікаючи, повідомив про його приїзд.

— Звісно, повідомлю, пане Вайсманне, — відповів колишній унтер. — А ви тим часом ідіть до будинку й почекайте в передпокої.

Знову це прозвучало як наказ. «Щоб тобі заціпило, старе хамло», — сердито подумав гість і рушив мощеною алеєю до високого ґанку. При цьому йому здалося, що крок його раптом зробився ритмічним і чітким, майже як стройовий.

У вітальні виявилося холодно, мов у погребі, тому Вайсманн залишив на собі пальто, знявши тільки кашкета, шарф і рукавиці. Камін тут не розпалювали, схоже, давно, чи то сподіваючись на весняне потепління, чи заощаджуючи дрова. Залишки попелу в ньому були схожими на закам'янілості з музею прадавньої природи, а довжелезна кочерга, що стояла поруч, здавалася непотрібним і випадково забутим тут предметом.

Попри те що у вітальні стояло кілька стільців, довкола прямокутного столу, призначеного, мабуть, для спільної трапези чи ділових обговорень, гість вирішив почекати на прийом стоячи. Він підійшов до вікна і трохи ширше відхилив важкі запилюжені портьєри.

З протилежного боку шибки був похмурий, але доглянутий сад. Кілька старих яблунь, розлогі вишні й акуратні кущі смородини. Найпевніше, за садом також доглядає сторож. Той самий жорсткий унтер у відставці. Щойно Вайсманн подумав про нього, як тієї ж миті той сам зайшов до передпокою.

— Пан майор чекає на вас, — коротко повідомив старий служака.

— Прекрасно, — відповів гість, і, не дивлячись більше на нього, зайшов до сусіднього покою.

Той, кого сторож назвав майором, не мав на собі військового мундира. Чоловік був одягнений у звичайний твідовий костюм з вузькою, нерівно зав'язаною краваткою. При появі гостя неспішно підвівся з-за столу й простягнув йому руку для привітання. Після цього вказав прибулому на стілець.

— Не чекав вас, — прямолінійно, проте без жодної неприязні сказав майор, знову сівши за стіл і відкинувшись на спинку стільця. Той жалібно заскрипів під його масивним атлетичним тілом.

— Не скажу, що й сам збирався покинути до дідька сьогоднішню роботу і пхатися в це задуп'я, пане Фішере, — з образою в голосі відповів ювелір, — приємності для мене в цьому вкрай мало.

— Ну-ну, пане Вайсманне, — примирливо промовив майор, — не ображайтесь. Я сказав, не подумавши. Бажаєте чаю?

Гість уявив, як чай готує той самий унтер, і поспішно відмовився. Фішер, здавалося, вгадав його думки.

— То, може, трохи бренді? — запропонував він. — Я попрошу Клавдію нам принести.

— Клавдія також тут? — здивувався ювелір.

— Так, пане Вайсманне. Скажу більше: ледь не весь Третій відділ* зараз під Баденом...

Майор на хвилину вийшов з кабінету. Власне, це справді був його кабінет, хоч це приміщення нагадувало радше бібліотеку.

Книжкові полиці стояли вздовж усіх чотирьох стін і навіть затуляли частину вікна за спиною Фішера. І зовсім не тому, що майор, заступник директора Управління прусської військової розвідки, полюбляв читати. Книжки добре поглинали звук, тож мовців у кабінеті було доволі важко підслухати ззовні. І, звісно ж, за книжковою полицею зручно ховати потаємні двері, а між самими фоліантами — документи та зброю.

Вайсманн також знав, що майор тільки на позір недбало вийшов за двері й лишив гостя самого в кабінеті. Чоловік майже фізично відчував, як його зараз свердлить уважний погляд звідкілясь з-за тих книжок. От хоча би з тієї щілини між масивним зібранням енциклопедистів** і раритетним виданням «Божественної комедії» Данте. Жоден, навіть найменший, рух прибулого не залишиться непоміченим. Що вже й казати про яку-небудь дію. Тому Вайсманн сидів нерухомо, як статуя, аж доки не повернувся Фішер. Майор знову вмостився на своєму стільці і вже тепер зосереджено глянув на гостя.

---

* Третій відділ (*Abteilung III b*) — служба прусської військової розвідки, заснована 1889 року. Існувала до закінчення Першої світової війни.

** Енциклопедисти — французькі інтелектуали XVIII ст., що працювали над виданням «Енциклопедія, або Тлумачний словник науки, мистецтва й ремесел». Серед них Дені Дідро, Вольтер, Луї де Жокур та ін.

— Вам не гаряче в пальті? — запитав він Вайсманна.

— Трохи, — відповів той і підвівся, аби зняти його з себе. — У вашому передпокої можна зберігати трупи... Там достатньо зимно.

Фішер засміявся.

— Вішак праворуч від вас, — по-господарському сказав він і встромив до рота цигарку. Пожувавши її своїми повними м'ясистими губами, майор запалив сірника й закурив. Після цього гостинно підсунув відкритий портсигар на край столу, аби ювелір міг пригоститись. Той не відмовився.

— То що трапилося, дорогий пане Вайсманне? — запитав Фішер, випускаючи в його бік густий струмінь диму. Своїми великими округлими щоками цей чоловік міг би завиграшки видувати скляні кулі, мов заправський склодув.

— Сьогодні вдень до моєї крамниці зайшов один молодий чоловік, — перейшов до справи гість, — він приніс на продаж дещо надзвичайно цікаве...

Ювелір потягнувся до кишені жилета, але тієї ж миті двері прочинилися й до кабінету зайшла чорнява жінка в темно-синій сукні, несучи в руках тацю з пляшкою «Ашбаху»* і трьома келихами-сніфтерами. Вайсманн смикнувся, як від болю, але тієї ж миті заспокоївся.

— Пані Шраґмюллер, радий вас бачити, — сказав він, ґречно підводячись.

— Я вас також, Альберте, — кинула жінка й, підійшовши до столу Фішера, поставила тацю на стільницю.

---

* «Ашбах» (нім. *Aschbach Uralt*) — марка німецького бренді. Одна з найстаріших.

— Дякую, Клавдіє, — промовив майор, — залишіться, будь ласка. Пан Вайсманн приніс нам якусь цікаву звістку.

Він підвівся й приніс жінці стілець. Потім розлив бренді у три склянки.

— І що ж мав при собі той молодик? — запитав Фішер, подавши кожному його порцію випивки.

— Дещо дуже цікаве, — повторив ювелір. Він випив бренді одним ковтком, а тоді відставив порожню склянку й витягнув з кишені перстень. — Гляньте...

— Яка гарна річ, — вихопилося у Клавдії.

— Ще б пак, — нервово посміхнувся ювелір, — але справжня цінність її в дечому іншому... — тут він виразно глянув на Фішера. — Ви здогадуєтеся, про що я, пане майоре?

— Хочете сказати, перстень з тієї самої колекції? — запитав той після паузи.

— Я не хочу сказати, я це стверджую, чорт забирай! — не стримався Вайсманн.

— Якщо ви вже дозволили мені залишитись, панове, то, може, відкриєте тему розмови? — сказала Клавдія.

Вона вперше усміхнулася, і усмішка її виявилася чарівною. Пані Шраґмюллер була вродливою жінкою приблизно сорока років. Той вік, коли жіноча краса досягає своєї повноти й досконалості. Поодинокі зморшки її не псували. Губи нехай не палали, як у дівчини, проте були тонкими й привабливими. Шкіра зберігала еластичність, хоч, може, обличчя й здавалося занадто блідим. Аристократичності додавали високі вилиці й акуратний ніс. Єдине, що вражало випадкового спостерігача, — це її погляд. Щось було в ньому холодне, крижане й убивче. І, здавалося, приховувати його жінці було вкрай важко.

Так само, як важко приховати в тонкому делікатному одязі гострий смертоносний ніж.

— Чи пам'ятаєте, Клавдіє, такого собі Якова Бобровського? Російського вельможу-втікача, який за дивних обставин зник рік тому в Берліні? Кажуть, він, попри своє благородне походження, таємно підтримував есерів-революціонерів* у Петербурзі і за це потрапив у немилість до царя, — сказав Фішер. — Бобровському вдалося втекти до Пруссії, прихопивши при цьому майже все своє золото. Це було трохи більше року тому, а зник він цієї зими, у січні. Разом зі своїм бісовим багатством... Звісна річ, за Бобровським тепер полює «охранка», і, крім того, російський консул вимагає від нашої поліції знайти його живим або мертвим. Краще, звісна річ, живим разом із багатством.

— Пригадую, — мовила Клавдія, — здається, мова йшла про доволі велику кількість золота?

— Велетенську, — кивнув майор, — росіяни стверджують, що Бобровський вивіз близько двох тисяч фунтів.

— Але ж не міг цей чоловік вивезти стільки коштовного металу за пазухою.

— Звісно. Поліція припускає, що золото було в ящиках з рудою, яка прийшла вантажним кораблем в Гамбург. Потім «руду» доставили в Берлін до власника. Де воно тепер, а головне — де сам Бобровський, лишається загадкою.

— А як до цього причетний наш любий Альберт? — жінка перевела погляд на ювеліра.

— Справа в тому, що князя Бобровського я знаю доволі давно. Йому належала копальня в Уральських горах, де

---

* Есери — партія соціалістів-революціонерів, заснована 1901 року.

я купував золото, — пояснив Вайсманн. — Природно, що, опинившись у Пруссії, він зв'язався зі мною.

— Чому?

— Просив допомогти йому оцінити коштовності й порадити надійний банк. Не підозрюючи, звісна річ, що я пов'язаний А III b.

— Тобто ви бачили цей скарб, Вайсманне? — здивовано вигукнула жінка.

Той кивнув.

— Не просто бачив, пані Шраґмюллер, а й склав детальний список усіх коштовностей, які на той час мав граф. Від мене він приховав тільки золоті злитки. Їх він міг оцінити й без допомоги ювеліра, — пояснив Вайсманн, — на щастя, копія цього списку залишилася в мене.

— А ви завбачливий чоловік, — похвалила його Клавдія.

— Я знав, що історія тільки розпочинається, тому одразу зв'язався з майором Фішером. Проте прусська таємна служба не встигла... — він з докором зиркнув на офіцера.

— І цей перстень... — промовила жінка, і в очах у неї зблиснули хижі вогники.

— І цей перстень я вже бачив, пані Шраґмюллер, — доповнив ювелір, — тримав у руках, оцінював, а потім заніс у список під номером 178... Саме тому, коли він вдруге потрапив мені на очі, я майже одразу його впізнав.

— Гаразд, — озвався Фішер, — якщо ви впевнені в тому, що цей перстень і справді зі скарбу Бобровського, то чи маєте якісь здогади, звідки він у того молодика, що приніс його вам?

— Я не запитую такого в клієнтів, пане майоре, — відповів ювелір, — ці питання відлякують, і тоді все йде псові під хвіст. Клієнт вирішує, що я працюю на поліцію, й забирається геть.

— Чорт забирай, Вайсманне! Саме в цьому випадку слід було зробити виняток. Або ж придумати щось, хай вам трясця! — викрикнув Фішер.

— А я і придумав, — сварливо відповів ювелір. — І, якщо дасте мені можливість договорити, то дізнаєтеся що саме.

Офіцер замовк і підпалив наступну сигарету.

— Це коштувало мені чималих грошей, — продовжив Вайсманн після паузи, — і я навіть не сподіваюся, що ви компенсуєте мені бодай частину... Від мене той молодик отримав боргове зобов'язання на десять тисяч марок. Він прийде за своїми грішми через два тижні.

— Ви взяли занадто багато часу, — вже спокійніше зазначив майор.

— Саме стільки потрібно, щоб провести банківську операцію. Якби я назвав коротший термін, він би щось запідозрив. Бо вигляд мав чоловіка недурного, — пояснив Вайсманн.

— Слід було сказати, що гроші у вас в іншому сейфі... — не вгавав Фішер.

— Годі вам, — перебила його Клавдія. — Пане майоре, ви занадто прискіпливі. Як на мене, наш друг чудово зорієнтувався в ситуації. І наш відділ мусить бути йому вдячним.

Вона підвелася, взяла зі столу пляшку і вправно долила бренді чоловікам і собі.

— Гаразд. Визнаю, ви маєте рацію, пані Шраґмюллер, — примирливо сказав Фішер. — У цій справі нарешті виявлено хоч якийсь слід, і це заслуга Вайсманна...

Він підвівся і підійшов до вікна, затуливши своєю громіздкою постаттю майже весь вид на похмурий сад. Замість нього над столом зависла хмара цигаркового диму, ніби четвертим співрозмовником був який-небудь дух із потойбіччя.

— А що можете сказати про того молодого суб'єкта? — не озираючись, запитав майор. — Звідки він? Чим займається? Де мешкає?

Вайсманн стенув плечима.

— Інтелігентний, стриманий... Можливо, інженер або вчитель. Думаю, мешкає тут, у Бадені.

— Або курортник, — припустила Клавдія. — Лікує шлунок, наприклад.

— Хтозна, хтозна... Стривайте, — раптом осінило ювеліра. — Від нього справді чувся запах медикаментів.

— Ну от, — вдоволено мовила жінка.

— А може, він просто доглядає хворого родича? — припустив Фішер.

— Або ж лікар за фахом, — додав Вайсманн.

— Словом... — Фішер повернувся до присутніх. — Нашим філерам є над чим працювати. І вже точно доведеться побігати.

Здавалося, майор вирішив таким чином завершити розмову, проте Вайсманн не поспішав іти геть.

— Мусимо обговорити ще одне питання, пане Фішере.

— До ваших послуг.

— Питання... грошей, — тут він покосився на Клавдію, — мені, зізнаюся, не надто зручно при дамі.

— Насамперед пані Шраґмюллер — наша з вами колега і моя права рука, — відповів майор, — тож забудьте про те, що вона жінка.

«Забудеш тут», — майнуло у Вайсманна в голові. Її вродою він обпікався, як гарячим залізом. І хоч був уже чоловіком в літах, з подивом помічав, як не в силах стримати сороміцькі фантазії, від яких червонів так, ніби розповідав їх уголос. Втім, справу слід було доводити до кінця, тому він продовжив:

— Я витратив п'ять тисяч марок готівкою на купівлю цього персня. І ще десять тисяч мушу викласти за два тижні. Все це зроблено в інтересах A III b.

— Хочете сказати, що загалом ваші видатки складають п'ятнадцять тисяч марок? — уточнив Фішер.

— Саме так.

— І це справжня вартість тієї коштовності? — майор вказав на перстень, який весь цей час ювелір не випускав з рук.

— Відверто кажучи, ні, — зізнався той. — Така річ коштує дорожче.

— Наскільки дорожче?

— Десь у півтора рази.

— От і чудово, тоді просто залишите її собі. Звісно, не зараз. А згодом, коли вона вже нам не знадобиться, — підсумував офіцер.

— Але ж це речовий доказ, — засумнівався ювелір.

— Ми не поліція, пане Вайсманне, — сказав Фішер, — тому просто заберете персня собі.

— Вам легко казати, — поскаржився ювелір. — Будь-що зі скарбу Бобровського притягує неприємності.

— Які ще неприємності? — майор потроху втрачав терпіння.

— Гадаєте, я зможу легко його продати? Так само легко, як продали мені? Шанси наштовхнутися на якого-небудь головоріза з російської «охранки» в мене будуть чималі.

— Послухайте, пане Вайсманне, — видихнув Фішер, — ви не штатний працівник Третього відділу, й гарантувати винагороду від Генштабу я вам не можу. Звісно, ми платимо своїм інформаторам, але ці гонорари значно менші, ніж сума, про яку йдеться. Я пропоную дещо інше... — чоловік підніс до рота склянку й вихилив звідти залишки бренді.

— Дещо інше? — нетерпляче перепитав ювелір.

— Коли ми відшукаємо золото, то, гадаю, зникнення невеликої частини злитків ніхто не зауважить. Саме злитків, а не прикрас, які можна впізнати. Там же є злитки, пане Вайсманне?

Чоловік кивнув.

— От і чудово, — промовив Фішер, — тож тільки після того, як ви візьмете зі скарбу свою винагороду, ми передамо його прусському Генштабу. Не раніше... Сподіваюся, тепер ми домовились?

Вайсманн, звісна річ, мав сумніви щодо цієї угоди, проте згодився. Ювелір потиснув на прощання руку Фішеру і вклонився Клавдії. «Нехай буде так, — думав він, прямуючи до свого автомобіля. — Наразі так... А далі — побачимо».

У той самий час Фелікс Краут блукав вулицями Бадена, почуваючись щасливим, але добряче розгубленим. Щасливим, бо мав у кишені п'ять тисяч марок, і марно намагався пригадати, чи колись у житті бачив таку суму. Думка про те, що за два тижні він отримає вдвічі більше, зводила його з розуму, змушуючи прискорювати крок і хаотично будувати в голові найсміливіші плани на майбутнє. На їхнє спільне з Ґретою майбутнє. А розгубленим — бо ця удача виявилася несподіваною, як Господнє диво.

До того ж він ще не виконав доручення, хоч це й здавалося дрібницею... Та, попри всі сумніви, одне Краут знав напевно — цих грошей він вже нікому не віддасть! Це, можливо, його єдиний шанс попрощатися із сірим існуванням. Стати кимось іншим, ніж звичайним асистентом психіатра в клініці для душевнохворих.

Десь за пів години блукань Фелікса врешті осінило, що вештатись містом з такими грішми небезпечно. Хоч і в білий день. Краще піти додому й заховати їх у надійному місці, лишивши в портмоне якусь там сотню-дві.

Опинившись знову в помешканні, чоловік довго вибирав схованок. Можна заховати поміж книжок, зашити в підкладку старого кожуха, зробити в шухляді подвійне дно... А хоча... Чому б їх не покласти просто в банк?

Розмірковуючи, Фелікс непомітно для себе вмостився на ліжку, підібгавши ноги, й заснув, обійнявши пачку купюр, наче своє немовля.

Прокинувся він, коли в кімнаті вже сіріло. «Котра година?» — це питання гучним дзвоном вдарило в його голові, й він злякано схопився на ноги. Пачка з грішми впала на підлогу, й чоловік рвучко їх підняв. У голові запаморочилося від надто різкого руху.

Фелікс сів на край ліжка, дочекався, коли минуть паморoки, й витягнув з кишені годинника. Була шоста. У клубі треба бути о сьомій. До того ж слід вийти з дому раніше, ніж повернеться Ґрета. Тоді він не муситиме пояснювати, куди йде, точніше, не брехатиме їй.

Де сховати гроші, він так і не придумав, тому запхнув їх знову в кишеню. Поки що це видавалося найнадійнішим місцем. Після цього Фелікс вмився холодною водою і сяк-так причесав волосся. Глянув на себе в дзеркало й скривився: вигляд мав стомлений, одяг зім'ятий, як у волоцюги. Проте гаяти часу більше не міг. Чоловік вийшов з дому й рішуче попрямував туди, де, як він пам'ятав, був клуб «Пігмаліон».

Ні він сам, ні жоден із його знайомих не могли похвалитися, що колись потрапляли всередину цього клубу. Загальновідомим був факт, що туди щовечора з'їжджається виключно богема: мільйонери, найблагородніші дворяни та політики найвищих рангів, кожен з яких за вечір протринькує цілі статки.

Як потрапити всередину, він також не думав аж до моменту, коли кремезний охоронець, одягнений у вечірній фрак, перегородив йому дорогу.

— Чи є у вас запрошення, шановний пане? — з награною люб'язністю запитав він у Фелікса.

— Я не збираюсь тут засиджуватися, тільки мушу виконати доручення, — відповів той.

— Яке доручення?

— Передати дещо певній особі, — твердо сказав Краут. — Даруйте, це вас не стосується.

— Мені шкода, але я не можу вас пропустити.

— Чому?

— Бо такі правила, — буркнув наостанок здоровань і відвернувся.

— Послухайте... — розгублено промовив Фелікс, але той не мав наміру його слухати.

— Гей, ви! — гукнув він різкіше.

Охоронець повернувся.

— Я вже пояснив вам, що не можу пропустити, — говорив він тепер сердито, і Фелікс зрозумів, що запас люб'язності в нього вичерпався.

— Тоді повідомте графа Орлова, що в мене для нього лист, — упівголоса сказав Краут.

Назване прізвище, схоже, справило враження на цього Голіафа. Він кивнув і попросив когось постояти замість нього. Фелікс полегшено відійшов убік. Запалив цигарку, але не встиг докурити до кінця, коли повернувся охоронець і заперечливо хитнув головою.

— Його світлість граф Орлов повідомив, що нікого не чекає, — сказав Голіаф.

— Ну звісно не чекає, але я мушу...

— Усього найкращого, шановний пане. Гарного вечора, — безцеремонно перебив охоронець.

Несподівано Фелікс відчув, як чиясь тендітна рука взяла його за лікоть. Він повернув голову й з подивом побачив перед собою молоду жінку в елегантному пальто й стильному французькому капелюшкові, прикрашеному темно-фіолетовими стрічками.

— Що сталося, Філіппе? — незнайомка, як не дивно, звернулася не до нього, а до Голіафа. — Чому ви не хочете пропустити цього гарного кавалера?

— Пані Шене... Мадам, — трохи розгублено промовив охоронець, — це для вас він гарний кавалер, а для мене — особа, що не має запрошення.

— Не турбуйтеся, мій друже, я маю два.

— Але пані...

— Ви мені не вірите? — жінка насупила брови.

— Ну що ви, мадам...

— Тоді не стійте на дорозі.

З цими словами вона впевнено рушила вперед, потягнувши Фелікса за собою. Одночасно вільною рукою послала спантеличеному Голіафові повітряний поцілунок.

Та щойно вони опинилися за масивними дверима, де починався яскраво освітлений коридор, як уся приязність цієї жінки несподівано зникла. Вона більше не тримала Фелікса за лікоть, а обличчя прибрало якогось знуджено-байдужого виразу. Тепер Фелікс не знав, що спантеличило його більше: її несподівана допомога чи ця разюча зміна.

Пані Шене квапливо рушила вперед, знаком наказавши йому йти слідом. Коридор впирався у сходи, застелені темно-зеленим килимом. Вона розстебнула пальто і, підібравши краї своєї вечірньої сукні, спритно збігла сходами вгору. Фелікс не встигав, і жінка мусила зупинитись на останній сходинці, аби його почекати.

— Дозвольте запитати куди... куди ми... йдемо? — важко дихаючи, запитав Краут, не витримавши цієї таємничої мовчанки.

— А куди ви збиралися, добродію? — насмішкувато запитала мадам Шене, дивлячись на нього згори, як антична богиня на смертного, що з останніх сил дерся на її Олімп. — Хіба ви не хотіли зустрітися з графом?

— Хотів...

— От до нього ми і йдемо. Покваптеся, мсьє Орлов не любить чекати.

Вона відвернулася від нього й рушила далі, зупинившись лише біля гардеробу, де зваблива білявка, одягнена в грецьку туніку, взяла в них верхній одяг. Коли ця німфа наблизилася, Феліксу вдруге забило дихання. Туніка її здавалася невагомою, груди жінка мала високі й гоструваті, а до Краута підійшла так близько, що майже ними до нього доторкнулася. Вловивши на собі черговий іронічний погляд мадам Шене, Фелікс відчув, як обличчя його спалахнуло вогнем, а по спині покотилися тонкі струмені бридкого поту. Гість послабив краватку й спробував усміхнутися — слід було себе опанувати. Він, зрештою, не який-небудь гімназист, а чоловік, що не вперше бачить напівоголену жінку.

До великої клубної зали Фелікс зайшов уже впевненіше. Мадам Шене провела його поміж столиками, потім уздовж сцени, на якій розігрувався піаніст і метушилася решта музикантів. Зрештою, вони підійшли до дверей ложі і, перш ніж постукати, жінка поспіхом поправила зачіску та бретельки сукні.

Коли чоловічий голос зсередини дозволив увійти, вона прочинила двері й зайшла першою. Орлов сидів у кріслі, боком до них, поставивши ноги на камінні ґрати. У каміні палахкотів слабкий вогник — очевидно, запалили недавно. Чоловік тримав у руках сигару й дивився кудись перед собою, де висів турецький килим, а під ним стояла канапа, обшита пурпуровим полотном. Поруч був столик з напоями: невідкоркована пляшка чорногорської ракії, метакса, місцеве баденське вино й графин з водою. Біля них склянки й гільйотинка для сигар.

Орлов перевів погляд на прибулих. Одразу ж усміхнувся мадам Шене.

— Дякую, моя люба, — промовив він, — сподіваюся, у цього пана і справді важлива справа до мене. Варта, скажімо так, ваших зусиль і мого часу.

Жінка усміхнулася у відповідь і вмостилася на канапі, закинувши ногу на ногу. У присутності Орлова вона почувалася вільно, певно, маючи для цього підстави.

— Я повідомив охоронця, коли прийшов, — озвався раптом Краут, якого зачепила ця зверхність. — Той відповів, що ви нікого не чекаєте, й не пропустив мене... Я зовсім не потребував допомоги мадам Шене. Якби ви дозволили мені зайти...

— Я не зустрічаюся аби з ким, — ліниво перебив Орлов. — Ми не знайомі з вами, юначе. Я гадки не маю, хто ви й що вам від мене потрібно. Можу назвати десяток цілком достойних людей, достойніших за вас, що місяцями чекають на авдієнцію у мене. Вони були б украй здивовані, що я прийняв вас із простої цікавості... Тож перейдімо до справи! Маєте дві хвилини.

Він і справді дістав з кишені золотого годинника, мовби підкреслюючи цим серйозність сказаного.

— Дві хвилини — надто багато, пане Орлов, — відповів гість, — я всього лише хочу передати вам листа. Від Яші... Це займе значно менше часу.

Фелікс витягнув з кишені конверта й простягнув його росіянину. Граф перемінився на очах. Відклав сигару й звівся на рівні ноги. Зросту він виявився чималого, втім, схоже, мав звичку горбитись. З обличчя чоловіка в одну мить зникла пиха, погляд більше не був знудьгованим і зверхнім. Орлов уважно глянув на співрозмовника, а потім на конверт. Причому дивився так прискіпливо, ніби хотів прочитати листа не розпечатуючи.

— Від Яші? — перепитав він, беручи послання до рук.

Прибулий кивнув.

— Люба пані Шене, — звернувся граф до жінки, стримуючи усміх, — чи могли б ви ненадовго нас залишити?

У відповідь жінка спочатку надула губки, проте за мить підвелася з канапи й вийшла за двері. Тільки тоді Орлов розірвав конверта й витягнув з нього невелику записку. Швидко прочитав, після цього знову опустився в крісло, тримаючи папір двома пальцями правої руки, точнісінько як перед тим тримав сигару.

— Як вас звати? — запитав він у гостя.

— Фелікс Краут.

— Сядьте, пане Крауте. Будь ласка.

Гість підійшов до канапи, де щойно сиділа мадам Шене, й сів на її місце. Йому прагнулося чимшвидше піти, проте несподівано Фелікс відчув, що сукно зберегло трохи тепла цієї жінки, а в повітрі довкола ще відчувався запах її парфумів. Це схвилювало його так сильно, наче вона ще була тут і якимось дивом опинилася в його обіймах. Краут навіть не одразу почув, що граф знову до нього озвався.

— ...відомо, що тут? — вловив він тільки уривок запитання.

— Даруйте? — червоніючи від вуха до вуха, перепитав Фелікс.

— Я запитав, чи знаєте ви, про що йдеться в цій записці, — повторив граф.

— Яша... Мій пацієнт пояснив, що просить вас про зустріч, — відповів гість.

— Отже, ви його лікар? — уточнив росіянин.

— Не зовсім. Я допомагаю доктору Ріцке. Чесно кажучи, ми вперше побачилися з Яшею сьогодні вночі.

— Он як...

Орлов згорнув записку й поклав її в кишеню фрака. Після цього знову взяв до рук сигару й задумливо підніс її до рота. Затягнувся, докладаючи трохи більше зусиль, ніж це зазвичай роблять курці. Видно, сигарний попіл встиг пригаснути.

— А чи знаєте ви, хто такий цей Яків?.. Тобто Яша? Маю на увазі пацієнта вашої клініки.

Фелікс заперечливо хитнув головою.

— Мені зовсім нічого не відомо про нього.

Орлов ще на хвилину задумався, присмоктавшись до своєї сигари, мовби звідти разом із димом витягував думки.

— У листі Яша повідомляє, що віддячив вам насамперед за вашу мовчанку, пане Крауте, — продовжив граф. — А також за те, що влаштуєте нам зустріч.

З першим Фелікс погодився, а от друге було брехнею. Яша ані словом не обмовився про те, що саме йому доведеться влаштовувати візит Орлова до клініки. Втім, пригадавши, яка сума лежала в його кишені, Краут вирішив не заперечувати. Чорт із ним! Зрештою, відвідини пацієнта — звична річ. І нічого протизаконного Фелікс не зробить. Хіба що знову приховає все від доктора Ріцке...

— То як? — продовжив Орлов. — Я можу на вас покластися?

— Можете, — підводячись, відповів Краут. — Післязавтра в мене знову нічне чергування. Буду до ваших послуг.

— Пропонуєте зустрітися з Яковом уночі? — здивувався граф.

— Ні, звичайно. Це викличе зайві підозри у випадкових свідків, — промовив Фелікс, — найкраще, якщо прийдете вранці. Скажімо, о сьомій. У цьому не буде нічого незвичного, деяких пацієнтів провідують о цій годині родичі.

— А як же доктор?

— До приходу пана Ріцке залишиться ще ціла година.

На обличчі Орлова прочиталося схвалення.

— Рівно о сьомій ранку я чекатиму на вас біля запасних воріт, крізь які можна потрапити одразу до нашого парку, — продовжив Краут, — у цей час санітари виведуть Яшу на прогулянку і залишать його під моєю опікою. Я відійду і дам вам можливість поговорити сам на сам.

— Прекрасно, — похвалив граф, — як на мене, задум чудовий.

Він підійшов до столика з випивкою.

— Хочете чогось? — люб'язно запропонував Орлов, вказавши на пляшки з алкоголем.

Фелікс випив би залюбки, але бажання завершити цю розмову й піти геть було сильнішим. Асистент відмовився, проте з жадібністю дивився, як співрозмовник відкорковує метаксу. Ніби не розчувши його відповіді, Орлов наповнив дві склянки.

— Ви нам дуже допомагаєте, пане Крауте, — сказав росіянин, подаючи йому келих. — Проте, мусите затямити одну річ... — Він зробив ковток. — Ані пари з вуст. Зрозуміло?

— Зрозуміло, — відповів Фелікс і вихилив свою порцію бренді одним ковтком.

— Тоді до зустрічі, — промовив Орлов і поплескав його по плечу. Зовсім як старого приятеля.

Поставивши порожню склянку на столик, Фелікс рушив до дверей.

— Якщо бажаєте, залишіться сьогодні в клубі, — сказав йому вслід Орлов, — у нас цього вечора чудова програма. Вам сподобається.

«Пішов ти під три чорти», — подумав Фелікс, але вдячно кивнув графу й поспіхом вийшов з ложі.

Так само поспіхом він збирався пройти через залу, проте несподівано спинився й витріщився на сцену. Там був той самий піаніст і ті самі музиканти, яких він помітив, ідучи до Орлова. Тільки цього разу поряд з ними стояла мадам Шене. Сцена була яскраво освітлена, і її дрібна постать, здавалося, от-от розтане у променях софітів, як грудка цукру в чашці з кавою.

Першим вступив піаніст, потім кларнетист. До них додалися звуки контрабаса і неспішний ритм барабанів. Грали «*Sweet sixteen*» з репертуару Гаррі Макдоно*.

Врешті залунав голос пані Шене:

When first I saw the love-light in your eyes,
I dreamed the world held not but joy for me.
And even though we drifted far apart,
*I never dream but what I dream of thee...***

Голос жінка мала приємний: грудний, але не надто низький. Такий серед вокалістів називається мецо-сопрано. Здивований і вражений до краю, чоловік сів за вільний столик, аби дослухати пісню до кінця. Зала заповнилася приблизно на третину, але публіка все прибувала. Очевидно, виступ пані Шене був своєрідним привітанням. Коли закінчилася пісня, він перший зааплодував. Причому так енергійно, що на нього позиралися слухачі з сусідніх місць. Краут вирішив бути стриманішим.

---

* Гаррі Макдоно (справжнє ім'я — Джон Скантлбері Макдональд; 1871–1931 — популярний канадський співак та менеджер звукозапису 1900-х та ранніх 1920-х.

** Коли любові світло вперше я побачив у твоїх очах,
То світ навколо віщував, здавалося, тільки радість.
Між нами відстань, ми в розлуці, але я
Про тебе мрію. Я у твоїй владі. — (*з англ.*)

Непомітно до його столика наблизився усміхнений кельнер.

— Чи бажаєте щось випити? — запитав він.

У питанні не було нічого незвичного, проте Фелікс глянув на нього зі здивуванням в очах, ніби той говорив латиною.

— У нас є чудовий «Ельблінґ»*, — вирішив допомогти йому офіціант, — може бути для початку.

— Так... будь ласка, — розгублено відповів той.

Кельнер, втім, не відходив, мовби розмова мусила продовжитись.

— Склянка «Ельблінґу» цілком пасує, — повторив Краут уже впевненіше.

— Звісно, — ще ширше всміхаючись, проказав офіціант, — однак мушу попередити шановного пана, що цей столик зарезервовано, починаючи з дев'ятої години. Тобто дослухати прекрасну мадам Шене ви зможете, а от коли розпочнуть танцювати наші німфи... — чоловік зробив виразну паузу, мовби даючи можливість гостеві краще уявити спокусливих танцівниць, — коли вони танцюватимуть, вам, на жаль, доведеться пересісти.

«Підходящий привід все це закінчити», — подумалося Феліксу, й він звівся на ноги. Слід було опанувати себе і піти врешті додому. Тим більше, що завдання виконано.

— Що ж, не щастить мені, — з награним жалем у голосі промовив Фелікс.

— О, запевняю вас, я знайду вільне місце... — розпачливо сказав кельнер.

---

* «Ельблінґ» — сорт білого вина з однойменного винограду, який здавна вирощують в долині річки Мозель.

— Ні-ні, не переймайтеся, — заспокоїв його гість. — Буде мені наукою. Наступного разу бронюватиму собі столика завчасно.

— А ваше замовлення?..

— Що ж, вип'ю «Ельблінґу» іншим разом. На все добре.

Чоловік стрімко рушив до виходу. Він встиг почути, як співачка своїм розкішним голосом почала «*Sweet Adeline*»*. Понад усе хотілося повернутися за столик і слухати. Замовити чогось міцного (до біса «Ельблінґ», такому голосу пасував би добрий бренді або ще краще — димне віскі), запалити цигарку і пити, потроху п'яніючи, а точніше втопаючи у цій чуттєвій розкоші. Втім, Краут розумів, що мадам Шене зараз для нього — мов сирена для моряка**. Якщо повернеться, то розіб'ється об скелі.

У коридорі та сама німфа здивовано віддала йому капелюха й плаща. Зазвичай так рано з клубу ніхто не йшов, адже вечір з усіма його принадами тільки починався. Хоч, мабуть, у цього молодика він сьогодні не вдався. Вона співчутливо усміхнулася йому наостанок і грайливо помахала рукою вслід. Такою була її робота. Мусила злегка розпалювати клієнтів, щойно ті приходили до гардеробу і на прощання, коли залишали клуб. Тоді додому вони потрапляли з відчуттям невтамованого голоду, а це чи не найліпша мотивація повернутися сюди знову.

Вранці домовленого дня, за чверть до сьомої, Краут сам розбудив чергових санітарів і наказав їм вести

---

* *«Sweet Adeline»* — популярна пісня на слова Річарда Джерарда, що в 1900-х рр. входила до репертуару багатьох виконавців.

** Сирени — в античній міфології — напівжінки-напівптахи, що своїм співом зачаровували моряків, змушуючи їх скеровувати кораблі на небезпечні скелі.

пацієнта з двадцять восьмої палати на прогулянку. Ті не ставили зайвих питань. Треба — значить треба. Лікарям видніше, як поводитися з цими вар'ятами...

Яша чекав, стоячи посеред кімнати одягнений і поголений. Тримався рівно, урочисто й дещо гордовито, мовби за хвилину мав виступити в Райхстазі. Ще опівночі, під час огляду, Фелікс потайки від санітарів попередив його, де й коли відбудеться зустріч з Орловим.

— Ви мій рятівник, — усміхнувся тоді Яша.

Асистент не відповів. Він думав про те, що вперше обдурює доктора Ріцке. І понад усе йому хотілося, аби це трапилося востаннє. Навіть якщо Яша знову запропонує йому таку саму щедру винагороду.

Як і було домовлено з Орловим, за чверть години, рівно о сьомій, санітари залишили пацієнта в парку під наглядом асистента Краута. Зрадівши можливості ще трохи подрімати, вони поспіхом подалися назад у приміщення, до своєї комірчини, знову без зайвих запитань. Нічні зміни робили їх байдужими. І навіть якби Яшу чорти вхопили одразу за їхніми спинами, або ж він почав корчитись у жахливих конвульсіях, ніщо, здавалося, не змусило б їх повернутися до парку.

Дочекавшись, доки за ними зачиняться двері клініки, Фелікс удавано безтурботною ходою підійшов до металевої хвіртки в паркані і, діставши з кишені чималого ключа, не без зусиль відчинив її. Орлов стояв за десяток метрів від огорожі, звівши очі догори й розглядаючи гілля столітнього дуба, по яких стрибала темно-руда білка. Схоже, він, як і Краут, намагався вдавати байдужість. Якого-небудь курортника, змученого відпочинком роззяву, що прогулювався неподалік після вранішніх вод. У його руках навіть виявилися два грецькі горіхи, і він постукував ними один об одного, щоб зацікавлена білка наблизилась і їх забрала. Так робили всі, кому були призначені гуляння міськими парками, причому з таким азартом, мовби годування білок — найцікавіше заняття в цілому Бадені, а то й в усій Німецькій імперії.

Втім, як виявилося, граф і справді був у доброму гуморі. Привітно усміхнувся Феліксові й поцікавився, як минув його вечір у «Пігмаліоні».

— Цілком добре, — відповів Краут, бо, зрештою, нічого поганого і справді не сталося. — У вас чудова співачка.

Йому хотілося, щоб це прозвучало як недбала репліка, сказана без жодних емоцій, проте граф, схоже, помітив його внутрішнє хвилювання.

— О, так, — відповів Орлов, усміхаючись ще ширше, — наша солоденька мадам Шене уміє завести публіку.

У голосі його зазвучали якісь огидні хтиві нотки, від яких Фелікса охопила злість. Приховати її було б ще важче, втім, Орлов, на щастя, не цікавлячись його реакцією на сказане, першим зайшов у хвіртку, трохи пригнувши голову в чорному мелоніку*, щоб не зачепити ним верхню частину прямокутного отвору в огорожі.

«Добре, що все це закінчується», — подумав Краут, ідучи слідом.

Він знову замкнув вихід і став здаля спостерігати, як росіяни радісно подалися один одному назустріч. Їхню розмову він чути не міг. Але навіть якби й чув, то не зрозумів би ані слова — ці двоє заговорили російською.

---

* Мелонік — вид капелюха, модного на початку XX ст.

— Яке щастя бачити вас при доброму здоров'ї, Якове Олександровичу, — сказав Орлов, беручи співрозмовника за плечі й тричі по-православному розціловуючи.

— Думаю, ви хотіли сказати «при здоровому глузді», — виправив його Яша, — зважаючи на місце, в якому я перебуваю вже стільки часу.

У голосі його почулися нотки якоїсь майже дитячої образи.

— На бога, Якове Олександровичу, — трохи спохмурнів Орлов, — ви ж самі знаєте, що ця лікарня — найбезпечніше для вас місце. І я задіяв чимало зв'язків, щоб вас помістити сюди інкоґніто...

— Знаю, знаю, князю, — перебив той. — Знаю й буду вдячний вам за це до кінця свого життя, скільки мені там ще залишилося.

— Ну, батєнька. Що за песимізм?

Він лагідно підвів Якова до лавки й жестом запропонував сісти. Коли вони вмостились, Орлов озирнувся довкола. Подвір'я клініки в цей час було безлюдним, не враховуючи, звісно, худорлявої постаті асистента Краута, що стежив за ними з відстані кількох десятків кроків.

— Для радощів у мене занадто мало підстав, Інокентію Михайловичу, — відповів Яків. — І в клініці, і в усій цій клятій Пруссії я можу довіряти тільки собі й вам.

— Я говорив, що доктор Ріцке — також цілком надійна людина.

— Я не певен.

— Запевняю вас...

— До біса ваші запевнення! — Яків несподівано перейшов на крик і схопився з місця, мовби побачив перед собою змію. — Готовий битися об заклад, він при першій нагоді здасть мене російським або німецьким шпигам! Залежить від того, хто більше заплатить!..

Орлов побачив, що Краут уже готовий кинутися до них, аби заспокоїти пацієнта, тому широко посміхнувся й знаком показав, що все під контролем.

— Сядьте, Якове, — з притиском сказав він співвітчизнику. — Сядьте і заспокойтесь.

Той ще якусь мить постояв, а тоді підкорився. Сівши, він вперся ліктями в коліна й закрив обличчя руками.

— Прошу мене вибачити, — голос з-під його долонь звучав приглушено й ледь розбірливо. — Живучи серед психів, сам врешті-решт перетворюєшся на психа...

— Все гаразд, мій друже, — Орлов поклав йому руку на плече, — недовго ще залишилося.

— Я, власне, тому й попросив вас про зустріч, Інокентію Михайловичу, — Яків опустив руки й повернув до співрозмовника розчервоніле обличчя. — Хотів сказати, що боюся.

— Ну, батєнька...

— Боюся, що ви про мене забудете, — продовжив пацієнт, — або до мене врешті-решт дістануться.

— Ніхто не знає, що ви тут, Якове Олександровичу, — твердо запевнив граф.

— Ви недооцінюєте імператорську розвідку, — гірко зітхнув Яків, — і так само прусський Третій відділ... Господи милосердний, та навіть есери, яких я всіляко підтримував рік тому у Петербурзі, воліли б бачити мене радше мертвим, ніж живим, щоб отримати мої гроші...

На цих словах пацієнт затнувся, схоже, не бажаючи вдаватися в деталі. Орлов витримав паузу. Якби Яків у цей момент уважно придивився до його обличчя, то зрозумів би, що ці слова зачепили графа.

— Наші дорогі товариші революціонери, Якове Олександровичу, і мене з великою охотою відправили б на той світ. Слідом за моїм братом... Ця їхня революція пролетаріату — ненажерливе чудовисько, яке заснуло колись у Франції, але прокинулося в Росії. І тепер щодня й щогодини хоче жерти. Уся ця наволоч: анархісти, есери, комуністи, всі ті, що оголосили себе вільними людьми, — насправді раби цього чудовиська. Щоб годувати його, вони й застосовують цю свою експропріацію* й терор, нічим при цьому не відрізняючись від звичайних грабіжників і вбивць. Інакше воно почне жерти їх самих... Через цих нелюдів кожного разу, повертаючись до Росії як титулована й багата особа, я ризикую своїм життям.

— Однак, цар погодився на реформи, — зазначив Яків, — якщо вони будуть доведені до кінця, все зміниться.

— Не будуть, — заперечив Орлов. — Для реформ потрібен надійний ґрунт, а Росія — це суцільне в'язке болото. На ньому прорости може тільки невігластво і насилля. От побачите, Думу, цей наш парламент**, створений на взірець французького, невдовзі розженуть. Усе тому, що народ сам хоче, аби ним правили, як скотиною.

---

* Експропріація — насильницький спосіб присвоєння майна, до якого вдавалися, зокрема, більшовики, грабуючи багатих «класових ворогів», щоб фінансувати свою революційну діяльність.

** Дума — законодавчий орган Російської імперії, створений 1905 року. Одна з поступок, на які пішов Микола II після січневих заворушень у Петербурзі.

— Бог з нею, з Росією, народом, Думою... — гірко зітхнув Яків, — я достатньо заплатив за свої вподобання.

— Радий це чути, — похвалив граф.

— Інокентію Михайловичу, Христа ради! Заберіть мене звідси, — гаряче сказав пацієнт, — у мене кепські передчуття. Нутром чую, якщо залишуся, то кінець мені. Або сьогодні, або завтра. Доберуться до мене!

— Тихо, тихо, сердешний ви мій, — лагідно проказав граф, — заберу, я ж не назавжди вас тут заховав. Щойно знатиму, що назовні безпечно...

— Заберіть мене звідси негайно!

— Ви чудово знаєте, що просто зараз це неможливо.

Пацієнт відвернувся й трохи помовчав.

— А якщо я скажу вам... — продовжив він сухим, приглушеним голосом. — Якщо скажу, де моє золото... Адже вам це також цікаво. Правда ж, ваше благородіє?

— Безумовно, — відповів Орлов, удруге озираючись на асистента Краута. Здавалося, він хотів переконатися, що той не підійшов до них ближче.

— Тоді завтра, щойно опинюся у вашому автомобілі, — твердо проговорив Яків, — до того ж не пізніше ранку. У цей самий час, перед восьмою, до приходу доктора Ріцке.

— Гаразд, я буду.

Почувши остаточну відповідь, Яша звівся на ноги й подав знак асистенту Крауту, що розмову завершено. Потім, не прощаючись з графом, швидкою ходою рушив до клініки, де назустріч йому вийшли двоє санітарів.

Орлов не збрехав. Наступного дня, о сьомій, його «*Panhard*»* зупинився в тому самому парку, де напередо-

---

* «*Panhard*» — марка французького авто, яке випускали з 1891 року.

дні він пригощав горіхами білок. Вийшовши з авто, він цього разу подався не до хвіртки, а до головного входу. Усе було залагоджено: санітари мусили передати йому пацієнта щонайпізніше за чверть години. Тобто о сьомій п'ятнадцять Яків, тримаючи в руках валізу, мав би чекати його біля лікарняного турнікета.

Так само, як і вчора, граф — для годиться — спочатку прогулявся алеєю, потім порозглядав псевдоантичні скульптури, що зображали Діану в оточенні вірних мисливських псів і Аполлона з арфою, якого обступили закохані в нього музи. Скульптури потроху зеленіли від часу, обростаючи мохом, і, без сумніву, потребували втручання реставраторів.

Врешті граф відгорнув полу плаща і дістався до позолоченого годинника на делікатному, проте надійному ланцюжку. Орлов перевірив час. Лишалося ще п'ять хвилин, отже, слід було йти до лікарні. Сховавши годинника назад до кишені й застебнувши плаща, чоловік жваво закрокував алеєю, ритмічно вдаряючи по бруківці тонкою лакованою тростиною.

Втім, опинившись за якийсь десяток метрів від клініки, граф зупинився й завмер від подиву. Замість Якова біля турнікета він побачив поліційного фельдфебеля. Схоже, тому було наказано охороняти вхід. Першою думкою Орлова було чимскоріше повернутися до свого автомобіля й вирушити звідси геть, але цікавість взяла гору. Закуривши цигарку, він повільною ходою підійшов до вартового, вдаючи з себе знудьгованого роззяву. Той зміряв його обережним поглядом.

— Доброго ранку, — привітався граф.

Постовий кивнув у відповідь.

— Нудна робота, еге ж? — продовжив Орлов.

— Чия? — не зрозумів той.

— Ваша, звісно. Стояти тут і охороняти психів... — кажучи це, граф дістав з кишені портсигара і, відкривши його, простягнув поліціянтові. — Закурите?

— Чом би й ні, — стенув плечима той і потягнувся за цигаркою. — О, єгипетські...

— Аякже. Турецькі деруть горло, — мовив граф, підносячи йому запалений сірник.

— А я смалю тільки наші, прусські, — відповів поліціянт, випускаючи перший струмінь диму. — О, справді добра річ, — похвалив він цигарку, розглядаючи її з усіх боків, наче та відрізнялася чимось від інших.

— Візьміть собі ще, — запропонував Орлов, знову розкриваючи портсигар.

— Ні, що ви, — почав відмовлятися постовий.

— Беріть, беріть, — наполіг граф, — ви ж тут, зазвичай, стоїте цілий день? Так?

— Ні, що ви, — засміявся поліціянт, ховаючи ще одну сигарету в кишеню шинелі. — Зазвичай поліція цих вар'ятів не охороняє. Це тільки сьогодні.

— Он як? — удав здивованого до краю Орлов. — А що сталося?

— Один псих утік, — тихо сказав поліціянт, — перебрався в санітара, і тільки його й бачили...

— Та що ви кажете! — цього разу здивування графа було непідробним. — А він небезпечний?

— Ні, кажуть, цілковито миролюбний вар'ят. Тільки ані слова нікому...

— Звісно, звісно... — пообіцяв граф, відчуваючи, як ноги самі почали відступати назад.

Він ще змусив себе люб'язно попрощатися з поліціянтом і побажати тому легкої служби. Після цього, не стримуючи себе, майже побіг до свого авта.

У готелі його зупинив рецепціоніст і передав чиюсь поспіхом і недбало складену записку. Розгорнувши її, Орлов швидко прочитав нерівний текст, хоча зміст знав наперед: «Яша втік. Що робити? Ріцке».

— Не знаю, що робити, сраний ти ідіоте! — сердито проказав граф і швидко рушив до свого номера.

III

Берн
10 квітня 1906 року

О восьмій тридцять ранку дещо огрядний добродій високого зросту, вбраний у темно-сірий плащ і чорний мелонік, неспішним, майже прогулянковим кроком звернув з Ратгаузґассе і через вузький безіменний пасаж вийшов на простору й шумну Крамґассе. Тут він рушив ще повільніше, мовби насолоджуючись людською метушнею довкола себе: армією клерків з товстими портфелями й порепаними папками в руках, котрі мчали кудись на службу, ледь не на ходу встрибуючи та вистрибуючи з трамваїв, міських екіпажів та поодиноких таксі, торговців, що якраз відчиняли свої крамниці, доверху набиті сувенірами, шоколадом, швейцарськими ножами та флягами, одягом, зброєю, екзотичним чаєм, сушеними фруктами, тютюном і винами. Крамниці поділялися на верхні й нижні. Верхні займали звичні місця на першому поверсі в будинках, над рівнем вулиці і на рівні очей перехожих. Нижні – знаходилися під ними, у підвалах, куди часто провадили карколомні сходи. Вхід до них здавався радше входом до погребу. Звісна річ, товар нагорі був дорожчим, а торговці багатшими, тому підземний світ здавався їхнім кривим відображенням. Місто потроху наповнювали туристи: чоловіки, вдягнуті здебільшого в короткі зручні куртки, легкі світлі капелюхи та вузькі штани, заправлені на армійський манер у похідні чоботи, жінки – в пальта з тонкого сукна, накинуті поверх щільних суконь, схожі на ті, що використовують для верхової їзди. Капелюшки невеличкі, якраз такі, щоб можна було заховати під ними туго зв'язане волосся. Туристів сюди зазвичай привозить ранішній поїзд із Парижа або Марселя. У місті вони затримуються заледве на кілька годин, швидко снідають в тутешніх кав'ярнях, купують сувеніри і вирушають далі, в ближні Бернські Альпи, щоб нарешті розважитись і відіспатись після виснажливої дороги.

Біля Церінґера* чоловік зупинився, зняв рукавиці й заховав їх до кишені плаща. Потім дістав з нагрудної кишені срібний портсигар і закурив. Уся його постать випромінювала спокій та умиротворення, на противагу войовничому ведмедеві у бойовому обладунку, що стояв над ним на задніх лапах, тримаючи передніми щит і спис. Помилувавшись трохи нескінченною перспективою Крамґассе, чоловік повернувся у протилежний бік, де височіла

* Фонтан Церінґера *(нім. Zähringerbrunnen)* – один з найстаріших фонтанів Берна, присвячений засновнику міста – Бертольдові фон Церінґеру. Фонтан відомий також як «Ведмежий» *(нім. Bärenbrunnen)* – оскільки фігура над ним зображає ведмедя-лицаря в обладунку.

Годинникова вежа*, якраз у той момент, коли на ній пробило три чверті до дев'ятої. Що ж, тепер слід було поспішати... Чоловік видихнув залишки диму з легень і, квапно загасивши недопалок, пожбурив його до сміттєвої урни. За десять хвилин швидкої ходи він опинився на Мюнстерґассе, перед триповерховим будинком, що належав банку «*Hottinguer*». Затримавшись на хвилину перед масивними дверима, ніби для того, щоб прибрати якнайповажнішого виду, чоловік врешті зайшов досередини.

Попри ранню годину, у вестибюлі вже очікувало з десяток клієнтів. Всі вони в одну мить перевели погляд на прибулого, понуро відповіли на його привітання й одразу ж втратили до нього інтерес. Одні знову втупилися поглядом у ранкову газету, інші — в простір перед собою. Атмосфера панувала тут важка й гнітюча.

Чоловік, однак, не збирався приєднуватись до їхнього товариства. Йому було призначено на дев'яту, він прийшов без запізнення, отож мав цілковите право проігнорувати це товариство.

— Вішак — ліворуч від вас, — вдруге відірвавшись від сторінок «*Tages-Anzeiger*»**, промовив до нього вусань у твідовому костюмі. — Ви в черзі вже одинадцятий або дванадцятий, тож знімайте плащ і чекайте. Раніше за нас усе одно туди не потрапите...

Він кивнув головою у бік темно-коричневих дверей з табличкою «*Empfang*»***.

---

* Годинникова вежа (нім. *Zytglogge*) — найвідоміша вежа в історичній частині Берна, на якій встановлено давній астрономічний годинник.

** «Tages-Anzeiger» — швейцарська німецькомовна газета, що виходить з 1893 року.

*** *Empfang* (нім.) — прийом.

— Не думаю, — коротко відповів прибулий.

— Якщо ви у кредитних справах, то мені повірите, — сердито буркнув «твідовий костюм», — я тут щопонеділка, і жоден розумник ще не переступив через мою голову.

Чоловік ще вирішував, як відповісти на цю грубість, коли ж прочинилися зовсім інші двері, з-за яких визирнув молодий банківський клерк у жилеті й нарукавниках поверх білої сорочки.

— Пане Вістович? — звернувся він до прибулого.

Той ствердно кивнув у відповідь.

— Прошу, заходьте, — запросив його клерк і прочинив двері ширше, мовби побоюючись, що кремезний гість інакше не пройде.

Знервований читач «*Tages-Anzeiger*» метнув сповнений ненависті погляд спершу на клерка, потім знову на Вістовича, а далі згорнув газету, ніби з остраху, що ненароком спопелить її своїм розгніваним поглядом, якщо буде дочитувати.

Клерк зачинив двері за новим клієнтом, узяв його плащ, капелюх і рукавиці.

— Прошу вибачення, сьогодні прийом наших позичальників, тому, як це завжди буває в такі дні, настрій у вестибюлі, мов у розстрільній камері, — проговорив він.

Вістович усміхнувся.

— Запевняю вас, що добродій за дверима — бездоганний взірець ґречності й добрих манер, порівнюючи з тими людьми, з якими я зазвичай маю справу, — сказав він.

— Ви також працюєте в банку? — поцікавився клерк.

— Ні, в кримінальній поліції.

Відповідь чомусь справила на клерка несподівано сильне враження. Він завмер і якийсь час не міг підібрати слів, дивлячись на Вістовича, як на статую, що несподівано ожила й побажала йому доброго ранку.

— Пан Освальд Пульманн чекає на вас, — молодий чоловік врешті прийшов до тями. Після цього наблизився до інших дверей, обережно постукав і, зачувши приглушене «Так», відчинив їх перед гостем.

— Ага, пан Адам Вістович! Правильно? — чоловік за масивним письмовим столом підвівся назустріч прибулому і простягнув руку для привітання через гору паперів, брульйонів і якихось відкритих довідників. Пульманн мав дещо комічну зовнішність: лису голову, маленькі поросячі очка за скельцями окулярів у дротяній оправі, рожеві щоки, гострий ніс і червоні, як у дівчини, вологі губи.

Вістович кивнув, удруге за сьогодні підтверджуючи свою особу.

— Прошу сідати, — Пульманн вказав на стілець. — Як довго ви в Берні? — знову запитав банкір, вишукуючи щось серед своїх паперів.

— Лише два дні, — відповів гість.

— Раджу вам лишитися на довше. Наше місто має чим здивувати навіть гостей із чарівної Австрії... Я, знаєте, родом із Базеля, але, приїхавши одного разу сюди, одразу вирішив залишитися тут назавжди... Хтозна, може, й ви, пане Вістовичу, підете моїм шляхом і переїдете, — банкір засміявся і глянув на гостя поверх окулярів.

— Тільки якщо хвилюватимусь за свої гроші, — віджартувався той.

— О, ні! Запевняю вас, такої причини ви не матимете, — Пульманн промовив це вже без жодних жартів. — Ага, ось і потрібна папка...

Банкір відкрив її, щоб дістати звідти кілька документів. Якусь хвилину чоловік зосереджено їх перечитував.

— Що ж, пане Вістовичу, — продовжив він, — перед тим як ми підпишемо договір, ще раз нагадаймо собі кілька важливих пунктів. Отже, ваш депозитний вклад становить сорок тисяч німецьких марок. Від конвертації в австрійські крони або швейцарські франки ви відмовилися... Що ж, рішення вважаю правильним. Річний відсоток буде менший, зате не доведеться платити комісію за цю операцію...

Він знову кинув на Вістовича короткий погляд з-над окулярів, а тоді продовжив:

— Угода наша діятиме п'ять років і, в разі відсутності взаємних претензій, буде продовжена автоматично на такий самий період... Відсотки з вашого вкладення ми виплачуватимемо щоквартально через австрійський банк у Лемберзі...

Банкір узяв до рук увесь стос паперу, з якого складався контракт.

— Решту, якщо бажаєте, перечитайте самі. Можете не поспішати, — сказав він, простягаючи угоду клієнту.

Клієнт узяв папери до рук і заглибився в пронумеровані пункти сухого банківського тексту. Десь за чверть години він повідомив банкіру, що заперечень не має і з усім згоден.

— Чудово! — з ледь помітним полегшенням відповів Пульманн. — Тоді підписуємо, і справу зроблено.

Уже ставлячи свій підпис чорним соковитим атраментом унизу сторінки, клієнт випадково глянув на титул папки, що наступною опинилася в руках банкіра. Погляд його затримався там, либонь, на десяту частину секунди, допоки Пульманн не відклав її вбік. Втім, комісар готовий був присягнути, що помітив на ній добре знайоме йому ім'я. Підписавши свій контракт, він передав його банкіру й спостерігав якусь мить, як той дмухає на чорнило, аби воно швидше висохло.

— Ну от, — врешті промовив Пульманн, — тепер можете підписати і свій екземпляр.

Він простягнув йому ідентичний примірник, де також уже стояла банківська печатка.

— А скажіть, пане Пульманне, — ніби знічев'я промовив гість, — чи багато у вас клієнтів-австрійців?

— О, так, звісно, — відповів той, — саме тому ми тісно співпрацюємо з Банком Австрії.

— А чи багато з них із Ґаліції?

— Думаю, кілька десятків я б нарахував.

Вістович небавом підписав свій екземпляр і так само, як хвилину тому Пульманн, подув трохи на чорнило. Після цього знову запитав:

— А чи є ще хтось з Лемберга, крім мене?

Прозвучало це геть невинно. Невинніше, мабуть, ніж запитання босоногого хлопчака, який розпитує діда-єгера про його пригоди на полюванні. Втім, банкір несподівано спохмурнів.

— Пробачте, пане Вістовичу, але я не можу вдаватися в такі деталі, — категорично заявив він. — Навіть таку інформацію про наших клієнтів ми старанно приховуємо.

Гість добре бачив, що насправді це була вистава для самого ж Вістовича. Пульманн щиро хотів продемонструвати, як добре він виконує свої обов'язки і як дбає про анонімність вкладників. Найпевніше — повідомити, скільки львів'ян тримають свої гроші в швейцарському

«*Hottinguer*» не було б жодним порушенням, але чоловік не наполягав. Він згорнув свій контракт і заховав до внутрішньої кишені піджака. Після цього попрощався з банкіром та, обмінявшись з ним побажаннями гарного дня, вийшов з кабінету.

За дверима його зустрів той самий молодий клерк, який одразу ж подав йому верхній одяг.

— На котру годину призначено сьогодні панові Альфреду Редлю? — несподівано запитав Вістович, уважно вдивившись тому в обличчя.

— На четверту дня... — розгублено відповів той.

Клерк не встиг подумати, навіщо його про це запитували і як цей чоловік дізнався, що інший клієнт з Лемберга також прибуде сьогодні, коли той подякував, приязно всміхнувся і вийшов у вестибюль. Тут він знову проігнорував сердитий погляд вусаня у твідовому костюмі, глибше насадив на голову мелоніка й рушив до дверей.

Ідучи по вулиці, відчув, як неприємно почало нити трохи нижче грудей. Так відбувалося щоразу, коли десь поруч змією звивалася небезпека. Від ранкового піднесення не залишилося й сліду... Комісар львівської кримінальної поліції Адам Вістович тепер почувався препаскудно. З одного боку, не було жодної загрози в тому, що вони з полковником Редлем користувалися послугами одного банку. Та ще й такого, що знаходиться за півтори тисячі миль від Лемберга. А з іншого...

Альфред Редль, як і Вістович, також походив з цього прикордонного галицького міста. Ще в чині майора служив у Генштабі, у Відділі збору інформації, проте невдовзі його підвищили до полковника й відправили з Відня назад до Львова, призначивши на посаду, начальника Галицького підрозділу *Evidenzbüro**.

Так само свого часу зі столиці до рідного Лемберга повернувся й Вістович, щоправда, в чині штабскапітана, будучи випускником елітної Терезіанської академії**. Щойно залишивши стіни своєї суворої *Alma Mater*, молодий львів'янин вирішив більше ані дня не залишатися в армії. Своє рішення він ніколи й нікому не витлумачував, навіть батькові, інженерові залізниці, який вже встиг потішитися майбутній військовій кар'єрі сина. На питання суворого й безкомпромісного Романа Вістовича про те, що той робитиме далі, Адам врешті-решт відповів: «Піду служити в поліцію, якщо так необхідно, аби я носив мундир!». Батькові це видалося жартом, він розсміявся, що й підбурило Адама того ж дня, не зволікаючи, подати клопотання до ц. к.*** Дирекції поліції з проханням прийняти його на службу. Адамові Вістовичу там не відмовили, лише для годиться перевіривши в поліційних архівах, чи не мав він або хтось із його родичів проблем із законом. Нічого такого не виявили, нічого такого, зрештою, в родині Вістовичів і не траплялося.

Ясна річ, нового мундира Адам не отримав. Поліційні однострої на щодень носили тільки постерункові, кінні або піші. А тодішній директор львівської поліції не був

* *Evidenzbüro* (*нім.*) — Управління австро-угорської військової розвідки та контррозвідки.

** Терезіанська академія (*Die Theresianische Militärakademie* (*нім.*) або скорочено *TherMilAk*) — військова академія, заснована імператрицею Марією Терезією 1751 року.

*** Цісарсько-королівську (нім. *Kaiserlich-königlich*) — скорочення, прийняте в Австрійській імперії, а згодом і в Австро-Угорській, для позначення австрійських державних установ..

дурнем, щоб відправити випускника Термілаку ганяти дебоширів на вулиці. Його приписали ад'юнктом до кримінального відділу, де вже за рік він став комісаром другого класу, а відтак і першого.

З перших днів служби Вістович зрозумів, що надто мало знав, як ведеться в поліції. Якби йому більше було відомо про нудну рутину, недалеке начальство й огидних суб'єктів, як-от убивць і маніяків, з якими доводилося мати щодня справу, то, може, і не зважився би на цю роботу. Але було пізно. Батько з його насмішками видавався йому гіршим за всіх цих небезпечних деліквентів разом узятих.

Служба в поліції зробила його стриманішим і холоднокровним. Від запального юнака, що в одну мить перекреслює кар'єрні можливості військового у Відні, не лишилось і тіні. Цей зашкарублий характер, зрештою, допоміг йому пережити подальші життєві біди: смерть батька, перед тим — тихий відхід матері, лагідної й люблячої Соломії Вістович, в дівоцтві Вільчківної. І нарешті розлучення з дружиною, львівською акторкою Анною Каліш, котру слава й амбіції поманили геть з провінційного Лемберга спочатку на сцену берлінського Шаушпільгаузу*, а далі в «Лобе-Театр» у Бреслау**. Поліційні розслідування комісар тепер сприймав, як шахові задачі, чітко й методично розв'язуючи одну справу за іншою. Невдовзі про успішного детектива з Лемберга вже знали у столиці, де в Міністерстві поліції він значився як «безумовно, найкращий слідчий Галичини».

---

* *Schauspielhaus Berlin* (*нім.*) — Берлінський драматичний театр.

** *«Lobe-Theater»* (*нім.*), *«Teatr Lobego»* (*пол.*) — неіснуючий тепер театр у Вроцлаві, тодішньому Бреслау.

З Редлем Вістович уперше зустрівся тільки 1903 року. Якимось дивом вони досі не зналися, хоча обидва походили з львівських сімей залізничників, навчалися у Відні та повернулися потім назад до свого міста. Тоді у Львові сталося вбивство провіденського депутата Сейму. Зі столиці Редлю надійшов наказ негайно розкрити справу. Зі свого боку, начальник Галицького *Evidenzbüro* вимагав швидкого розслідування від директора поліції, той — від свого найкращого детектива. Це службове коло замкнулося й перетворилося для комісара на коло пекла. Йому зрештою вдалося знайти вбивцю, але вся слава й винагорода одноосібно дісталися Редлю. З тих пір Вістович полковника недолюблював.

Ця справа, може, і забулася б, але якихось пів року тому комісар і полковник зіштовхнулися в Позені. Тоді Вістович спільно з прусською контррозвідкою провадив справу, в якій були замішані перші політичні особи Німецького Райху. Власне, у тракті цього розслідування він і отримав гонорар у сорок тисяч марок, які сьогодні успішно розмістив у швейцарському «*Hottinguer*».

Проте особливістю цих грошей було те, що прусський А III b на знак вдячності дозволив йому вивезти їх із Пруссії, не сплативши ані пфеніга податку. Так само без проблем йому вдалося розмістити цю чималу суму в австрійському банку, звідки гроші було перераховано до Швейцарії. Австрійські й прусські таємні служби були давніми союзниками, Редль знав про позенське розслідування Вістовича, а отже, й знав про цей дозволений «сірий» капітал комісара. Ясна річ, опинитися з полковником в один день у Берні й стати клієнтом одного банку — здавалося дурнуватим вибриком долі.

Втім, виникало питання, що в Берні робить сам полковник? Звичайно, Швейцарія — не Росія або Франція, чиїм розвідкам австро-прусський союз протистоїть віддавна. Ця країна з часів Віденського конгресу* зберігає залізний нейтралітет. Але саме завдяки нейтралітету її територія перетворилася на театр для шпигунських ігор. І оскільки начальник галицького *Evidenzbüro* — особа знана й важлива, то, перебуваючи тут навіть інкоґніто, він добряче ризикує потрапити в руки потенційного ворога. Що ж у такому разі змусило його не зважати на ризик? Невже тільки турбота про конто в банку? Можна було припустити, що полковник виконує тут професійне завдання. Але цю думку Вістович одразу відкинув. *Evidenzbüro* зазвичай відряджає за кордон пересічних безликих агентів. Невідомих ані пресі, ані контррозвідкам інших держав.

Роздумуючи, що робити тепер, коли цей бісовий полковник так само може дізнатися про його перебування в Берні, комісар дійшов до свого готелю на Мюнстерплац. Біля входу він зупинився й мимоволі озирнувся. Площа виглядала по-міському звично: торговці смаженими каштанами вигукували щось на тутешньому діалекті, либонь заохочуючи покупців. Молода квітникарка дрімала у своєму крихітному павільйоні, підставивши обличчя першому по-справжньому теплому весняному сонцю. Жебраки тупцювали перед катедральним

---

* Конгрес, що відбувався у Відні з листопада 1814 до червня 1815 року після розгрому Наполеонівської Франції, його ціллю було встановлення нових кордонів у Європі. Тоді ж представники Швейцарії підписали кілька міжнародних правових актів, що проголосили неучасть держави у жодному союзницькому військовому чи політичному формуванні.

собором, окрасою й гордістю Берна. Чувся дитячий галас. Це зграя хлопчаків ганялася за голубами біля фонтана, прикрашеного фігурою Мойсея. Пророк стояв над ними, звівши погляд угору, а в руках тримаючи розгорнуту книгу з десятьма заповідями. «У Швейцарії шпигуном може виявитися навіть святий, — подумалося раптом Вістовичу. — А щодо грошей, то краще б я залишив їх у австрійському банку, чорт забирай...»

У готелі комісар замовив у номер пляшку «Фрапену». Кельнер приніс його за кілька хвилин, і, щойно за ним зачинилися двері, Вістович зняв піджак, черевики, розв'язав краватку і розстебнув верхні ґудзики сорочки. Відкоркував коньяк, налив собі у склянку невелику порцію і, вмостившись у кріслі навпроти вікна, запалив цигарку. Він любив миті, коли не треба було поспішати й можна було спокійно обдумати навіть найскладніші ситуації. І навіть якщо рішення не знайдеться, то добра випивка й запашна цигарка безумовно поліпшать настрій. За кілька хвилин Вістович загасив у попільничці недопалок і відставив порожню склянку. Потім заплющив очі, не опираючись легкій дрімоті. Тінь сну пробігла по його виразному, чисто виголеному обличчю: міцному носі, блідих щоках і тонких губах. Коли за двадцять хвилин він прокинувся, то почувався бадьорим, а головне — остаточно вирішив, що робити далі, мовби рішення прийшло до нього у сні. Насамперед слід попросити рецепціоністів унизу повернути в залізничну касу його сьогоднішній квиток на нічний поїзд і продовжити перебування в готелі ще на добу.

За чверть до шістнадцятої Вістович стояв на Мюнстреґассе, на відстані приблизно тридцяти кроків від банку «*Hottinguer*». Він знайшов зручний завулок, звідки міг спостерігати за входом до будівлі, сам при цьому зостаючись непоміченим. Якщо Редлеві, як повідомив сьогодні вранці клерк, і справді призначено на четверту по полудні, то полковник от-от з'явиться. Пунктуальність австрійським військовим вбивали цвяхом у голову ще в академіях, після чого вона залишалася їхньою незмінною рисою впродовж усього життя.

Полковник з'явився через десять хвилин. Попри те що вбраний він був у цивільне: темний плащ і модний англійський капелюх — Вістович одразу впізнав його довготелесу постать і меланхолійну ходу. Редль зупинився на секунду біля дверей, роззирнувся, а тоді зайшов досередини. Пробувши там сорок хвилин, впродовж яких комісар ні на мить не залишив свого сховку, полковник вийшов назовні й помітно було, що перебуває той у чудовому гуморі. Більше він не роззирався довкола з підозрою, а навпаки — випрямився і, високо несучи голову, попрямував кудись углиб міста. Відрахувавши кілька секунд, Вістович рушив за ним.

Полковник вийшов до міської оглядової тераси, звідки відкривався прегарний вид на долину Ааре* з гігантським Кірхенфельдбрюке** та на далекі засніжені Альпи. На терасі були розставлені столики поближньої кав'ярні, звідки час від часу до клієнтів вибігали кельнери. Людей за столиками не бракувало, і Редль спішно зайняв єдине вільне місце. Кельнера не кликав, здавалося, вирішивши дочекатися, коли той підійде до нього сам. «Якщо

* Ааре — ріка, що протікає через Берн.

** Кірхенфельдбрюке (нім. *Kirchenfeldbrücke*) — залізничний та пішохідний міст через Ааре, збудований 1883 року.

так, — подумалось комісару, — то зробити замовлення полковнику вдасться зовсім не скоро». Офіціантів не вистачало, а тому обслуговували вони дуже повільно, хоч і старалися з усіх сил. Не минало й хвилини, щоб хтось не здійняв догори руку, вимагаючи до себе уваги. Ці руки спершу нерухомо стриміли над головами інших клієнтів, а потім нервово тріпались, коли їх не зауважували, і — як наслідок — не залишали бідолашним кельнерам ані сантима чайових.

Вістович тим часом зауважив, що на лавці під платаном, звідки зручно було б і далі спостерігати за полковником, двоє шахістів закінчили свою гру. Після цього один із них підвівся, потиснув супернику руку й пішов геть. Не довго роздумуючи, комісар підійшов до лавки й став навпроти вакантного місця.

— Ви дозволите? — запитав він у літнього пана, що грав досі за білих.

Шахіст усміхнувся у відповідь і радо погодився на нову партію. Суперники заходилися розставляти фігури, хоча Вістович, ясна річ, увесь час скоса поглядав убік полковника, який так і сидів без жодного замовлення, дивлячись кудись удаль перед собою. Комісар був добрим гравцем. Ще нікому в усій Дирекції поліції не вдалося обіграти його, а тому, якби хтось записував сьогоднішню партію, вона б стала його ганьбою до кінця життя.

— Вам слід трохи повчитися, — поблажливо промовив швейцарець, забираючи у Вістовича королеву.

— Мені шкода, — пробурмотів той у відповідь, роблячи черговий безглуздий хід.

Тим часом Редль підвівся з-за столика. Можна було подумати, що він просто не дочекався кельнера і, як десятки інших знервованих відвідувачів, йде геть. Проте Вістович добре розумів, що це не так. Усе було б занадто просто... Зовсім забувши про свою гру, комісар ловив кожен рух полковника. Бачив, як той підійшов до краю тераси й, милуючись горами, закурив. Вістович перевів погляд на порожній столик і несподівано помітив на стільниці залишений конверт. Тієї ж миті на місце Редля сів інший суб'єкт: широкоплечий чоловік у картатій кепці й альпійській куртці, яку зазвичай вдягають лижники або велосипедисти. Він, мовби знічев'я, накрив конверт долонею, а далі непомітно заховав його до кишені. Редль тим часом зник...

— Гра не має сенсу, — долинув до Вістовича розчарований голос шахіста. Чоловік прибрав з дошки фігури й почав складати їх у невеликий полотняний мішечок, вочевидь, втративши будь-яку надію заволодіти увагою свого візаві.

— Мені дуже шкода, — повторив комісар, підводячись зі свого місця, але тільки тому, що з-за столика підвівся той, за ким він спостерігав. Якби цей тип продовжив сидіти, у Вістовича не забракло б нахабства вимагати від швейцарця реваншу.

— На все добре, — сказав комісар на прощання й поволі рушив за незнайомцем.

Крок за кроком вони разом спустилися людними сходами униз до набережної, де за кількома вулицями починався річковий порт. З кожною хвилиною комісарові здавалося, що він цього типа уже десь бачив. Вістович сказав би це напевно, якби той повернувся й показав обличчя, але, на щастя, незнайомець ішов, дивлячись увесь час перед собою. Втім, в одному комісар був переконаний: бачитися з цим суб'єктом вони могли тільки за звичних для Вістовича обставин, тобто, швидше за все, той був яким-небудь пройдисвітом.

Біля порту було вже не так людно, як нагорі, в Старому місті, тому виправу з переслідуванням слід було припиняти або закінчувати в якийсь інакший спосіб. Комісар подумки ще раз поспіхом усе зважив: Редль не мав би бути в Берні, не мав би зв'язуватись із злочинцями, а найголовніше — не мав би знати, що Вістович у цьому місті також має свій інтерес. Проти Редля треба було шукати важливий козир, хай навіть здобути його буде ризиковано. Цей козир, власне, щойно вийшов на дерев'яний портовий поміст і почав роглядатися довкола себе, мовби шукаючи когось. Комісар ледве встиг заховатися за старою поламаною огорожею. У ту ж мить в ніздрі йому вдарив сильний запах кінської сечі. Озирнувшись, Вістович побачив порожнього фіакра і візника, що стоячи неподалік, гриз сушену рибу. Вістович підійшов до нього і якомога спокійніше, долаючи внутрішнє хвилювання, запитав:

— На Мюнстерплац завезеш?

— А чом би й ні? — стенув плечима той.

— Тільки не напряму, а так, щоб покружляти передмістям.

Візник криво всміхнувся і з підозрою глянув на цього клієнта. Тоді комісар вирішив перейти до вагоміших аргументів і тицьнув йому п'ять франків.

— Дам ще десять, якщо мене дочекаєшся.

— Як вам завгодно, дорогий пане, — запопадливо відповів той.

Тоді Вістович, більше не гаючи часу, стрімким кроком подався в бік незнайомця, який все ще стояв на тому самому місці спиною до комісара. Зачувши чиїсь швидкі кроки, він сполохано озирнувся і від здивування роззявив рота:

— Вістовичу? Що ти, в біса, тут ро?..

Комісар не дав йому договорити. Правою рукою він висмикнув з-під його куртки конверта, чий білий край по-зрадницьки визирав із внутрішньої кишені, а лівою щосили зацідив йому в пику. Цей бездоганний лівий прямий добре знали у Лемберзі та околицях. Тамтешні батяри були б здивовані, якби хтось зумів устояти на ногах і лишитися при свідомості, отримавши такий удар від Вістовича, та ще й як зараз — прямісінько в нижню щелепу. Тип у альпійській куртці винятком не став. Навіть не змахнувши руками, він повалився у воду, ніби мішок із піском, здійнявши довкола себе цілу гору бризок. І доки нечисленні свідки цієї події не прийшли до тями, Вістович щодуху кинувся до фіакра, де візник, чесно його дочекавшись, погнав свій скрипучий екіпаж чортзна-куди, в тутешні села, обіцяючи, як було домовлено, тільки за годину щонайраніше дістатися до Мюнстерплацу.

Всередині фіакра, трохи віддихавшись, комісар придивився до відібраного конверта. Той був невеликий, прямокутний, приблизно п'ятнадцять на двадцять сантиметрів. Ззовні не мав жодних написів, крім однієї літери N, виведеної темно-бузковим чорнилом в одному з кутів. Склеювальна смужка тягнулася вздовж коротшої сторони, і Вістович з радістю зауважив, що клей не встиг як слід засохнути. Отже, конверт вдасться відкрити, не пошкодивши.

Він дістав з кишені складаного ножа й, незважаючи на те, що фіакр трусило на розбитій передміській дорозі, обережно виконав цю делікатну операцію. Потім акуратно витягнув з конверта вміст. Це виявився канцелярський аркуш, складений вчетверо. Листок приблизно наполовину був заповнений, здавалося, випадковими буквами й цифрами, а насправді — добре продуманим шифром, покликаним приховати зміст. Трохи поміркувавши, комісар дістав записника і рядок за рядком переписав у нього невідоме послання. Далі вклав аркуш знову в конверт і, загнувши клейкий край, кілька разів провів по ньому рукою. За хвилину паперовий трофей мав такий самий вигляд, як тоді, коли вперше потрапив йому до рук.

Врешті, знову опинившись у Старому місті, фіакр зупинився, й Вістович простягнув візникові обіцяні десять франків. Далі вийшов з екіпажу, з приємністю відчувши під ногами нехитку надійну опору. Вже темніло, й на вулицях Берна то тут, то там спалахували електричні ліхтарі. Містом, як злий пес, блукав холодний гірський вітер, що розганяв перехожих по кпайпах і власних оселях. Теплий весняний день закінчився, наставала крижана квітнева ніч.

Комісар застебнув плаща на всі ґудзики й підняв комір. Це трохи рятувало, проте понад усе хотілося якнайшвидше опинитися в готелі. Зайшовши до вестибюля, він швидко пройшов повз стійку рецепції, не помітивши, яке враження справила його поява на двох адміністраторів. Зрештою, якби й помітив, то навряд чи здогадався б про причину такої реакції.

Щойно відчинивши двері, Вістович зрозумів, що всередині хтось є. У ніздрі вдарив сильний запах дешевого тютюну й пасти для взуття. Комісар зупинився у передпокої, вирішуючи, що робити далі: піти геть чи зайти в кімнату. Зброї він при собі не мав. Вирушаючи з Лемберга у «відпустку» (а саме відпусткою пояснювалася його теперішня відсутність у документах поліційної канцелярії), брати з собою службового «Ґассера»* не мав права. Приватного ж браунінга** залишив удома, щоб уникнути зайвих питань і можливих проблем на кордоні. Рішення, втім, з'явилося вже за хвилину, коли на іншому боці передпокою з'явився полковник Редль з націленим на нього револьвером у руці.

— Ви довго, Вістовичу, — промовив військовий, — ми вас зачекалися.

«Хто це, в біса, "ми"?» — подумки запитав комісар.

— Ну ж бо, проходьте, — нетерпляче додав полковник.

Вістович підкорився й зайшов до кімнати, одразу побачивши іншого суб'єкта, який разом із Редлем складав суть цього множинного займенника «ми». Невідомий сидів у кріслі, заклавши ногу на ногу, й уважно спостерігав за прибулим. Він, як і полковник, тримав у руці зброю, трохи витягнувши вперед кисть, щоб у разі стрілянини не схибити. Попри свій тандем, ці двоє мали вигляд двох протилежностей: полковник — високий з продовгуватим блідим обличчям, з яким контрастували короткі вусики і близько посаджені темні очі, незнайомець — опасистий, червонолиций, з густою, давно не стриженою бородою.

Комісар, звісна річ, знав, чим накликав на себе їхній візит, а проте був щиро здивований, як полковнику вдалося так швидко його відшукати. Редль помітив його подив і не стримав єхидної вдоволеної посмішки.

---

* «Ґассер» — восьмизарядний револьвер, який виготовляла австрійська компанія *«Rast-Gasser»* з другої половини XIX ст.

** Браунінг — загальна назва пістолетів, які в той час випускала бельгійська фірма *«Fabrique Nationale d`Armes de Guerre»*.

— Познайомтеся, пане Вістовичу, це — інспектор Клебер з кантонської поліції, — представив полковник незнайомця в кріслі.

Той недбало відсалютував лівою рукою, ні на секунду не опускаючи праву, в якій стискав, як тепер зміг роздивитися комісар, стару модель шестизарядного «Шамело-Дельвінь»*.

— Пан Клебер тут для того, — продовжив полковник, — щоб пред'явити вам звинувачення у викраденні надзвичайно важливого документа, що належить безпосередньо посольству Австро-Угорщини в Швейцарії.

Комісар чекав, що той скаже щось і про напад у порту, але Редль на цих словах замовк, даючи зрозуміти, що цього факту досить для того, аби у Вістовича з'явилися величезні неприємності з тутешньою поліцією.

— Саме так, — вперше озвався поліціянт, напрочуд жваво підводячись з крісла. Він виявився доволі невисокого зросту, більш ніж на голову нижчий за комісара. — Втім, якщо повернете полковнику згаданий документ, покарання буде не настільки суворим, — продовжив він, — думаю, обмежимось видворенням з країни.

Вістович якийсь час помовчав, дивлячись спочатку на поліціянта, що цілився тепер зі свого револьвера йому прямісінько в живіт, а потім перевів погляд на полковника, який, очікуючи на його відповідь, почав помітно нервуватися. Врешті комісар був готовий до контрвипаду:

— Пане Клебере, — звернувся він до інспектора, — якщо згаданий документ настільки важливий, як стверджує

---

* «Шамело-Дельвінь» (фр. *Chamelot Delvigne*) — армійський револьвер, який випускали з 1865 року спочатку в Бельгії, відтак у Франції та Швейцарії.

полковник, то як австрійський підданий, а надто як представник закону в своїй країні прошу добродія Редля пояснити, чому він власноруч передав його сьогодні приблизно о пів на п'яту злочинцеві на ім'я Карел Грумм.

Перед очима в комісара знов промайнула здивована фізія чоловіка в похідній куртці, якого він відправив у нокаут в порту і чий перекривлений рот так і не закінчив фразу «Що ти, в біса, тут робиш?». Авжеж, не тільки Грумм, до того як звалитися у воду, впізнав поліціянта. Побачивши перед собою його мармизу, Вістович не мав жодного сумніву, хто перед ним.

Карел Грумм походив звідкілясь із Богемії і, перш ніж стати злочинцем, навчався на гірничого інженера у Празі. Невідомо, чи закінчив цей чоловік свої студії, але здобуті знання з піротехніки вирішив використовувати для підриву залізничних колій, банківських будівель і автомобілів. За ним полювала ледь не вся імперська поліція, і тільки комісару прикордонного Лемберга Адаму Вістовичу вдалося впіймати його й відправити до в'язниці. Рішення суду для підривника виявилося надто м'яким. Подейкували, це сталося через те, що анонімно втрутилися впливові родичі, котрі хоч і соромилися Грумма, а проте не втрачали надії, що той коли-небудь покається й візьметься за розум. Замість смертної кари, що присуджувалася зазвичай у таких випадках, він отримав лише десять років в'язниці. Та вже за рік стало відомо, що під час етапування ув'язнених залізницею десь у Карпатах Грумм змайстрував саморобну вибухівку, підірвав двері свого вагона й вистрибнув на ходу з поїзда. З тих пір — а сталося це близько десяти років тому — про втікача ніхто не чув. Тільки раз прийшла неофіційна звістка, що

Грумма помітили з іншого боку кордону, десь під Києвом. Втім, ніхто не надав цьому жодного значення. Якщо це й правда, то втікач тепер — проблема царської поліції, а не цісарської.

Тепер же в бернському готелі тінь підривника Грумма мовби прошмигнула між цими трьома чоловіками, двоє з яких тримали в руці зброю й не мали наміру її опускати. Якийсь час тривала мовчанка.

— Мені повторити запитання? — сказав Вістович, звертаючись одночасно до Редля і Клебера.

Інспектор Клебер здавався дещо розгубленим. Вочевидь, слово «злочинець» справило на нього очевидне враження.

— Не треба, — буркнув полковник, — я добре його почув.

— Тоді буду вдячний за відповідь.

— А чи не здається вам, Вістовичу, що я не зобов'язаний відповідати якомусь провінційному комісару? — з притиском сказав полковник. — Я звітую виключно Генштабові, а не вам.

— Гадаю, Генштабові буде ще цікавіше, ніж мені, що пов'язує вас із Карелом Груммом, — зі спокоєм у голосі зауважив комісар.

Знову нависла тягуча пауза. Інспектор не витримав і, відклавши вбік зброю, закурив. Тютюн був до біса смердючий, а дим від нього виїдав очі. Саме цей сморід видав інспектора, щойно Вістович зайшов до свого номера.

— Де конверт? — з ненавистю запитав Редль. — Скажіть, і я обіцяю, ми розійдемося з вами мирно.

Вістович дуже повільно опустив руку в кишеню і так само повільно витягнув звідти листа. Редль вхопив його й відійшов на два кроки назад. Потім підніс до очей і якусь мить оглядав паперові краї.

— Відкривали його? — запитав він у комісара.

— Ви ж бачите, що ні, — не моргнувши й оком, відповів той.

— Інспекторе Клебере, — промовив полковник, опускаючи послання кудись у безодню внутрішніх кишень свого пальта, — оскільки в мого співвітчизника вистачило глузду повернути вкрадений документ, вважаю конфлікт вирішеним. Я не подаватиму жодної заяви, а ви не матимете пекельного клопоту, який неодмінно з'являється, коли у справі замішані іноземні громадяни.

Той розвів руками, поставив револьвера на запобіжник і запхнув його за пояс штанів.

— Як бажаєте, панове, — коротко промовив він. — Я, як і моя країна, завжди готовий дотриматися нейтралітету.

— А я, дорогий інспекторе, завжди дотримуюсь обіцянок, — сказав полковник і, підморгнувши поліціянтові, простягнув йому темно-сіру картку з витисненим невідомим гербом і позолоченим текстом. — Ось візитівка винної крамниці Геклерів. Там для вас відкладено кілька пляшок відмінного «*Moët & Chandon*»*.

— Ах, — видихнув Клебер, і його широке обличчя розпливлося у вдоволеному усміху, ніби кавалок масла на гарячій пательні. — Їй-богу, полковнику... Ви не мусили.

— Звісно, що не мусив, — відповів той, — тому зробив це єдино з приємності. Крім того, сподіваюся, що у вас буде безліч причин, аби розпити його в доброму товаристві.

---

* «*Moët & Chandon*» — легендарний французький виробник шампанського. Компанію засновано ще в XVIII столітті.

— Ваші слова Богові до вух, — весело підсумував інспектор, вдягаючи на голову капелюха. — Що ж, якщо справу залагоджено, то я піду. Зичу гарного вечора, полковнику... А вам, добродію, — інспектор зупинився на хвилину біля Вістовича й зміряв того останнім підозрілим поглядом, — вам я раджу не затримуватися в Берні. Та й взагалі у Швейцарії. Чим швидше ви поїдете звідси, тим краще буде для вас... Мені, старому тутешньому вовкодавові, можете повірити на слово. Всього найліпшого!

Клебер вийшов нарешті з номера, залишивши двох львів'ян наодинці.

— Отже, тепер ви підкуповуєте поліцію, — єхидно зауважив комісар, щойно двері зачинилися.

— Облиште, Вістовичу. Клебер — мій давній знайомий, і кілька пляшок шампанського — це зовсім не підкуп, — відповів Редль, — крім того, іншого способу легально сюди проникнути я не мав. Мусив скористатися з його допомоги.

— Звідки ви дізналися, де я зупинився? — далі допитувався комісар.

— З реєстраційної книги в банку. Домовляючись про візит, ви мусили вказати тимчасову бернську адресу, — пояснив полковник.

— Отже, конфіденційність, яку декларує і обіцяє банк «*Hottinguer*», насправді існує лише на папері, — зауважив Вістович.

— Чому ж? Просто герр Пульманн — також мій друг.

— Сподіваюсь, ви і його не обділили шампанським.

— Банкіри зазвичай полюбляють міцніші трунки, — сказав Редль, — мабуть, через нервову роботу. Ще нервовішу, ніж робота в поліції.

— А що п'ють злочинці на кшталт Грумма? — підвищив голос комісар.

Редль замовк на якийсь час, мовби підбираючи правильні слова. Врешті, підійшовши до вікна і не дивлячись на комісара, спокійно промовив:

— Послухайте, Вістовичу, я розумію, це все виглядає дивно, але чому б вам не повірити, що я зараз на службі й усі мої дії мають під собою службовий ґрунт? Чи ви забули, який відділ я представляю?

— Аж ніяк не забув, полковнику. Хоча б тому, що ви й мені пропонували посаду в *Evidenzbüro*.

— І все ще чекаю на вашу відповідь.

— Якщо в цій службі офіцери не гидують співпрацею з мерзотниками штибу Карела Грумма, то відповідь моя очевидна.

— Не будьте таким категоричним, Вістовичу. Ви, зрештою, також не святий. Узяти хоча б ваш рахунок в «*Hottinguer*». Не забувайте, мені відоме походження цих грошей. Залишати їх у Банку Австрії було ненадійно, чи не так? Хтозна, яких перевірок може зазнати конто комісара поліції.

— Як і ваше.

— Як і моє, — погодився Редль, — через це всі свої заощадження я тримаю тут, у Берні... І погодьтесь, є щось символічне в тому, що ми обидва виявилися клієнтами одного банку.

— Радий був би обійтися без цих узагальнень, полковнику, — сказав комісар.

— Як буде завгодно.

Вістович тим часом вирішив, що тепер настала його черга переходити в рішучий наступ:

— То як почувається добродій Грумм? — вимовив він, хоч насправді чхати хотів навіть на те, чи сучий син живий.

— Думаю, з ним усе гаразд, — відповів Редль, ніяк не виказуючи те, наскільки ця тема для нього дражлива, — у воді він одразу прийшов до тями, а випадкові свідки інциденту допомогли йому вибратися на берег. Після цього Грумм негайно повідомив, що конверт перейшов у ваші руки.

— І вам достатньо було потурбувати знайомого інспектора, щоб проникнути в мій номер і чекати на мене тут.

— Бачите, як усе просто?

Вістович криво всміхнувся у відповідь.

— Повертаючись, однак, до Грумма, пане Редль, — сказав він, — в Австро-Угорщині й союзній Пруссії його б заарештували як злочинця. А якщо зважити, що він, за чутками, перебрався до Росії, то вийти на міжнародну шпигунську арену цей суб'єкт міг би лише як агент царської розвідки. А якщо це так, то ви, полковнику, пов'язані з...

— Не поспішайте з висновками, пане Вістовичу, — перебив його Редль, — запевняю вас, дійсність не така жахлива, якою ви її змальовуєте. Ми з вами знаємо один про одного невеличкі таємниці, тож це певним чином зрівноважує наші взаємні звинувачення. Пропоную перебратися з цього, даруйте за прямоту, бридкуватого номера куди-небудь в краще місце й випити по чарці.

— Те, що я дізнався, полковнику, заледве чи можна назвати «невеличкою таємницею», — зауважив комісар.

— Гаразд. Отже, пити ми також будемо щось направду вартісне, — Редль перейшов на цілком дружній тон.

Здавалося, це не він ще кілька хвилин тому цілився в комісара із зарядженої зброї.

— То що, їдемо? — повторив він запрошення. — Обіцяю, до кінця вечора багато речей ви розумітимете краще.

— Гаразд, — погодився комісар.

Зрештою, жодних інших планів на вечір у нього й так не було. Як і чіткого бачення, що робити далі в цій ситуації.

На вулиці вже зовсім стемніло, проте полковник впевнено рушив до неосвітленого провулка, що тягнувся від Мюнстерплац кудись у глибину вечірнього міста. З темряви несподівано виринули обриси автомобіля. Редль навпомацки відкрив дверцята й заліз на сидіння водія. Потім завів двигун і ввімкнув фари.

— Сідайте! — гукнув він комісару, вказавши на місце праворуч від себе.

Той обійшов авто спереду, затуляючи очі від сліпучого автомобільного світла, і приєднався до полковника.

— Куди ми їдемо? — запитав комісар, щойно авто поводі рушило нічними вулицями.

— Я замовив столик в ресторані готелю «*Bellevue*», — відповів полковник, не відриваючи погляду від дороги, — збирався повечеряти сам, але, сподіваюся, ви не проти скласти мені компанію? Повірте, це найкращий ресторан в усьому Берні. До того ж у них чудовий бар з випивкою.

«*Bellevue*» знаходився на узвишші, звідки можна було милуватися розкішним краєвидом. Зрештою, про це свідчила сама назва готелю й однойменного ресторану*.

Редль назвав своє ім'я метрдотелю і, коли той відшукав його в списку гостей, попросив столик у барі, поруч

---

* *Belle vue* (*фр.*) — прекрасний вид.

з більярдними кімнатами. Там збиралися виключно чоловічі товариства, замовляючи здебільшого міцну випивку і відповідну закуску.

— Рекомендую тутешній антрекот, — тоном знавця сказав полковник, коли вони зайняли віддалене місце під стіною. Звідти Вістовичу добре було видно шинквас і перехід між рестораном та баром. За старою звичкою комісар непомітно оглянув цей простір, подумки запам'ятовуючи деталі, а надто — відвідувачів.

— Або печеню з кролика, якщо хочете чогось делікатнішого, — продовжив Редль.

— Антрекот, — згодився комісар, хоч зовсім не відчував голоду.

— Чудово... — полковник на хвилину занурився в читання меню, але майже одразу відклав його, — собі я замовлю те саме... Бажаєте вина чи віскі?

— Віскі, — не задумуючись, зробив вибір Адам Вістович.

— Тоді дванадцятирічний «*Dalmore*» вам сподобається. Це мій улюблений сорт. М'ясо готують доволі довго, тож цей скотч прикрасить наше очікування.

Сказавши це, полковник гукнув кельнера й повторив йому замовлення. «*Dalmore*» опинився на їхньому столі за лічені хвилини разом з невеличкою металевою посудиною, наповненою кубиками льоду. Полковник попросив залишити цілу пляшку.

— Ніколи не думали про те, щоб піти з поліції? — раптом запитав Редль, щойно кожен з них відпив по ковтку. Віскі смакувало й справді розкішно.

— Мені важко уявити себе деінде, — зізнався Вістович, — я цілковито присвятив себе службі.

— Як і я, — Редль запалив цигарку і, почастувавши співрозмовника, продовжив: — А тим часом, зовсім поруч струменіє цілком інше життя.

Полковник вказав рукою на сусідню залу, яку заливало м'яке світло, що струменіло з велетенських жирандолів під стелею та перелискувало на гранях ресторанного кришталю й дорогих прикрасах на жіночих шиях, грудях і пальцях. Зі сцени почулися перші акорди квінтету, а соліст м'яким баритоном звернувся до публіки, закликаючи до танців і музичних замовлень.

— Коли-небудь, — коротко промовив комісар і випив ще один ковток. Подумки він намагався уявити, скільки коштувала пляшка на їхньому столі. Підозрював, що не менше ста франків.

— «Коли-небудь» — це як постріл у голову, комісаре, — засміявся Редль. — Після такої відповіді зазвичай вже нічого не відбудеться.

— Свого часу я міг обрати Відень, — сказав Вістович, — залишитися там, збудувати кар'єру. Але покинув усе й повернувся до рідного Лемберга.

— Що ж, а я обрав столицю. Тримався за неї з усіх сил, намагався вислужитись перед начальством, тільки б там залишитися. Врешті, одного дня разом із підвищенням отримав наказ перебратися назад в Ґаліцію. Як бачите, моя історія — наче дзеркальне відображення вашої.

— Думаю, таких історій можна назбирати тисячі по всій імперії.

— Згоден. Але не завжди випадкова примха начальства повинна визначати наше майбутнє. А доля тих, що служать і в армії, і в поліції часто напряму залежить від зверхників.

— Так вже влаштовано й армію, і поліцію. Ми з вами знали, на що погоджувались.

Вістович збрехав. Він і гадки не мав, у якому опиниться болоті, коли 1885 року переступив поріг Дирекції на Академічній. Проте зараз волів опонувати всьому, що скаже полковник, потроху розуміючи, куди той хилить.

— Все ж, комісаре, вам притаманне цілком здорове грошолюбство. Погодьтесь. Інакше ви б не приїхали до Берна, опікуючись своїм позенським гонораром.

— Тут я не буду заперечувати. Не хочеться, коли постарію, поволі гнити в якомусь притулку при монастирі.

— От, нарешті! — Редль на радощах плеснув у долоні. — Нарешті притомна думка!

Він ухопив пляшку й знову наповнив їхні спорожнілі склянки.

— За здоровий глузд! — запропонував він тост.

Комісар підтримав, і чоловіки випили, після цього одразу заповнили легені тютюновим димом.

— Тепер, гадаю, час перейти до справи, — посерйознішавши, сказав полковник. Він загасив недопалок і пильно подивився на комісара. — Чи не хотіли б ви, Вістовичу, отримувати час від часу деякі гонорари, що значно б доповнили ваш теперішній рахунок у банку «*Hottinguer*»? Ніхто в Австрії цього не знатиме. Про це буде відомо лише мені, вам і вашому банкіру. Скажімо, тому самому Освальдові Пульманну, з яким ви й так маєте справу.

Комісар подумки щиросердно вилаявся. Чому цей горе-вербувальник заговорив напряму саме тепер? Чому не дозволив випити ще бодай склянку цього направду чудового віскі? Зрештою, міг почати розмову вже тоді, коли принесуть антрекот. Від хорошої випивки у Вістовича прокинувся апетит, і з'їсти бодай шматок добре зготованого м'яса він би не відмовився. Вголос комісар тільки важко зітхнув і поклав на стіл серветку.

— Ви розумієте, полковнику, що, почувши це, я повинен вас або заарештувати, або пристрелити? — запитав він.

— Чому ж? — той старанно приховував емоції, що зародилися в ньому після такої відповіді.

— Бо не досить того, що ви самі працюєте на росіян, то ще й схиляєте до цього мене.

— Звідки висновок, що я працюю на росіян? — Редль здавався щиро здивованим.

— Усі свої здогади я представив ще в готелі.

— Це через Грумма? Так, він тепер агент. Але щодо росіян ви помиляєтеся, комісаре, — твердо вимовив Редль.

— Тоді на кого я повинен працювати, щоб отримувати «деякі гонорари»? — Вістович говорив тепер, мов на допиті. У його тоні змішувалися роздратування й злість.

— Був би вдячний, якби ви говорили тихіше, — сказав Редль, роззираючись довкола. Ніхто, втім, не звернув уваги на надміру емоційну репліку комісара.

— З ким ви пов'язані, полковнику? — повторив запитання Вістович.

— З одним приватним розвідувальним бюро тут, у Швейцарії. І не роблю нічого, що шкодило б інтересам Австро-Угорщини, — відповів той.

— Он як? — здивувався комісар. — Існують, виявляється, приватні шпигунські агенції.

— А чому б ні? Адже існують приватні детективні служби?

— І разом з вами в цій агенції служить Карел Грумм?

— На жаль, так. Якщо гадаєте, ніби я про нього іншої думки, ніж ви, то помиляєтесь.

— Що було в конверті, який ви йому сьогодні передали?

— Прикро, але я не можу вам сказати, Вістовичу. У будь-якому разі, запевняю, що нічого навіть близько пов'язаного з Росією.

Комісар не втримався і сам собі наповнив склянку. Потім випив одним ковтком. Редль сприйняв це як добрий знак і вигідніше розвалився в кріслі.

— Тепер ви бачите, що ваші висновки про мене були дещо поспішними? — запитав він, запалюючи нову цигарку.

— Тепер я бачу, полковнику, що мій антрекот будете їсти ви, — сказав комісар, підводячись з-за столу, — сподіваюся, додаткова порція вам ніяк не зашкодить.

— Стривайте...

— Дякую за віскі, — додав той.

— Останнє, комісаре, — попросив Редль, притримавши його за рукав. — Коли ви повертаєтеся до Лемберга?

— Не знаю. Я здав квиток, а іншого не взяв, — сказав Вістович.

— І не візьмете. На найближчий тиждень у бік Ґаліції немає жодного поїзда, — повідомив Редль, — проте у мене зарезервовано два на завтрашній експрес. Він уже вирушив сьогодні з Венеції, завтра в полудень буде в Берні, потім через Страсбург, Прагу і Відень прямує до Лемберга. Один квиток я залишаю собі, а інший — якщо до завтра не зміните адреси — надішлю вам. Що скажете?

— Буду вдячний, — сухо промовив комісар і, кивнувши на прощання, вийшов із бару, а відтак і з ресторації.

IV

Лемберг
10–14 квітня 1906 року

Антоні Самковський, ад'юнкт львівської кримінальної поліції, не любив весни. Точніше, не любив той час, коли тільки починав танути сніг, з-під якого на світ Божий з'являлося дрібне сміття, трупи здохлих тварин і просто мотлох, що його не встигли прибрати восени. Зима цьогоріч відступила пізно. Якихось два тижні тому ще трималися морози, мовби невідомі чари перенесли ціле місто кудись далеко на північ.

Лемберг у такий час мав потворний вигляд. По закінченню дня вони з шефом, комісаром Вістовичем, зазвичай ішли кудись перехилити по чарці, але шеф уже тиждень перебував у відпустці. «Яка, до біса, може бути зараз відпустка? За такої погоди?» — думав Самковський, дивлячись у вікно їхнього спільного кабінету, звідки проглядалася брудно-сіра смуга вулиці Академічної*, що тягнулася до однойменної площі з пам'ятником Александеру Фредру** посередині.

Втім, відсутність шефа його насправді тішила. Яка б причина не змусила Вістовича вибратися з міста на цілий тиждень, Самковський мав добру можливість відпочити від його важкого й часом непередбачуваного характеру. Шеф був гарним співрозмовником за чаркою, але нестерпним начальником на службі.

До knайпи ад'юнкт тепер заходив лише повечеряти. Здебільшого в «Тлусту рибу», непримітний заклад на Підзамчі. Як можна було виснувати з назви, головними тут були страви з риби: зупа з линів, печені карасі, мариновані плітки, а також оселедці, подавані на стіл з цибулею, вареною картоплею і чорним замарстинівським хлібом. До них, ясна річ, клієнт міг замовити келишок місцевого аквавіта. Приміром, холодної житньої «Балабанівки» або добірної, знаної на цілу Галичину, горілки «Baczewski». Щодо цієї горілки, то господар, невисокий лисуватий Моріц Зайґельт, наливаючи клієнтові трунок до склянки, неодмінно промовляв знану в усіх кнайпах «конклюзію»:

Jeśli jechać to już sanną
Jeśli kochać się to z panną

---

* Тепер — проспект Шевченка.

** Граф Александер Фредро (1793–1876) — польський драматург, поет, громадський діяч. Пам'ятник Фредрові був на місці теперішнього пам'ятника Грушевському. Згодом цей пам'ятник був перевезений до Вроцлава.

Gdy się bawić to z kolegą,
*Jeśli pić to Baczewskiego.**

Сьогодні, знову вислухавши цю приповідку від пана Зайґельта, Самковський усміхнувся й перехилив половину келишка до рота. Решту він вирішив випити, коли принесуть замовлених на вечерю карасиків. Вмостившись за столиком біля стіни, під гасницею**, він розгорнув свіжий випуск «*Wieku Nowego*»***, який купив ще вранці. Неуважно переглянув новини Галицького сейму, далі двічі прочитав оголошення про те, що вартість проїзду в трамваях невдовзі підвищиться до 20 гелерів. Скрипнув зубами, бо якраз трамваєм щодня діставався на службу, а потім зі служби. Отже, тепер це коштуватиме йому сорок гелерів на день замість тридцяти, як було досі. А з огляду на те, що на підвищення наразі можна було не сподіватися, такі новини не додавали гумору. Втім, наступна новина мовби пропонувала рішення: «Товариство львівських роверистів уже цього літа отримає власний стадіон для змагань!». Чудово! Замість трамвая можна пересісти на велосипед.

Самковський гмикнув і, не втримавшись, надпив ще трохи аквавіту з чарки. На наступній сторінці анонсувалися перші перегони на іподромі. «Звісно, якщо тільки Господь буде добрим, — зазначав автор статті, — і не нашле на місто негоду. Бо в минулі роки кінні забіги

---

* Такий вірш, під назвою «*Konkluzja*», тобто «Підсумок» було вміщено на рекламних буклетах лікеро-горілчаної продукції «Бачевського».

** Гасова лампа.

*** «*Wiek Nowy*» — львівська польськомовна газета, що виходила в період 1901–1939 рр.

починалися вже в останній декаді березня, а цьогоріч весна добряче забарилася...».

— Якщо тільки Господь буде добрим, — пошепки повторив ад'юнкт.

Йому часто доводиться бувати в таких дільницях Львова, про які Господь, здається, зовсім забув. А може, ніколи й не пам'ятав. Наостанок залишив собі кримінальну хроніку. Передивився уважно, хоча, звісна річ, знав набагато більше, ніж там було написано. На окремій шпальті, де містилися виключно міжнародні новини, встиг помітити повідомлення, що «в Росії вбито одного з лідерів революції, православного попа Георгія Гапона. Сталося це, правдоподібно, ще в березні, але кореспонденти з-за кордону дізналися про це лиш тепер...», коли за спиною почулася чиясь надміру гучна розмова.

Самковський спочатку вирішив не зважати. Для будь-якої кнайпи — звична річ, коли хтось, перебираючи зайвого, починає горланити. Однак тут його увагу привернув предмет розмови. Грубий підхмелілий голос розповідав, як 1894 року зумів утекти з поїзда, що перевозив ув'язнених.

— Але ж як, до ясної холєри, вдалося вивалити ті вагонні двері? — допитувався у нього співрозмовник.

— Кажу ж, Грумм їх підірвав, — роздратовано відповів бас, — цей скурвисин може змайструвати вибухівку з чого завгодно. Навіть з мотлоху під ногами. Навіть з лайна!..

— І що, ви стрибнули на ходу? Ти й він?

— Ми разом, майже одночасно. А з нами ще троє відчайдухів...

— А чого було не влаштувати вибух на якій-небудь станції. Під час зупинки?

— Здурів? Ну, гримне... А далі що? На станціях купа дідів і янців![*]

На якийсь час ці двоє замовкли, й чути було тільки голосне ковтання, з яким вони відправляли до нутра пиво.

Самковський не належав до числа сміливців, але і боягузом не був. Такі зазвичай не кидаються сторчголов у вир небезпеки, проте якщо вже доля кидає виклик, то знаходять у собі відвагу його прийняти. Ад'юнкт допив решту горілки й, витягнувши з кишені хустинку, протер чоло й окуляри.

— Чув, що тих трьох спіймали, — продовжилася тим часом розмова.

— Спіймали одного, — виправив бас, — двоє інших зламали собі карк... Грумм також добряче покалічився. А я родився в сорочці! Завдав його собі на рамена й поніс.

— Куди поніс?

— Куди очі світили... Знайшли якусь порожню гавіру[**], там пересиділи... А потім добрі люди допомогли перейти кордон.

Язик мовця заплітався, і балаканина, здавалося, от-от увірветься, проте розпитувач не здавався:

— А повернувся ти чого, Берле?

— Як то чого? — спалахнув той. — Як то чо-г-о-о-о?.. Я тут народився! Це моє місто!..

— Тебе тут замкнути можуть... Вас із Груммом досі шукають!

---

* На злодійському жаргоні кінця XIX — початку XX століття «дід» (пол. *dziad*) — означало «поліціянт», «янцьо» (пол. *jancio*) — «солдат», «жовнір».

** Гавіра (пол. *Hawira*) — хата, будинок (*злод. жарг.*).

— Е-е-е, ні! — загрозливо протягнув він. — До Відня я більше не піду*. І Грумма не візьму до млину**. Ми з ним тепер, як брати... А тих скурвисинів, що за нами полюють, я голими руками... Я їх, курва, душитиму...

Самковський підвівся й повернувся до них обличчям, перед тим помітивши, що господар стояв за шинквасом блідий, наче місяць удень, і короткими жестами спілкувався з принишклими клієнтами, очевидно, намагаючись пояснити їм ситуацію. Співрозмовник Берла поволі встав і залишив утікача самого за столом. Самковський сів замість нього. Спільник Грумма виявився здоровилом з чорною густою бородою, що ховала пів обличчя. Одразу над нею були горбатий ніс і пара чорних важких очей. Ці очі глипнули на худорлявого, трохи сутулого незнайомця в окулярах, обмацали його субтельні риси, високе чоло й недбало зачесане темно-русяве волосся. Самковський мав ледве за тридцять, тож воно в нього було ще без сивини й залисин.

— Даруйте, підслухав ненароком вашу розмову, — ад'юнкт раптово відчув, що від його хвилювання не залишилось і сліду. Тепер він був упевненим в собі, мовби за спиною мав усіх ад'юнктів, комісарів і надкомісарів з Дирекції, а за дверима кнайпи чатували з десяток офіцерів та унтерофіцерів військово-поліційної служби. Насправді ж сподіватися Самковський міг тільки на себе і свій старий службовий револьвер у кишені.

— А ти що за ґаврук*** один?

— Щирий ваш шанувальник, — відповів

---

* «Піти до Відня» — означало «піти до в'язниці» (*злод. жарг.*).

** «Взяти (спільника) до млину» — означало «видати поліції» (*злод. жарг.*).

*** Ґаврук (пол. *gawruk*) — могло означати «пан», «особа», «тип» (*злод.*

ад'юнкт, — подивляюся з ваших пригод.

— Думаєш, юри стругаю*?

— Боже збав! Я вам вірю. Але хотілося б почути більше.

— Замов мені гари**, — видихнув Берл.

Самковський подав знак Зайґельту, і той, швидко наповнивши дві чарки, поставив їх перед ними на стіл. Утікач випив одним духом свою порцію, тоді втер бороду і, стиснувши свій велетенський кулак, підсунув його співрозмовнику під ніс.

— Ось цією рукою одним ударом я розлупив його довбешку, як гнилий гарбуз, — промовив Берл.

— Чию? — перепитав Самковський, про всяк випадок відсовуючись на деяку відстань.

— Того діда на кордоні, що збирався мене затримати.

— Ти вбив поліціянта? — перепитав ад'юнкт, відчуваючи, як у горлянці в нього пересохло, а серце збільшилось до розмірів легенів і калатало тепер, наче церковний дзвін.

— І не одного, — стишивши голос, проказав утікач. — Я б інакше сказав...

— Як? — прохрипів Самковський.

— Я б сказав: «І не останнього»... І не останнього, курва!

На цих словах бородань зайшовся гучним п'яним реготом, який, щоправда, несподівано урвався на найвищій ноті, коли той помітив у руках Самковського націлений на нього револьвер.

— Це що таке? — запитав він, мовби вперше в житті

жарг.).

* Стругати (пол. *strugać jur*) — брехати (*злод. жарг.*).

** Гара (пол. *hara*) — ґорілка (*злод. жарг.*).

бачив зброю.

— Вставай, — коротко наказав ад'юнкт, — ти під арештом.

— То ти сраний хатрак*, — здивовано промовив Берл, миттю тверезіючи.

— Можеш випити й мою чарку наостанок, — поліціянт вказав поглядом на свою порцію горілки, до якої не торкнувся.

— Стерво! — раптом загорланив Берл і, перш ніж Самковський зрозумів, що коїться, підняв край столу догори й пхнув його на поліціянта.

Гримнуло два постріли з револьвера, проте перша куля влучила в стільницю, навряд чи діставшись крізь неї до злочинця, а друга — кудись у стелю.

— Затримати його! Затримати злочинця! — кричав Самковський, намагаючись вибратися з-під важкого дубового столу. Проте ніхто його не послухав. Усе тому, що за спиною ад'юнкта були не поліціянти, а вечірні відвідувачі «Тлустої риби», вкрай розімлілі від пива й горілки.

Звівшись нарешті на рівні ноги, Самковський щодуху кинувся до відчинених дверей, крізь які, очевидно, хвилину тому втік Берл. Однак несподівано відчув, що втрачає рівновагу, ніби хтось підставив йому ногу. Останнє, що побачив ад'юнкт, — брудну зачовгану підлогу просто в себе перед носом. Після цього страшенно заболіло трохи вище потилиці, і світло перед очима згасло.

Коли прийшов до тями, то найперше почув стишені голоси, чоловічий і жіночий. Чоловічий давав лікарські настанови, а жіночий тільки промовляв короткі фрази:

---

* Хатрак (пол. *chatrak*) — поліційний агент (*злод. жарг.*).

«так, пане лікарю», «добре, пане лікарю», «скільки крапель, пане лікарю?» тощо.

— І чоло йому протирайте. У воду можете додати трішки оцту, — почув ад'юнкт.

— Зрозуміла, пане лікарю. Ой, гляньте...

Вигук, очевидно, був пов'язаний з тим, що ад'юнкт раптом поворухнув головою і закліпав очима.

— А, з поверненням, *mein Freund**, — уже трохи гучніше сказав лікар.

Самковський розплющив очі, але через те, що був без окулярів, бачив украй погано. Втім, достатньо, щоб впізнати силует поліційного лікаря Ебергарда Фельнера. Точніше, поліційного патологоанатома...

— Невже я вмер, і ви робите мені розтин? — запитав ад'юнкт, відчуваючи, що слова ледь вдається видушити з себе, наче риб'ячі кістки, що застрягли в горлянці.

Фельнер засміявся.

— Жартуєте, Самковський, — промовив він. — Що ж, це добре... Ні, ви живий-живісінький, і я не маю жодного бажання зазирати вам усередину.

— Тут десь є мої окуляри?

— Ох, прошу вибачення...

Фельнер за мить насадив Самковському на носа його «додаткові очі». Ліве око бачило добре, а правому заважала дрібна павутина тріснутої лінзи.

— Окулярам також дісталося, — промовив лікар.

Все ж поліціянт тепер значно краще бачив його міцну присадкувату постать у білому халаті, накинутому поверх темно-сірого гарнітура, широке обличчя з крупним

---

* Мій друже (*нім.*).

носом, акуратно підстриженою бородою і окулярами, значно масивнішими, ніж у нього. Волосся Фельнер мав кучеряве і всуціль сиве, проте воно міцно трималося черепа, на заздрість тим, хто в його віці — а доктору було під шістдесят — мав голову лису, як військова каска.

Самковський крутнув головою, шукаючи своїм єдиним видючим оком володарку ніжного голосу, якій Фельнер давав розпорядження, проте від різкого руху в цьому самому оці потемніло від болю.

— Не вертіться, дідько б вас узяв! — сердито промовив лікар і заходився поправляти йому компрес десь на маківці. — Ще бодай кілька днів мусите рухатися повільно, як канатоходець над прірвою. Затямте це.

— Що зі мною сталося? — запитав Самковський, переводячи погляд з доктора на бридко-зелену стіну за його спиною, а потім на сіру, місцями пожовклу стелю.

— Хтось добряче вперіщив вас по потилиці чимось важким, — відповів Фельнер, — усе, що можу наразі сказати.

— Як це «хтось»? — Самковський відчув, як обличчя його багряніє від обурення, — у кнайпі була купа свідків...

— Юначе, — перебив його доктор, — ви, мабуть, забули, що я не слідчий і не постерунковий! Переказую те, що чув, коли мені вас доставили сюди непритомного. Думаю, невдовзі до вас прийде хто-небудь з Академічної, от його й розпитаєте.

— Було б добре, щоб прийшли зараз, — вже спокійнішим тоном, в якому чулося більше прохання, ніж ствердження, сказав ад'юнкт, — я маю повідомити дещо важливе в Дирекцію.

Фельнер відхилив полу халата, за якою зблиснув

срібний годинниковий ланцюжок, що тягнувся від борта піджака до кишені. Доктор дістав годинника і перевірив час.

— Заледве восьма, — промовив він, — але, гадаю, це не проблема.

— Восьма вечора? — перепитав Самковський.

— Восьма ранку, — всміхнувся Фельнер, — сутичка в кнайпі сталася вчора. *Morgenstund hat Gold im Mund**.

Доктор був галицьким німцем**, родом десь з-під Злочова***, тому рідною німецькою послуговувався часто і залюбки. Попри те, ніколи не приховував, що має насправді «жидівське походження».

— Отже, я пролежав тут цілу ніч?

— Виходить, що так. Але, погодьтеся, краще тут, ніж у морзі.

Самковский стрепенувся від цього жарту, як від укусу.

— Зосю, люба, — доктор з несподіваним теплом у голосі звернувся до своєї асистентки, — спустіться, будь ласка, вниз до телефонного апарата. Зателефонуйте в Дирекцію і повідомте, що пан ад'юнкт прийшов до тями. Нехай пришлють когось.

— Так, пане докторе, — почув Самковський ту саму фразу. Вона пролунала в нього десь над лівим вухом, отже, Зося сиділа біля його голови. Почулося, як вона підвелася зі стільця й рушила до дверей. Цього разу ад'юнкт

---

* Хто рано встає, тому Бог дає (*нім.*).

** У Галичині у XVIII столітті виникло понад сто німецьких колоній. Німецькі робітники переселялися сюди на запрошення імператора Йосифа II в рамках його аграрної політики. Під Злочовим (Золочевим) існувало поселення Унтервальден (нім. *Unterwalden*).

*** Злочів (пол. *Złoczów*), або Золочів — місто на Львівщині.

вирішив усе-таки її побачити. Втім, доки повертав до неї зболену голову, асистентка вийшла. Самковський встиг зауважити лише тендітну постать у білому з дурнуватим сестринським чепчиком на голові.

— А доки хтось доповзе сюди з Академічної, дуже рекомендую вам поспати, — озвався Фельнер, вимикаючи десь електричну лампу.

Світла в палаті поменшало. Штори на вікнах тут розтуляти, видно, було не заведено.

— Зовсім я не хочу спати, — промовив ад'юнкт і одразу ж після сказаного провалився в пекучу дрімоту.

Розплющивши очі знову, Самковський побачив перед собою тонку пелену диму. В ніздрі вдарив запах тютюну. У палаті, крім Фельнера, був ще хтось, кому доктор описував стан пацієнта:

— ...струс мозку, тому дайте йому бодай тиждень, — долинуло до його вух.

— Курва, в Дирекції й так бракує рук! — розпачливо відповів співрозмовник.

Самковський спочатку впізнав голос, а вже потім зрозумів, що ці двоє говорили німецькою.

— Пане директоре, — промовив він, спираючись на лікті й надіваючи на носа свої напіврозбиті окуляри, й вдруге за сьогодні почув:

— О, з поверненням, Самковський.

Фельнер та директор і далі сиділи собі за столом навпроти нього, тільки винувато загасили цигарки, ніби школярі, яких застукали за курінням у класі. Вільгельм Шехтель, начальник львівської поліції, був схожої з доктором статури, але, на противагу до нього, лисий і з виразним черевцем.

— Як почуваєтеся? — запитав він у підлеглого, хоча відповідь була написана в ад'юнкта на блідому виснаженому обличчі.

— Вам треба нові окуляри, — зазначив він ще за якусь мить.

— Головне, що не знадобиться новий череп, — промовив Фельнер, — його власний, на щастя, вцілів.

— Пане директоре, чи впіймали того типа, якого я хотів арештувати? — запитав Самковський, пропускаючи повз вуха їхні зауваження.

— На жаль, ні, ад'юнкте, — відповів Шехтель. — Але ми взяли сучого сина, що вдарив вас по голові. Це його колишній співкамерник. Він поки мовчить, але, я певен, невдовзі заговорить і виведе нас на нього.

— Того здоровила називали якось на ім'я... Здається, його звали Берл, і він вихвалявся втечею...

Директор кивнув.

— Берл Брюкнер, ми вже встановили. Колись утік з поїзда разом із Карелом Груммом. Вас ще не було тоді в поліції. До речі, обидвох їх заарештував колись Вістович. У тисяча вісімсот дев'яносто п'ятому чи шостому році.

— Четвертому, — сказав Самковський. — Він назвав цей рік.

— У покидька добра пам'ять, — скривився Шехтель.

Ад'юнкт, розчарований до краю, поклав голову на подушку. Директор це, схоже, помітив.

— Не впадайте у відчай, — заспокоїв він підлеглого, — спіймаємо ми вашого Брюкнера. Якщо він повернувся до Лемберга, то ховатися йому особливо ніде. Усі спільники його давно по в'язницях.

Шехтель підійшов до його ліжка й поклав поруч на тумбу щось важке, загорнуте в брудно-білу шмату.

— Ваш револьвер, — промовив він і додав: — Цілком імовірно, що ви поранили Брюкнера. Ми знайшли кров на тому місці, де стояв цей скурвисин. Моя вам подяка, Самковський. Обіцяю, в поліції не забудуть ваш мужній вчинок.

— Спасибі, пане директоре, — ад'юнкт раптом відчув, що слова начальника додали йому сил.

— Відпочивайте, — по-батьківськи усміхнувся той. — Лікар каже, вам потрібно не менше тижня спокою...

— Я повернуся, щойно триматимусь на ногах, — пообіцяв ад'юнкт, — думаю, знадобиться значно менше часу.

— Гаразд, — кивнув Шехтель. — Будемо чекати. А наразі — на все добре.

Директор попрощався також із Фельнером, потиснувши йому руку й нагадавши про домовлену партію в шахи на наступних вихідних.

«У поліції не забудуть» — ця фраза тепер весь час крутилася в ад'юнкта в голові, доки врешті-решт не приспала його.

Наступного дня поліційний автомобіль відвіз Самковського додому, де, пролежавши ще добу під наглядом щиросердної домовласниці, пані Рози Абрекової, на третій день, як і обіцяв Шехтелю, з'явився на службу. Біль у голові більше не тривожив, і нудити перестало. Залишилося тільки це препаскудне відчуття слабкості, через яке навіть прості завдання, як-от піднятися вгору сходами, здавалися йому надважкими.

Настрій у Дирекції панував гнітючий. Звісна річ, в такій установі зазвичай небагато причин для радощів, проте сьогодні всюди, від місця чергового аж до їхнього з Вістовичем кабінету, напруга відчувалася майже фізично. Декотрі колеги стримано привітали його з одужанням, після чого хутко бралися до роботи. У місцях для куріння не було ні душі, запах кави ширився між поверхами за цілковитої тиші, мов привид, хоча в інші дні гучних розмов, балачок і просто галасу, який би долинав з кабінетів, не бракувало. Можливо, тому, що за кілька днів надходив Великдень, а отже, й працювати в Страсний тиждень нікому не хотілося... Самковський намагався пригадати, чи рік тому тут панувала така ж атмосфера, але жодних спогадів із пам'яті не виринуло.

Повітря в кабінеті було затхлим і важким. Зрештою, нічого дивного. Провітрювати було нікому. Не знімаючи плаща, ад'юнкт прочинив вікно і, сівши просто на свій стіл, кілька хвилин спостерігав за людською метушнею на Академічній: рота піхотинців місцевого гарнізону пройшла стройовим кроком кудись далі в бік Стежкової*, торговець кошиками, обвішаний своїм крамом, почвалав з площі до вулиці Фредра, прямуючи, либонь, до Галицького ринку. Нечисленний гурт студентів затримався на хвилину поруч скверу і, обмінявшись конспектами, подався далі до Університету**. Квіткарки з первоцвітами в кошиках неспішно пофалювали у зворотний бік — кудись до площі Ринок. Сніг усе більше танув, сміття з-під нього потроху прибирали, й міське життя ставало на наступне, весняне коло свого цілорічного обороту.

---

* Тепер — вулиця Саксаганського.

** У час розповіді Львівський університет розміщувався на теперішній вулиці Грушевського, поруч з тодішньою площею Фредра.

У двері постукали, й Самковський, відірвавшись від споглядання, вигукнув звичне в таких випадках «Прошу!». Зайшов черговий. Відмельдував, що за квадранс директор поліції чекає ад'юнкта у себе в кабінеті. «Це добре, — подумалося Самковському, — отже, має щось для мене...» Відповів черговому, що зрозумів, і глянув на годинник, аби точно відміряти час до авдієнції.

Шехтель прийняв його, сидячи за своїм столом, на якому височіло кілька стосів паперу, стояла переповнена попільничка, а поруч з нею — відкоркована пляшка коньяку.

— Вип'єте, Самковський? — одразу запитав директор.

Ад'юнкт відмовився. Пити алкоголь після недавніх пригод було ризиковано.

— Що ж, а я вип'ю... — промовив директор і, діставши звідкись з-під столу склянку, плеснув у неї порцію бурштинового трунку. — Гівняний день, — сказав Шехтель, зробивши довгий затяжний ковток, — гівнянішого й не вигадати... І це ледь не напередодні Великодня. І це за тиждень до приїзду в Лемберг міністра поліції...

Самковський стояв навпроти нього, все ще не розуміючи, про що йдеться.

— Ви не читали вранішніх газет? — здивовано запитав директор.

— Не встиг, — зізнався Самковський, — боявся спізнитися сьогодні на службу.

— Дарма, — відмахнувся Шехтель, роблячи наступний ковток, — ніхто б вам і слова не сказав...

Він витягнув з-під паперів свіжий випуск «*Kurjera Lwowskiego*» й простягнув його ад'юнктові.

— Ось, подивіться...

«Жорстоке вбивство поліціянта!» — виднівся заголовок одразу на першій шпальті.

«Вранці 13-го квітня неподалік станції Клепарів знайдено тіло 29-річного віцекапрала Симеона Шварца. Вбитий повертався додому після служби, коли ж зазнав нападу невідомого. Нападник завдав кілька смертельних поранень ножем або військовим багнетом, у тому числі вибрав бідоласі очі. Поліція просить зголоситися можливих свідків...» — прочитав далі Самковський.

— І де цей чортовий Вістович, коли він потрібен? — почулося зітхання директора. — Щоб його холєра взяла у тій відпустці...

Ця згадка про шефа неприємно вколола Самковського. Він повернув газету і, вирівнявшись, як жовнір, промовив:

— Я можу взятися за цю справу, пане директоре. Зрештою, я вже за неї взявся.

— Що ви маєте на увазі? — не зрозумів той.

— Дозвольте висловити припущення, що вбивця — це той самий Берл Брюкнер.

— Облиште ви цей свій протокольний тон, Самковський! — гримнув Шехтель. — Говоріть по-людському.

— Тоді у кнайпі я чув, як він обіцяв, що вбиватиме поліціянтів. Думаю, справа в помсті за себе й Грумма, — промовив ад'юнкт.

Директор помовчав якусь хвилину, дивлячись кудись у вікно, а тоді заговорив знову:

— Що ж, якщо дві справи можна об'єднати в одну — це, звісно, добре... Поцілити двох птахів одним каменем... Гаразд, ад'юнкте. Будете відповідальним слідчим. Вістович обіцяв повернутися в понеділок, 16-го. Якщо до того часу не впораєтеся, він вам допоможе... Тільки Великодня, як бачите, у вас цьогоріч не буде.

Самковський не стримав усмішки. Для нього не було гіршого покарання, як щороку на Різдво й Великдень вирушати на кілька днів додому, до рідного Дрогобича. У тісному будинку на Заваллє*, де, крім його пияка-батька і згорьованої матері, мешкало ще дві молодші незаміжні сестри і дванадцятирічний брат, ніколи не було по-родинному затишно.

Батько щоразу сідав за святковий стіл уже напідпитку. Він був поштарем, тож завжди мав привід вийти з дому, а вийшовши, не втрачав нагоди закласти за комір у якому-небудь дешевому генделику. Мати починала плакати через свою бідацьку долю, тицяючи пальцем на облізлі стіни, де-не-де порослі цвіллю, потріскані двері, а найголовніше — в бік порожньої спіжарки, де запасів лишалося на день-два. Батько не витримував і гримав на неї, щоб та замовкла. Після цього починали голосити сестри. А далі Антоні з братом підводилися з-за столу й виходили на подвір'я.

Самковський курив, а молодший Ігнацій пильно за ним стежив, ловлячи кожен рух, аж врешті наважувався попросити:

— Дай мені папіроску, Антосю.

Старший брат у відповідь вліплював тому потиличника.

— А більше нічого не хочеш?

— Ну, Анто-о-сю-у-у, — просив далі той, розтираючи забите місце.

---

* Заваллє — вулиця в Дрогобичі.

За кілька хвилин Самковський здавався й простягував йому свою викурену до половини цигарку.

— На, шмаркачу. Але швидко тягни, щоб з дому не побачили.

Малий тягнув у легені дим і одразу закашлювався.

— Яка ж міцна...

— А ти що думав? — підсміхався з нього ад'юнкт. — У поліції інших не курять.

— Піду, коли виросту, в поліцію, як ти, — повідомляв молодший.

— Ну, йди, — стенав плечима брат.

— Або до війська... Куди завгодно, тільки з цього пекла.

Самковський розумів його. Зараз батько постарів і вже трохи вгомонився. А раніше, повертаючись п'яним додому, вчиняв такий рейвах, що збігались сусіди.

— Добре, заберу тебе до Лемберга, — казав він малому й куйовдив йому чуприну.

— Обіцяєш? — перепитував той.

— Пф-ф, буду тут перед малим гівнюком обіцянками сипати.

— Ну, Анто-о-о-сю-у-у, — молодший починав нити, аж поки не отримував від брата виразне слово честі.

Врешті з будинку виходила мати й кликала їх назад до столу. Батько, мовляв, заспокоївся. «Заспокоївся» — означало, почав куняти за столом. Родина бралася до їжі, не зважаючи на нього, і лише тоді наставала коротка мить свята.

Саме тому, стоячи зараз перед директором поліції, Самковський повідомив, що може без проблем залишитись у Львові. «Шкода тільки малого, — подумалось йому, — він мене завжди чекає з нетерпінням. Але нічого, прийду після свят».

— Що ж, добре, — промовив Шехтель, встаючи з крісла.

Було видно, що така відповідь підлеглого припала йому до душі.

— Сьогодні зайдіть у канцелярію, — продовжив директор, — заберіть документи на отримання позачергової премії. Вчора я все підписав. Гроші вам зможуть видати десь через тиждень після Великодня. Ще через місяць якусь виплату зробить наша Страхова спілка...

— Дуже доречно, бо проїзд у трамваї дорожчає, — спробував пожартувати Самковський.

Директор, втім, не звернув уваги на цю репліку.

— Клопотатиму про ваше підвищення до комісара другого класу, але обіцяти не можу... Самі розумієте, доки хтось не піде на емеритуру або не вмре, місце не звільниться, — продовжив він.

Самковський кивнув. Звісно, він не вчора почав службу і з таким станом речей був добре ознайомлений.

— Втім, якщо розкриєте справу, для вас я переверну гори, — раптом сказав Шехтель. — І не тільки тому, що готуюся до приїзду міністра... Убито поліціянта. Для нас знайти вбивцю — справа честі.

Повторювати двічі не довелося. Вони попрощались, і Самковський вийшов з кабінету шефа.

«Що зробив би зараз Вістович?» — подумалось йому, проте ця думка одразу ж викликала роздратування. Ні, чорт забирай! Це його власне розслідування. І озиратися на шефа він не буде. Найпевніше, коли комісар повернеться, справу вже буде зроблено, і цей скурвисин Брюкнер сидітиме за ґратами, чекаючи на суд і повішання.

Самковський зайшов до свого кабінету, але тільки для того, щоб узяти плаща й капелюха. На якусь мить зупинився і, znявши окуляри, розтер вказівним пальцем червонуватий відбиток на носі. Нова оправа була важка, незручна і вдавлювалася в обличчя, мов середньовічна маска, призначена для покарань за підглядання чи пхання носа не в свої справи. Власне, за все, що було для поліціянта службовим обов'язком.

Ад'юнкт вирішив найперше вирушити до доктора Фельнера на Пекарську, де була міська мертвецька*. Фельнер, безумовно, встиг бодай поверхово дослідити труп жертви, отже, матиме що розповісти слідству. Навіть дещиця потрібної інформації могла б зараз допомогти.

Ад'юнкт намагався спершу зателефонувати доктору, проте в його кабінеті ніхто не піднімав слухавки. Тоді він попросив чергового підготувати службовий фіакр, прихопив нотатника, олівець і кілька вранішніх газет, аби перечитати їх по дорозі.

Газети подавали новину про жорстоке вбивство на Клепарові переважно однаково: «Загинув поліціант в чині віцекапрала», «Був добрим батьком, зоставив сиротами двох малолітніх дітей», «Убивцю не знайдено, жодних заяв у Дирекції не зробили», ліва преса, як-от «Робітник» та «Селянин», іронічно зауважувала, що і не знайдуть, бо «галицька поліція здатна хіба що розганяти мирні демонстрації трудящих і трусити їхні помешкання, шукаючи зброю та друковані видання з братньої Росії...». Самковський криво посміхнувся і заховав газети до кишені. Екіпаж зупинився біля «Царства мертвих» на Пекарській, як називав це місце сам Аїд-Фельнер.

---

* Мертвецька – морг.

Зрештою, це й було, мабуть, найкращим порівнянням. І не тільки тому, що тут зберігалися тіла небіжчиків. Низький коридор з бетонними стінами, який провадив до головних приміщень, ледь освітлювавсяількома лампами. Тиша, що панувала в ньому, давила на вуха, а сирість проникала під одяг і, здавалося, навіть під шкіру.

Самковський не знав достеменно, за якими дверима знаходиться кабінет Фельнера, тому зупинявся перед кожними, щоб прочитати на них таблички. Врешті, побачивши на одній з них напис «*Dr. Fehlner*», зітхнув з полегшенням і, вже збираючись смикнути за ручку, щоб відчинити, завмер. Зсередини кабінету почувся сміх. Спершу тонкий жіночий, потім хриплий чоловічий. Услід за цим — притишені голоси. Слова розчути було важко, але добре відчувалося збудження, з яким вони промовлялись.

Самковський спершу кашлянув кілька разів, а потім гучно постукав. Голоси затихли, проте почулось шурхотіння, наче хтось приводив до ладу одяг. За якийсь час зсередини повернувся ключ і двері відчинились. На порозі постав розчервонілий доктор Фельнер у картатій камізельці, сорочці з розтріпаним коміром і без краватки.

— Сам... Самковський? — здивовано витріщився він на прибулого. — Що ви тут робите?

— Я у справах слідства, — відповів той.

За плечима доктора промайнула жіноча постать у білому халаті.

— Але ви... Хіба ви... розслідуєте щось? — доктор говорив, бентежно озираючись назад, мовби господар, який не впевнений, чи в домі прибрано і чи можна пускати всередину гостя.

— Звісно, розслідую, — в ад'юнкта уривався терпець. — Директор призначив мене відповідальним слідчим у справі вбивства на Клепарові.

— Ах, ви про це... — доктор відступив нарешті, пропускаючи його досередини. — Бідолаха капрал, що тут скажеш.

— Віцекапрал, — виправив його Самковський і ґречно вклонився його асистентці, що ні в сих ні в тих сиділа на кріслі поруч столу. На столі поміж паперів стояла тарілка з над'їдженими канапками і кількома шматочками шоколаду. Поруч — дві порожні філіжанки.

— Зосю, зробіть гостеві кави, якщо ваша ласка, — звернувся Фельнер до помічниці.

Та схопилася з місця й випурхнула за двері. Зося! Самковський пам'ятав це ім'я. Саме цю жінку він намагався роздивитися, коли прийшов до тями в лікарняній палаті. Що ж, тепер це йому вдалося: невисока чорнявка, великі виразні очі, делікатний ніс і губи. Нижня прикушена, чи то від сорому, чи то від того, що асистентка стримувала сміх. На вигляд мала біля двадцяти п'яти або тридцяти років.

— Ви не подумайте нічого зайвого, Самковський... Я одружений чоловік, — пробелькотів Фельнер.

«Старий кнур», — подумав ад'юнкт, але промовив інше:

— Думаю, часу на каву в мене не буде, пане докторе.

— Як скажете, — з неприхованим полегшенням у голосі відповів той.

— Чи *мали ви час* обстежити тіло вбитого? — ад'юнкт, сам того не бажаючи, зробив у сказаному надто виразний і нескромний наголос.

Фельнер кивнув.

— Ходіть, я вам дещо покажу.

На цих словах чоловіки вийшли за двері, опинившись у тому самому бетонному коридорі, яким блукав ад'юнкт кілька хвилин тому.

— Зосю, кави не треба! — гукнув доктор, і голос його моторошно відлунився десь у темній порожнечі.

Вони пройшли коридором, далі звернули в якийсь лабіринт, де освітлення було трохи більше, проте стіни від цього не ставали привітнішими. Врешті опинилися перед дверима, до яких Фельнер довго шукав ключа у своїх кишенях. Знайшовши, видихнув з полегшенням і відчинив. Потім впевнено зайшов у темне приміщення, де намацав на стіні ручку вмикача. За мить яскраве світло залило невелику кімнату з двома столами посередині. На одному з них лежало тіло, вкрите простирадлом.

— Це так звана секційна, — діловим тоном сказав Фельнер, — тут я роблю розтини.

Він дістав з продовгуватої шафи халат і одягнув його, прибравши звичного для себе в цих стінах вигляду. Обличчя його також змінилося: перед Самковським тепер стояв не підстаркуватий Казанова, що забавляється з асистенткою, а добре знаний в Галичині судово-медичний експерт, фахівець своєї справи.

Фельнер відгорнув простирадло до половини. Небіжчик був без одягу, проте розтин ще не проводився.

— Смерть настала близько десятої вечора. Вбито ножем із широким лезом, який зазвичай мають мисливці, — почав доктор.

Самковський дістав блокнот і зробив першу нотатку.

— Удари було завдано згори, точно в шию... Судячи з усього, вбивця чималого зросту і доволі дужий...

— А це що, в біса, таке? — з жахом перепитав поліціянт, вказуючи пальцем на обличчя трупа.

Там, де в небіжчика мали бути очі, лишилися тільки дві чималі рани.

— Спосіб приховати сліди, — відповів доктор.

— Якийсь ритуал?

— Не зовсім.

— Тоді що?

Доктор важко зітхнув, наче йому довелося згадати щось мерзенне.

— Деякі вбивці переконані, що їхнє відображення залишається в очах жертви, як на фотографічній пластинці, — пояснив він. — Отже, його треба знищити. Я вже стикався з таким колись...

— Ніколи про таке не чув, — промовив ад'юнкт, повертаючись до своїх нотаток.

— Це ваша перша серйозна справа, чи не так, Самковський? — запитав раптом доктор.

Поліціянт кивнув у відповідь.

— Жаль, що зараз немає Вістовича, — додав Фельнер.

«Я дам раду і без вашого Вістовича!» — ледь не вирвалось у Самковського, проте ад'юнкт вчасно стримався.

— Мені відомо, хто вбивця, докторе, — сказав він натомість. — Цей огляд — лише формальність.

— Ну, коли так... — Фельнер знову накрив тіло простирадлом. — Коли так, то мені лишається тільки побажати вам успіху, пане ад'юнкте. Як зроблю розтин, пришлю результати вам на Академічну. Обіцяю, що не пізніше, ніж завтра.

Попрощавшись із ним, Самковський повернувся в Дирекцію, де піднявся до свого кабінету й кілька хвилин дозволив собі перепочити. Відчував жахливу слабкість. Наслідки травми ще давалися взнаки. Крім того, з пам'яті не йшов труп віцекапрала на столі в мертвецькій Фельнера.

Ад'юнкт відкинувся на спинку крісла й заплющив очі. Спробував розслабитись, але не вдалося. Йому раптом подумалось, як паскудно себе почувають зараз ті, що служать у військово-поліційній службі, адже загинув їхній безпосередній колега. Усі вони, від постерункового до капітана, очікують результатів розслідування. Хоча, по щирості, ці люди можуть зробити більше, аніж кримінальна поліція. Брюкнер може потрапити їм на око де-небудь на вулиці, поруч з борделем або дешевою кнайпою. Одразу після події в «Тлустій рибі» кожному постовому описали його портрет.

Врешті Самковський підвівся й знову спустився до чергового, наказавши йому привести в кімнату допитів затриманого спільника Берла. Спускаючись у підвал, ад'юнкт відчув, що тілом його пробігли крижані мурахи. Нутро переповнило дивне відчуття. Мовби суміш страху, злості й цікавості. Ще ніколи йому не доводилося провадити розмову з тим, хто не так давно ледь не проломив йому голову.

Нападника з кнайпи звали Альбертом Зарембою. Самковському спало на думку, що таке ім'я і прізвище могли б належати якому-небудь інженерові чи депутатові Галицького сейму, але натомість так звали пройдисвіта, який допоміг утекти злочинцю.

Утім, Заремба й був схожий радше на інтеліґента, що за повелінням долі чи власним невезінням опинився на дні суспільства. Поставу мав рівну, в очах світилася зверхність і насмішкуватість. Шкіра на обличчі й руках була, вочевидь, колись доглянутою, але тепер потріскалася і вкрилася дрібними виразками. Світло-руда щетина потроху переростала в недбалу бороду, а волосся, що також давно не знало руки перукаря, сягало плечей. На плечах висіла подерта камізелька поверх брудної картатої сорочки.

Двоє міцних поліціянтів пхнули його до кімнати й наказали сісти за стіл навпроти Самковського. Один із них — вусатий капрал без кітеля, в сорочці із закоченими рукавами — став за спиною Заремби, інший — молодий постерунковий — лишився біля дверей. В'язень несподівано посміхнувся, оголивши ряд жовтих зубів зі зламаними різцями.

— Як ваша голова, пане слідчий? — запитав він у Самковського.

Тієї ж миті капрал зацідив Зарембі кулаком у вухо. Той звалився під стіл і важко закректав. Тюремник вхопив його за комір і знову посадив на стілець.

— Дякую за турботу, як бачите, все гаразд, — спокійно відповів ад'юнкт.

Заремба все ще не міг оговтатися від удару, тому навряд чи почув його відповідь. Самковський знаком наказав капралові більше його не лупцювати. На якийсь час запанувала мовчанка, доки в'язень приходив до тями.

— А як вам тут ведеться? — запитав у нього Самковський.

Капрал іронічно гмикнув і схвально подивився на ад'юнкта. Потім перевів погляд на Зарембу.

— Файно, як у пансіоні, — процідив той у відповідь. Було видно, що ад'юнкт потрапив у десятку.

— Годують добре? — не вгавав Самковський.

— Аякже.

— Може, приносять забагато тлустого? Чи не слід переглянути ваш раціон? Адже ж піст...

Двоє поліціянтів реготнули. Самковський знав, що в цю мить його авторитет підскочив догори, а в курилках від сьогодні переповідатимуть ці його жарти. З якимсь диким завзяттям він тепер готовий був знищити людину навпроти. Не так через бажання помсти, як для того, аби ще більше ствердитись у жорсткому поліційному колективі.

Заремба кинув на нього погляд, сповнений ненависті.

— Чого вам треба? — запитав він.

Самковський кивнув капралові, й той виклав на стіл два чисті аркуші та олівець.

— Все, що вам відомо про Брюкнера, має бути відомо мені. Де може переховуватися, чи має спільників, де бере гроші, — чітко промовив Самковський. — Викладіть усе письмово. Мовби на уроці граматики, пане Зарембо... Що краще напишете, то кращу дістанете оцінку. З оцінки буде видно, як складуться ваші справи в подальшому.

— Як на уроці граматики? — в'язень скривив презирливу посмішку. — То, може, написати латиною? Ви знаєте латину, пане слідчий?

— Якщо знань моїх не вистачить, пане Зарембо, то я передам вас у руки кому-небудь менш терплячому... Скажімо, капралові Шимону. Не гарантую, що латину він знає краще, зате пояснить вам ваше становище значно зрозуміліше, ніж я.

— Моє становище? — спалахнув Заремба. — Яке, в біса, моє становище? Я винен тільки в тому, що вперіщив вас по голові. Таке трапляється у кнайпах. Ви були не на службі й випивали так само, як і я. Кілька місяців арешту або пів року яких-небудь громадських робіт — от і все, що мені загрожує.

Самковський дістав з кишені портсигар. Неквапно витягнув з нього цигарку й закурив.

— Щойно ви вдарили капрала Шимона, пане Зарембо, — холоднокровно проказав ад'юнкт, випускаючи перший струмінь диму.

Йому раптом подумалося, що саме таку тактику обрав би на його місці Вістович. Метод брудний, але ефективний... Що ж, комісар усі роки був для нього добрим учителем.

— Що? — обличчя в'язня почервоніло, а від зверхності, з якою він зайшов кілька хвилин тому до кімнати, не лишилося й сліду.

— Я сказав, ви щойно вдарили поліціянта, який стоїть поруч з вами, — повторив слідчий, вдруге затягуючись цигаркою.

— Я нікого не бив!

— Тут двоє свідків, які бачили, як ви підхопились і вперіщили капрала кулаком в груди. Правда, капрале?

— Саме так, пане ад'юнкте, — підтвердив той і театрально застогнав.

— Ось вам ще пів року, добродію, — повідомив Самковський.

— Ну ви й паскуди, — просичав Заремба.

— Потім ви кинулися на постерункового Вільху, — продовжив ад'юнкт, — і жорстоко почали його душити. Та у вас наче демон вселився! Ледве вдалося заспокоїти...

Самковський якийсь час мовчки курив, аж доки цигарка не перетворилася на недопалок. Ад'юнкт загасив його і, оскільки Заремба також не озивався, підвівся з-за столу.

— Бачу, писати ви не збираєтеся, — промовив слідчий. — У такому разі ставлю вам «*незадовільно*» і прощаюсь.

— Чекайте, — понуро вимовив той.

Самковський подивився на нього з удаваною байдужістю.

— Ви щось сказали? — перепитав він.

— Нехай ці двоє вийдуть, — Заремба кивнув на капрала й постерункового. — Писати я нічого не буду, краще розповім, але тільки вам. Ніхто інший не повинен чути.

Шимон спохмурнів і запитально подивився на Самковського. Той кивнув, віддаючи наказ. За хвилину двоє поліціянтів лишили їх сам на сам.

— Що ж, слухаю, — дещо настороженим голосом сказав ад'юнкт, щойно двері за ними зачинилися.

— Дайте цигарку, — попросив Заремба.

Обличчя його вже стратило червону барву і тепер вид мало спокійний, як на початку допиту.

Самковський знову витягнув з кишені портсигар і, відкривши його, поклав на стіл. Поруч кинув сірники. В'язень жадібно встромив одну цигарку до рота, а дві інші запхнув за вухо.

— Ви не заперечуєте? — перепитав він.

Слідчий похитав головою. Спостерігав якусь мить, як той затягується димом і блаженно відкидається на спинку стільця. Потім забрав свій портсигар, закрив і сховав до кишені.

— Бачу, як ви прагнете вислужитися, — промовив раптом Заремба. — Для вас ця справа не менш важлива, аніж для мене. Чи не так, пане Самковський?

— Схоже, я дарма витрачаю час і куриво, — відповів той, рвучко повертаючись до дверей.

— Я допоможу спіймати Брюкнера, — зупинив його в'язень. — Він довіряє мені. Зрештою, ви самі чули в тій кнайпі, що ми розмовляли дружнім тоном.

— Чув, — кивнув Самковський.

— Тоді я напишу йому листа. Повідомлю, що зібрав для нього певну суму грошей, але хотів би передати особисто. З рук в руки.

— Отже, в нього є адреса.

— Не адреса, пане Самковський, а так звана «поштова скринька». Місце, де ми залишаємо один одному листи...

Заремба відвів очі, ковзнув поглядом по брудних стінах, а тоді знову глянув на поліціянта.

— Коли Берл з'явиться на зустріч, схопите його, — додав він сухим здавленим голосом. — Мене ж натомість відпустите і, що найважливіше, знищите мою справу... Все, що є на мене в архіві.

Не кажучи ні слова у відповідь, Самковський підвівся, підійшов до дверей і постукав, даючи знати вартовим, що допит закінчено.

Близько сьомої вечора поліційний архіваріус приніс йому до кабінету папку з написом «Справа No 364 від 1894 року». Ад'юнкт розписався про отримання й зобов'язання повернути документи не пізніше, ніж за добу. Службовець архіву забрав розписку й полегшено зітхнув. Його зміна закінчилася, і подумки, очевидно, він уже вибудовував плани на вечір.

Самковський же нікуди не збирався. Відчував, як докучає голод, але вирішив залити в порожній шлунок порцію кави. Їсти на якийсь час перехочеться, і можна буде спокійно попрацювати.

«Справа No 364» стосувалася арешту двох підривників-убивць: Карела Грумма і Берла Брюкнера. Слідство провадив комісар другого класу Адам Вістович за поміччю військово-поліційної служби, яка, зі свого боку, запросила в армії дві роти піхотинців. Обох злочинців було взято на гарячому просто в центрі Львова під час спроби пограбування Галицької Ощадної Каси. Кількох їхніх спільників було вбито. Двом вдалося втекти. Поранено поліційного фельдфебеля і одного солдата.

Організатором цього та ряду інших злочинів указувався Карел Грумм. Виходець із Богемії, інженер. Людина чималої фізичної сили й розуму. Брюкнер був помічником. Хитрим, жорстоким і цілковито йому відданим. Зазначалося, що народився й мешкав цей суб'єкт у Львові, на Замарстинові. Батьки рано померли, будинок згорів, коли той служив у війську. Більше жодних притомних даних про нього Самковський не знайшов.

Остання сторінка справи містила в собі невелике досьє про Альберта Зарембу. Лікаря за освітою й симпатика лівих радикальних рухів...

Самковський скривив посмішку. От звідки, виявляється, його псевдоінтеліґентність і знання латини. За прикладом російських революціонерів Альберт вважав, що здобуття коштів через експропріацію для блага справи — спосіб допустимий і необхідний. Це й привело його в спілку зі злочинцями. За допомогу в пограбуваннях ті обіцяли йому частку. Так принаймні стверджували затримані, але на суді причетність лікаря довести не вдалося.

«Що ж, — подумав Самковський, — теоретично, в Зареmби може бути зуб на Грумма й Брюкнера, якщо ті справді свідчили проти нього в суді».

Після ще однієї чашки кави і коротких роздумів ад'юнкт впевнено вирвав з папки його сторінку і, склавши учетверо, заховав до кишені. Поруч лежала інша підшивка — актуальна справа Альберта Заремби, нападника на поліціянта Антоні Самковського у кнайпі «Тлуста риба» на Підзамчому. Взявши її, він вийшов з кабінету і знову рушив у кімнату для допитів.

Заремба його чекав, сидячи за столом. Перед ним лежав складений удвоє листок. Очевидно, з написаним усередині текстом.

Ті самі капрал і постерунковий отримали від Самковського наказ вийти за двері.

— Не збагну, що приваблює таких людей, як ви, у цих кровожерних лівих ідеях, — промовив він, кладучи перед в'язнем його справу і вирваний з архівної справи листок.

— «Чимало є, Гораціо у світі, що неспроможна мудрість осягнути...»* — відповів той. — Бачу, ви уважно прочитали мою справу.

— Там про вас небагато.

— І все ж, я волів би, щоб і цього не було.

Заремба потягнувся до принесених паперів і з цікавістю їх переглянув.

— Я дуже ризикую, ідучи на змову з вами, — промовив раптом Самковський загрозливим тоном, якого навіть сам від себе не сподівався. — Тому, якщо підведете мене,

* Цитата з трагедії В. Шекспіра «Гамлет, принц данський».

стрілятиму вам просто в лоба. Чи будь-куди... Але не сумніватимусь і не схиблю.

Якусь мить вони дивились один одному в очі.

— Я також ризикую, ад'юнкте. І повірте, якщо припущуся помилки, то мене очікує значно важча кара, ніж куля з поліційної зброї, — холодно відповів Заремба. — Утім, — продовжив він вже піднесено, — впевнений, усе вдасться. Вже завтра ви схопите Брюкнера й отримаєте схвалення начальства. Вас підвищать, чи не так, Самковський?..

— Покажіть лист, — перебив ад'юнкт.

— Прошу, — з якоюсь байдужістю в голосі проказав той і простягнув йому складений папір.

Самковський розгорнув аркуш і прочитав коротке послання: «Маю ґельди*. Приходь завтра. Випив кварту».

— Це все? — здивовано перепитав ад'юнкт.

— Повірте, Самковський, там більше інформації, ніж ви можете собі уявити, — посміхнувся в'язень.

— Що за «Випив кварту»?

— Означає, що мене відпустили.

Поліціянт все не міг відірвати очей від листа, мовби шукав у ньому прихований зміст. Його не покидало відчуття нерівноцінності обміну. Він видер з архіву усі дані про нього, вчинив, фактично, злочин. А цей тип у відповідь написав кілька слів.

— Мою актуальну справу ви мені також віддаєте? — запитав в'язень.

— Звісно, ні, — Самковський рішуче схопив зі столу папери.

— Але знищите її?

---

* Ґельди (пол. *geldy*) — гроші (*злод. жарг.*).

— Щось придумаю після того, як Брюкнер буде в нас. Заремба нервово пожував губами.

— Ну, гаразд. Повірю вам.

— Коли ви плануєте віднести листа до «поштової скриньки»? — запитав поліціянт.

— Найкраще сьогодні. Хтось від Брюкнера перевіряє її щоночі.

— Тобто не він сам?

— Звісно, ні, Самковський, — до Заремби повернувся його насмішкуватий тон, і він говорив тепер з ад'юнктом, як із дурником. — Це надто небезпечно для нього. Зазвичай відправляє туди когось...

— Гаразд, а що значить «приходь завтра»? Це о котрій? — поліціянт не стримував роздратування і говорив, мабуть, голосніше, ніж слід було.

— Між четвертою і шостою, — відповів Заремба, — саме тоді вам слід влаштувати на нього засідку...

— Пора самогубців, — вирвалось у Самковського.

— Пора обережних людей, — виправив його співрозмовник, — у такий час украй рідко хтось вештається навіть там, де знаходиться «поштова скринька».

— І де ж вона знаходиться?

— У покинутій броварні на Погулянці.

— А точніше?

— Вам не потрібно знати точніше, ад'юнкте, — сказав раптом Заремба, — тому що лист я повинен віднести сам.

Чоловіки знову стрілися поглядами.

— Ми про це не домовлялися, — зазначив Самковський.

— Якби ви трохи задіяли ваші мізки, пане слідчий, то допетрали б самі, що за тим місцем, а також за кожним, хто туди приходить, можуть стежити, — відповів Заремба, — у Берла завжди були спільники. І не виключено, що є й тепер. Якщо з'явлюсь я, жодних сумнівів у нього не виникне.

Ад'юнкт відчув, як усе його тіло кинуло в піт. Якусь мить, знявши з носа свої незручні окуляри, він протирав їх давно непраною хустинкою. Закінчивши з цим, повернув їх на місце, але відвернувся від Заремби, щоб подумати без його притиску. Хоч насправді думати вже не було про що. Зважившись на таку небезпечну гру, слід було йти до кінця. Одне тільки нестерпно гризло свідомість — усе це він робить без дозволу начальства, таємно. Власне, знову так, як зробив би його шеф. Чи вагався б Вістович? Можливо. Але точно не пасував би, зробивши такі високі ставки. Комісар ішов би ва-банк.

— Гаразд, — видихнув Самковський. — Сьогодні опівночі виїдемо на Погулянку.

В'язень кивнув.

— Де у вас відбуваються зустрічі? — запитав ад'юнкт.

— Не надто далеко звідти, на правому березі Пасіки*. Найкраще буде облаштуватися там вже о третій. Місцина малоприємна: гнила й багниста, але довкола чимало корчів і пагорбів. Ваші люди матимуть де сховатися...

За кілька хвилин Самковський вийшов з кімнати допитів і розпорядився, щоб Зарембу протримали там до одинадцятої. Сам вирішив повечеряти в якомусь із найближчих локалів або ресторацій. Найкраще з огляду на ціни й розміщення пасував «Локаль Шнайдера». Йти

* Один з міських потоків, що впадає в річку Полтву. Більша частина Пасіки, як і Полтви, в межах міста протікає тепер підземними колекторами.

було заледве дві-три хвилини, а добра горохівка з кавалком хліба, помащеним смальцем і складеними на ньому кружальцями цибулі, коштувала п'ятнадцять гелерів. Ще за двадцять можна було замовити чарку «Варшавської» чи «Балабанівки», але пити сьогодні було ризиковано. Перед такою ніччю краще мати свіжу голову.

З'ївши вечерю, Самковський довго курив за столиком, а кельнер, очікуючи, що той замовить випивку, крутився довкола, як муха. Врешті, на подив офіціанта, клієнт попросив принести йому міцну каву і новий випуск «*Gazety Wieczornej*». Знову на першій же сторінці йшлося про вбивство віцекапрала Симеона Шварца: «Мусимо визнати перед нашими чительниками ту прикрість, що жодних новин від поліції ми не отримали. Повідомлено тільки, що слідство очолив досі незнаний громадськості пан Антоні Самковський, що має чин ад'юнкта. Рішення ц.к. Дирекції видається нам дивним, бо до такої справи мав би бути залучений слідчий на посаді щонайменше комісара. А те, що інші детективи зайняті, навряд чи може слугувати виправданням...».

Самковський стиснув кулаки від злості, трохи зім'явши краї шпальти, втім, змусив себе дочитати статтю. Далі в ній переповідали обставини, за яких було знайдено тіло поліціянта, а наприкінці матеріалу автор ставив уїдливе питання: «Тож чи можемо ми, звиклі громадяни свого міста, почуватися безпечно, якщо бачимо безпорадність поліції? Чи має нас заспокоювати лише те, що постерункові сьогодні ходять і їздять кінно по троє, маючи при собі карабіни?».

— Можна подумати, що від убивства минув тиждень, — тихо проказав Самковський, — сучі діти ці писаки. Всі, як один...

Була тим часом уже восьма. Заплативши за вечерю, ад'юнкт вийшов з «Локалю Шнайдера» й подався знову в Дирекцію. Скоро починалися зміни в тих, кого він вибрав собі в помічники для нічної акції. Лишався час, аби переговорити з ними, ще раз все обдумати й підготувати зброю.

Альберт Заремба мав спокійний вигляд. Намагався навіть жартувати. Чи то щоб підбадьорити поліціянтів, чи то щоб укотре вколоти Самковського. Той врешті наказав йому стулити пельку і сісти в поліційний фургон. Виїхати вирішили з господарського двору Дирекції, щоб не притягувати зайвої уваги ані перехожих, ані начальства, оскільки хтось із зверхників міг затриматися до такої пізньої години.

Була одинадцята. Фургон викотився на Баторія*, відтак попри безлюдний Галицький ринок, перетнувши Панську**, в'їхав на Пекарську.

Коли, як можна було припустити, вони минали «Царство Мертвих» доктора Фельнера, Самковський не втримався й визирнув у шибку екіпажу. Звісна річ, розгледіти йому вдалося тільки самотній гасовий ліхтар, що розсіював довкола себе невеликий конус тьмяного світла. Ад'юнкт, проте, знав, що ліхтар стоїть поруч металевої огорожі. За нею парк Медичного університету, на теренах якого знаходиться мертвецька. Як не дивно, але пригадався йому в цю мить не Фельнер і навіть не вбитий віцекапрал, котрого той вже, мабуть, розітнув, щоб до ранку передати в Дирекцію свій остаточний висновок. Самковський подумав

---

* Тепер – вулиця Князя Романа.

** З 1871 року до 1929-го так називалась частина теперішньої вулиці Франка – від площі Соборної до повороту на Зелену.

про Зосю. Чи справді вона віддається тому хтивому стариганю-доктору просто в його кабінеті? Чи не заважає їй думка, що поруч з ними лежать мертвяки? Цікаво, як вона це робить? Задирає халат, спідницю, знімає білизну, сідає на стіл і розсуває ноги? Чи їй зручніше на той стіл спиратися ліктями, дозволяючи доктору брати її ззаду? *A tergo**, як пишуть у книжках з медицини. Ад'юнкт мусив прикусити нижню губу, щоб через біль позбутися несподіваної ексцитації.

— ...коли підніму руку, ніби збираюся поправити на голові капелюха, — долинуло до нього тільки закінчення фрази, яку промовив Заремба, що сидів навпроти, затиснутий з обох боків поліціянтами.

— Прошу вибачення, я не почув, — промовив Самковський, — трясе...

— Кажу, підете на Брюкнера в той момент, коли підніму догори руку, — повторив в'язень, — буде схоже, ніби я хочу поправити на голові капелюха. Місяць сьогодні у повні, ви добре будете мене бачити. Тим більше, на руках з-під пальта в мене виступають білі манжети.

— Гаразд, — відповів ад'юнкт.

Тепер уже роздивитися дорогу в шибці спробував Заремба.

— Чи орієнтуєтеся, де ми знаходимось, пане слідчий? — запитав він. Схоже, він занервував.

— Наближаємось до кладовища на Личакові, — відповів хтось із поліціянтів.

— Отже, ще трохи... — сказав в'язень і захрускотів пальцями.

---

* Ззаду (*лат.*).

— Припиніть, — сказав йому Самковський, і до самої Погулянки вони їхали вже мовчки.

Фургон зупинився в понурому місці, між кладовищем і руїнами старої вілли. Повний місяць, що вигулькував час від часу з-за хмар, витягував сірі тіні людей, запряжених коней і предметів, надаючи їм гостроти й химерності. Далі починався ліс, що був колись парком, проте останні кілька років здичавів. Лише в теплу пору на Погулянці облаштовували літні ресторації та розчищали місця для променадів, а на трав'яних галявинах — для гри в копаного м'яча.

Втім, до тепла ще було довго. Чоловіки, що повиходили з фургона — двоє поліціянтів, візник, ад'юнкт і Заремба, — одразу ж почали хукати собі на руки й розтирати щоки. Було до біса холодно. Хтось чиркнув сірником, закурив, присвітивши одночасно циферблат годинника.

— Пів до півночі, — промовив хриплий голос.

— Можна йти, — сказав на це Заремба, — дістанусь туди рівно в дванадцятій.

— Ліхтар потрібен? — перепитав Самковський.

— Ні, тільки заважатиме. Я добре знаю цю місцину.

Якусь хвилину всі мовчали.

— Зніміть з мене кайданки, — сказав нарешті в'язень, — чи ви думаєте, я піду зі скутими руками?

Поліціянти звернули обличчя до Самковського, чекаючи його наказу.

— Що ж, Зарембо, востаннє нагадую, — видихнув ад'юнкт, — якщо обдуриш, тобі кінець.

— За годину повернуся, — коротко відповів той.

— Зніміть кайданки, — наказав слідчий.

Брязнули ключі в руках одного з конвоїрів. Інший націлив на нього зброю. Невдовзі скрипнув замок, і звільнений Заремба з приємністю розтер зап'ястя. Потім, не кажучи ні слова, зник у темряві.

— Довіряєте йому, шефе? — запитав поліціянт, закидаючи кайданки до фургона.

— Хочу довіряти, — відповів той.

— Начальство з вас шкуру здере, якщо він одурить...

Ад'юнкт не відповів. Звісно, що здере. І не одну.

Втім, Заремба повернувся. Не минуло й години, як його постать виникла з темряви і наблизилася до поліціянтів. Коні, досі запряжені у фургон, стривожено зафиркали, відірвавшись від мішків з вівсом.

— Ну, все, — промовив прибулий, заспокоюючи дихання, — лист я залишив.

Самковський зітхнув з полегшенням. Щось навіть схоже на радість зігріло його серед весняного холоду. Інші ж поліціянти, здавалося, навіть не зауважили цього повернення. Вони сердито тупцювали на місці й без упину курили, мовби намагаючись зігрітися теплом від цигарки.

— Їдемо назад, — наказав Самковський, — зігріємось і повернемся сюди за дві години.

Ніхто, ясна річ, не заперечував.

Коли о третій ночі фургон зупинився на тому ж місці, нічний краєвид мовби змінився. Місяць піднявся вище, від чого тіні покоротшали. Жоден з чоловіків не зронив ані слова. Двоє конвоїрів тепер мали на плечі карабіни, а Самковський тримав у руках службового «Штаєра»*.

Заремба впевнено повів їх уздовж Пасіки, чиї води ледь чутно шелестіли зовсім поряд. Понад чверть години вони йшли стежкою, а потім звернули кудись у хащі,

* Штаєр (нім. *Steyr*) — самозарядний пістолет, розроблений в Австро-Угорщині наприкінці XIX ст.

з кожним кроком глибоко провалюючись у торішнє й позаторішнє листя. В'язень жодного разу не зупинився, ані щоб перепочити, ані щоб звірити дорогу. Йшов так, мовби навпомацки розрізняв кожне дерево й кущ.

Врешті біля поваленого граба, чиє гігантське коріння стриміло в темряві, мов змії на голові Медузи*, їхній провідник підняв догори півзігнуту руку й знаком наказав принишкнути. Потім підкликав до себе ад'юнкта.

— Ось там ми зустрінемося з Берлом, — пошепки промовив Заремба, вказуючи пальцем перед собою, де за десяток метрів, трохи нижче від їхньої схованки, виднівся берег потічка з чималим насипом каміння. — Зараз я піду туди й буду чекати. Не зводьте з мене очей, Самковський. А своїм людям накажіть сидіти тихо і не курити. У Брюкнера нюх, як у звіра. Зачує щось — і все пропало.

Ад'юнкт протер окуляри, уважно роздивився вказане місце і кивнув у відповідь.

— Коли подам знак, миттю на нього кидайтеся. Не зволікайте ні секунди, — продовжив Заремба. — Такого, як він, можна взяти, тільки заскочивши зненацька. Тікати Брюкнер зможе лише вгору, вздовж потічка. Іншої дороги для втечі немає, тож ви й ваші люди матимете безсумнівну перевагу...

Самковський з подивом помітив, що в'язень перехрестився. Лівак і злочинець виявився віруючим католиком.

— Чувайте, — повторив він і рушив на місце зустрічі.

Поліціянти прикипіли очима до його постаті, що скрадливо спустилася до потічка і завмерла, стоячи посеред німого темного каміння. Хвилина йшла за хвили-

* Медуза — в античній міфології — чудовисько зі зміями на голові.

ною, доки зрештою не минула ціла година. Самковський відчув, як сирість від землі проникла йому, либонь, до кісткового мозку, від чого суглоби почали нити, як на грозу. І вже коли терпець, здавалось, от-от урветься, внизу навпроти Заремби виникла ще одна постать у чорному вбранні.

Ад'юнктові сперло дихання. Він затиснув руків'я «Штаєра» і так широко вирячив очі, боячись проґавити домовлений знак, що вони ледь не торкалися скелець окулярів. Заремба, однак, зволікав. Вони про щось перемовлялися з Берлом, але жодне слово до поліціянтів не долітало. Відчувалося тільки, що розмова в них точиться нервова, а тон потроху підвищується. Врешті Зеремба потягнувся до кишені. Самковський знав, що там у нього конверт, який він зобов'язався принести Брюкнеру. Тільки замість грошей у ньому лежав акуратно порізаний газетний папір. Так, аби навіть на дотик здавалося, що всередині банкноти.

Заремба простягнув конверта Брюкнеру.

«Ну ж бо, не дай йому зазирнути всередину, — подумки промовив ад'юнкт, — піднімай свою гівняну руку...»

Берл, утім, не збирався перевіряти вміст. Чоловіки продовжили розмову, але вже спокійніше, мовби в одну мить порозумілись. Конверт зник десь у Брюкнера в кишені, хоч, може, той і далі тримав його в руках, просто згорнувши вдвоє.

Заремба раптом смикнувся усім тілом і відступив крок назад. Замість підняти вгору правицю, як було домовлено, він підняв обидві руки, трохи виставивши їх перед собою. Ад'юнкт побачив, як Брюкнер підскочив до нього й щосили вдарив кілька разів блискучим лезом, а тоді кинувся навтьоки. У ту ж мить поліціянти зірвалися з місця. Хтось вистрілив з карабіна, Самковський сам кілька разів смальнув зі свого револьвера услід втікачеві. Проте момент було втрачено. Ще кілька хвилин поліціянти намагалися переслідувати його, але темна постать швидко пропала з виду. Стало зрозуміло, що ловити вони можуть хіба що передранковий туман...

Самковський, ледве дихаючи від бігу й злості, повернувся до місця, за яким вони спостерігали із засідки. Заремба нерухомо лежав, розпластавшись на камінні. Голова була відкинута назад, а злощасний капелюх, який він так і не поправив на ній, потопав у багнюці за кілька кроків від власника. Ад'юнкт нахилився над тілом і спробував намацати пульс. Заремба був мертвим.

За кілька годин розпочався найжахливіший день у кар'єрі Самковського. Директор, дізнавшись про невдалу нічну операцію, був на службі вже о сьомій і негайно викликав ад'юнкта до себе. Майже сорок хвилин той слухав добірну лайку й прокльони у свій бік. Потім директор замовк, випив склянку води, розчинивши в ній заспокійливий порошок.

— Те, що вас звільнено з поліції, Самковський, — це майже доконаний факт. Усі папери будуть оформлені вже сьогодні, — промовив він. — Але не думайте, що це єдине покарання за такий службовий злочин. Буде суд.

Ад'юнкт слухав його, дивлячись прямо перед собою, де на стіні висів чималий герб монархії. Пазурі імперського орла тепер видавалися йому уособленням правосуддя, і він майже фізично відчував їх у своєму тілі.

— Забирайтеся, — почув Самковський наостанок і, не зволікаючи, вийшов за двері.

Все ще брудний від лежання в засідці на Погулянці, його руки були чорними від пороху, він пішки дістався до свого помешкання на Підзамчі й, не роздягаючись, звалився на ліжко.

У той день і в наступний Самковський не читав свіжих газет, тому й не знав, що у Львові знову сталося вбивство поліціянта. Бувалого фельдфебеля, міцного й загартованого, знайшли мертвим на Верхньому Личакові.

V

Експрес до Ґаліції
11–13 квітня 1906 року

Вістович завчасно дістався на Бернський двірець. Потяг з Венеції мав прибути лише за годину, ще стільки ж часу він стоятиме тут, доки висадить пасажирів і прийме наступних. Тих, що вирушать до Страсбурга, Праги, Відня або, як і він, до самого Лемберга.

Комісар за звичкою вкотре перевірив документи, які тримав у внутрішній кишені маринарки з теплого гарусу. Маринарку він купив сьогодні вранці у крамниці поруч готелю. В ній зручно буде подорожувати й не шкода, якщо до неї випадково вчепиться вагонний чи вокзальний бруд, оскільки коштувала вона якихось два франки. Під маринаркою Вістович мав свіжу накрохмалену сорочку, яку вчора забрав з готельної пральні, пристебнутий чистий комірець, що приємно лоскотав шию, і тонку краватку.

У лівій руці тримав плаща, оскільки в полудень у Берні потепліло і він мусив його зняти, у правій — свою невелику валізу.

Документи передбачувано виявилися у тій самій кишені, куди він їх поклав, розрахувашись за готельний номер. Паспорт, поліційне посвідчення, банківський контракт, складений учетверо й захований між сторінками нотатника. В іншій кишені лежав портсигар і єдиний сувенір із Швейцарії — бензинова запальничка «*Ronson*».

У двірцевій почекальні виявився більш-менш пристойний ресторан, де комісар вирішив пообідати перед дорогою. Замовив печеню з гуски і бокал червоного ельзаського вина. Очікуючи на замовлення, закурив, з цікавістю вуличного хлопчака підпаливши край своєї львівської цигарки американською запальничкою. Вогонь вистрибнув з неї і зашкварчав, лизнувши тютюн і делікатний цигарковий папір.

Тонке клацання на короткий момент привернуло до Вістовича увагу інших відвідувачів. Кілька чоловіків одночасно подивилося в його бік, чи то оцінюючи ще не надто поширене бензинове кресало, чи то самого курця. Одним із них виявився полковник Редль, якого комісар, зайшовши до ресторації, не помітив. Схоже, він також вирішив прибути завчасно і, як на злість, обрав те саме місце, щоб пообідати. Понад усе комісару не хотілося, аби той зараз підвівся й підійшов до його столика. І байдуже, щоб лише привітатись чи потеревенити. Але полковник, мовби відчуваючи нехіть спілкування з боку Вістовича, тільки кивнув йому й знову занурився поглядом у газету.

Втім, самої присутності його вистачило, щоб отруїти цей простір. До того ж принесена гуска виявилася недопеченою, а вино кислим, мовби Редль якимось чином зумів проникнути на кухню і втрутитися у роботу кухаря, а потім підступно долити в ельзаське, яке Вістовичу завжди смакувало, добрячу порцію оцту.

За якісь чверть години комісар підвівся, заплатив і вийшов, не залишився ані сантима чайових. Він досі не знав, що робити з таємницею, яку дізнався про полковника. Як порадити собі з власним сумлінням, знаючи, що разом з ним до Лемберга от-от вирушить імовірний російський шпигун. Так само не знав, як бути з тим, що він сам залежить від цього імовірного шпигуна. Адже бісовий Пульманн, з яким Вістович підписував контракт, — його друг. А отже, розповість Редлю все, що той забажає. Але найгірше те, що в комісара можуть бути неприємності з імперською фінансовою владою. Лишалося тільки сподіватися, що вони з полковником мовчатимуть навзаєм. Редль не заважатиме йому користуватися грішми на швейцарському конто, тримати їх на старість, отримувати відсотки через Банк Австрії, якщо він дозволить Редлю шпигувати з поміччю таких покидьків, як Грумм.

Комісар згадав про лист, який він змушений був віддати полковнику. І що зміст листа переписано в нотатник. Прикметно, що саме там, у записнику, зберігався й банківський контракт. Потайки навіть від самого себе Вістович сподівався, що в тому листі не було нічого важливого. Або щось, що, навпаки, не шкодить, а слугує інтересам Австро-Угорщини. Це означало би, що Редль не порушив військової присяги. І це звільнило би Вістовича від докорів сумління. Треба тільки розшифрувати написане. Найпевніше — доведеться зробити це самому. Адже довіритись якому-небудь криптографу в цій справі він не міг.

З такими думками Вістович спостерігав, як до перону поволі прибуває поїзд. Чорний локомотив з велетенською трубою, чахкаючи й скрегочучи своїм масивним сталевим тілом, підтягував до перону десяток сіро-брудних вагонів, серед яких було два, приналежних до першого класу, — один слугував ресторацією, а решта мали на собі маркування другого класу.

Завдяки полковнику Вістович отримав одномісне купе у вагоні номер два, що на своєму сталевому боці мав бронзові літери «KkStB»*. Дочекавшись, коли кондуктор, вусатий італієць у темно-зеленому однострої, запросить ламаною німецькою заходити досередини, комісар піднявся кількома вагонними сходинками і, пройшовши трохи тіснуватим коридором, зупинився біля дверей з написом «XII». Згідно запису в квитку, тут він проведе найближчі два з половиною дні, доки експрес не прибуде до Лемберга.

Впевнено смикнувши двері купе, Вістович зайшов досередини і одразу ж завмер, а на обличчі в нього з'явились одночасно подив і відраза. На оксамитовій канапі з півкруглою спинкою і дерев'яним різьбленим обідком спав якийсь чоловік. Цей тип мав лису голову, яку вмостив на подушку з вишитою емблемою Австрійської залізниці. Своє громіздке тіло він укрив ковдрою з таким же візерунком. З-під ковдри стирчали дві чималі ступні у темно-синіх шкарпетках і могутня п'ятірня з напівзігнутими пальцями, мовби сплячий тримав у ній невидиму склянку або м'яч для гри в теніс. На столику, вкритому світлим обрусом (з тією всюдисущою емблемою

* *Kaiserlich-königliche österreichische Staatsbahnen* (*нім.*) — Цісарсько-королівська австрійська державна залізниця.

посередині), поруч із маленьким вагонним світильником лежав стосик італійських газет і попільничка з горою недопалків. Незнайомець сопів напіврозкритим чималим ротом і трохи скривленим носом та, здавалося, видихав уже весь кисень, від чого повітря всередині було важке й смердюче.

Комісар зачинив двері й рушив до кондуктора. Той привітно усміхнувся назустріч пасажиру.

— Я маю місце в купе під номером дванадцять, — сказав Вістович, показуючи йому квитка.

— О, так! Дванацать, дванацать, — кивнув той, — прошу сахотити...

— Я б охоче, але там хтось спить, — пояснив комісар.

— Спит? О, неторозумінна, неторозумінна... *Mi scusi, mi scusi, mi scusi...*[*]

З цими словами італієць кинувся до купе, з якого щойно вийшов комісар. Вістович рушив слідом і побачив, як той, однією рукою затиснувши носа, другою почав обережно торсати сплячого. Виглядало це доволі кумедно, й комісар не стримав сміху.

— Я не можу його росбутити, — з образою і безсиллям у голосі промовив кондуктор.

— Дозвольте мені, — сказав Вістович і підійшов до незнайомця.

Львів'янин з силою термоснув того за велетенське, мов гора, плече. Сплячим тріпнуло, як у лихоманці, а його лиса голова лунко вдарилася об стінку.

— *Mamma mia!* — вирвалося у перестрашеного кондуктора.

---

* Вибачте, вибачте, вибачте... (*італ.*)

Такий несподіваний струс, утім, розбудив сплячого. Він розплющив очі й одразу схопився на ноги, ставши навпроти Вістовича в довгій до колін спальній сорочці й кальсонах.

— Що це, в біса, означає? — запитав він німецькою, і його сонний голос подібний був на звіриний рик.

Здавалося, тільки те, що комісар виявився однакового з ним зросту і такої ж міцної статури, стримало його від удару у відповідь. Хоч, може, насправді незнайомець просто не збагнув зі сну, що сталося.

— Ви зайняли моє місце, добродію, — Вістович відповів з усією лагідністю, на яку тільки був здатний.

— Що ви верзете? — рикнув той. — Йдіть під три чорти!

— Будьте ласкаві, покажіть ваш квиток, — попросив комісар.

Незнайомець відвернувся до гардеробу, відчинив дверцята й витягнув з кишені плаща складену картку.

— Ось! — тицьнув він її Вістовичу.

Той, не розгортаючи, передав папір кондуктору.

— Тринацать! У вас тринацать, сеньйоре Салтіні! — вигукнув італієць. — Це насупне купе! Насупне!

Пасажир у кальсонах сердито скрипнув зубами.

— Це ваша помилка, — гримнув він тепер вже на кондуктора. — Вчора у Венеції ви мали б помітити, що я розмістився не на своєму місці.

— Неторозумінна, — розвів той руками, — *mi scusi...*

— Дайте мені чверть години, я одягнуся, а тоді перейду, — звернувся Салтіні до Вістовича, — не йти ж мені в спідньому.

— Куди прямує цей пасажир? — запитав Вістович у кондуктора.

— Лемберґ, — зазирнувши у квиток, прочитав італієць.

— Нехай залишається тут, — промовив комісар, — я просто займу його місце.

Не чекаючи відповіді, львів'янин вийшов у коридор і відчинив сусідні двері. У тринадцятому, також одномісному купе було чисто, на полиці для одягу виднівся комплект свіжої постільної білизни, на столі чекала порожня попільниця. Вістович з полегшенням умостився на канапі. Поїзд вирушить лише за годину, отже, можна вийти й прогулятися пероном, але йому не хотілося. Краще посидіти в тиші.

Ввечері поїзд зупинився в Базелі, де простояв знову годину. Після цього попрямував до німецького кордону. Знаючи, як довго триває прикордонна перевірка, Вістович вирішив повечеряти ще у Швейцарії. Як виявилося, така ідея спала на гадку не тільки йому, і в ресторації було людно. Точніше, вільним залишився тільки один столик, який комісар поспіхом зайняв. Кельнер нагодився за мить і вручив меню в цупкій картонній оправі. Не відпускаючи його, Вістович замовив м'ясний салат і чарку горілки.

— Чи можна мені звернутись до вас із проханням? — раптом сказав офіціант.

Комісар здивовано поглянув на нього.

— Про що мова? — перепитав він.

— Усі окремі столики зайняті, і одному добродію ніде повечеряти. Чи дозволите йому приєднатися до вас?

— Звісно, що цей пан дозволить, — почулося в кельнера за спиною.

Той відхилився вбік, і Вістович побачив перед собою пасажира, якого будив у полудень.

— Якщо вже я вторгся в його купе, то вторгнення за стіл він мені точно пробачить, — у голосі Салтіні відчувалася примирлива наполегливість.

Чоловік впевнено відсунув стілець і сів навпроти комісара.

— Мені те саме, що замовив пан Вістович, — недбало кинув він офіціанту.

— Не полінувалися дізнатися моє прізвище? — промовив львів'янин, коли кельнер пішов.

— Щоб перевірити реєстр пасажирів, немає нічого складного, — сказав прибулий і, простягнувши руку співрозмовникові, представився: — Мене звати Доменіко Салтіні.

— Як на італійця, у вас добра німецька, — зауважив комісар, відповідаючи потиском.

— Я швейцарець. Мав справи у Венеції, а тепер знову у справах їду до Лемберга.

Вістович кивнув, але водночас придивився до співрозмовника уважніше. Звісна річ, тепер на ньому вже був зовсім інший одяг, ніж при їхній першій зустрічі: добре скроєний гарнітур з двобортним піджаком і золотою шпилькою в петлиці, шовкова сорочка та високий комір з елеґантним краватом, зав'язаним, щоправда, дещо недбало. Обличчя мав старанно поголене, й усміхався з усією приязністю, яку тільки міг із себе витиснути.

— Ви підприємець? — комісар допитувався радше за звичкою, аніж з цікавості.

— Скажімо, деякий ґешефт я таки проваджу, — трохи подумавши, відповів той. — Наразі займаюсь паперами. Рукописами, якщо точніше.

Вістович не стримав посмішки.

– Рукописи – це, мабуть, небезпечно? – запитав він.

– Що ви маєте на увазі?

– Те, що у вас при собі зброя.

Обличчям Салтіні майнула тінь. Якусь секунду воно могло здатися здивованим, але вже наступної миті цей подив минув.

– Не бачу нічого дивного в тому, що людина мандрує зі зброєю, – зазначив він, – часи зараз непевні.

– Згоден, хоч сам я залишив пістолет удома, – промовив комісар, – не хочу проблем на кордоні.

– Прикордонна поліція необов'язково її знайде. А якщо й знайде, то я готовий надати всі супутні документи, – сказав Салтіні. – Як бачите, у вашому відкритті немає нічого незвичайного, й дивуватися тут нічому. Так, у мене з собою надійний *«Zig-Zag»**, який вже не раз виручав у різноманітних ситуаціях.

– Мене це не дивує, пане Салтіні. Точніше, дивує інше... Навіщо, йдучи до ресторації, ви перевірили вміст барабана вашого револьвера і навіть доклали набоїв у порожні камори? Остерігаєтесь тут когось?..

Чоловік не встиг відповісти. До їхнього столика підійшов кельнер із тацею, на якій стояли дві чарки з горілкою. Поставивши випивку перед клієнтами, він відійшов, пообіцявши за хвилину принести замовлений салат.

– Як ви дізналися? – з цікавістю запитав Салтіні.

– На вказівному і великому пальці правиці у вас ледь помітний слід від мастила. Револьвер ви тримали в лівій руці. Барабан повертали вказівним пальцем правої,

---

* *«Zig-Zag»* – шестизарядний револьвер *Mauser M 1878*.

великим запихали набої в порожні отвори. Так робить кожен, якщо він не шульга. Ви — не шульга.

— Маєте рацію, — засміявся той, подивившись на свої пальці.

— У Венеції вам довелося стріляти, чи не так? — раптом доволі різко запитав комісар, і вся привітність на обличчі його співрозмовника розтанула, мов цигарковий дим.

Підійшов кельнер і поставив перед ними дві порції м'ясного салату. Знову відійшов, побажавши смачного.

— Не треба так лякатися, пане Салтіні, — сказав Вістович, — це ж просто здогад. Якщо у вас є звичка завжди тримати при собі заряджену зброю, то, виходить, йдучи сюди, ви згадали, що там бракує патронів. Можливо — одного, можливо — двох... Так чи інакше, але ви стріляли. Далі припущення: стріляли у Венеції, звідки їдете.

Салтіні одним ковтком випив свою горілку.

— Одразу зрозумів, що ви поліціянт, — видихнувши алкогольне повітря, сказав він. — З першого погляду.

Комісар вирішив розділити свій трунок на кілька ковтків.

— Я служу в поліції, але в поліції австрійській. Тож не маю тут жодних повноважень... — сказав він після першого. — Хіба що можу перевірити, чи траплялись у Венеції останнім часом убивства. Чи не знаходили десь у міських закутках трупи з вогнепальними ранами. Але не робитиму цього.

— Чому? — поцікавився Салтіні, занурюючи ножа й виделку у свою холодну страву.

— Бо не знаю італійської, — пояснив комісар і зробив те саме. — Крім того, хтозна, можливо, ви стріляли, щоб захистити себе. Закон це дозволяє, наскільки мені відомо, у всіх цивілізованих країнах.

Кілька хвилин вони мовчки вечеряли, а тоді Салтіні промовив:

— А що ви скажете, пане Вістовичу, якщо я запропоную вам невелику, проте вигідну для вас угоду?

— Відмовлюся, — не відриваючись від їжі, сказав комісар.

— Не поспішайте. Хіба вам не цікаво бодай дізнатися про що йдеться?

— Про що б не йшлося, пане Салтіні. Я ні в чому не допомагатиму вам у Лемберзі. Там у мене служба, а отже, там я живу за чіткими правилами.

Подумки Вістович зауважив, що відмовляється вже вдруге. Спершу відмовився співпрацювати з Редлем, а тепер — з цим типом. Так, мовби ця подорож була навмисне для того, щоб перевірити його на стійкість до сумнівних пропозицій.

— Я пропоную вам гарний відсоток від надзвичайно прибуткової справи, пане Вістовичу, — мов не почувши його відповідь, сказав Салтіні. — А натомість проситиму лише бути моїм провідником у цьому незнаному для мене місті. Лемберг, щиро кажучи, має темну репутацію. А тому, щоб ходити його вулицями, мені поруч потрібен хтось зі світлим розумом. Як-от ваш.

— Ви не зрозуміли мене, добродію, — відповів комісар. — Щойно ми опинимося в Австрії, я змушений буду вас заарештувати. Просто в поїзді або на пероні.

— З якого дива?

— Хоч би з припущення, що у Венеції ви спровадили когось на той світ.

— Облиште. Ви забудете про обов'язок, щойно дізнаєтеся розмір вашого гонорару.

Салтіні заговорив із підкресленою байдужістю, як людина, що безмежно впевнена в силі своїх слів і в силі грошей. Доївши свою страву, він витер губи серветкою, після чого дістав з кишені шкіряний етуі, в якому зберігав візитки. Витягнувши одну з них, простягнув Вістовичу.

— Це щоб мої слова не розходилися з ділом і ви знали, з ким маєте справу, — додав він.

Взявши в руку світло-сіру картку з дорогого картону, комісар прочитав текст у золотистій рамці:

«Єнс Ебербах, приватний детектив.
Зальцбург, Леопольдґассе, 23»

— Доменіко Салтіні, як на мене, звучить краще, — зауважив комісар.

— Мої рідні з вами б не погодилися, — скривив посмішку псевдоіталієць, — втім, на їхню думку можемо не зважати. Називайте мене, як хочете, але пам'ятайте про мою щирість. Адже я відкрив перед вами свою найважливішу карту.

— І все тому, що вам у Лемберзі потрібен помічник? — не вгавав Вістович.

— Провідник, — уточнив той. — Такий самий провідник, якого беруть собі дослідники нових земель. Їм потрібен хтось із місцевих, щоб не заблукати в хащах і не загинути.

— Якщо так потрібна моя поміч, то викладайте інші карти, — сказав комісар. — Що ви плануєте робити в цій небезпечній і темній Ґаліції.

Детектив хвилину подумав, ніби збираючись з думками, а тоді перехилився через стіл і майже пошепки проговорив:

— Мова про одну давню делікатну справу, в якій був замішаний теперішній дуже важливий посадовець, а тоді — дрібний чиновник. Усе сталося близько тридцяти років тому, але наслідки проявилися тільки тепер... Моє завдання — запобігти крахові його репутації... Наразі це все, що я можу сказати. Решту, все до найдрібніших деталей, знатимете, щойно погодитеся на співпрацю.

— Я мушу подумати, пане Ебербах, — відповів Вістович.

— Звісно, — з ледь чутним піднесенням чи радше полегшенням сказав той. — Ми ще дві доби будемо в дорозі, тож часу маєте вдосталь. А тим часом дозвольте мені пригостити вас...

Еберебах-Салтіні знаком покликав кельнера і попросив принести дві склянки десятирічного бренді.

— Я дотримуюсь переконання, що цей благородний напій сприяє роздумам і приводить до правильних рішень, — пояснив він комісару.

Вістовичу здавалося дещо дивним бути зараз за одним столом, а тим більше пити з тим, кого не так давно він ледь не лупцював сплячим, проте відмовитись комісар не встиг. Кельнер на подив швидко приніс замовлення, мовби давно його передбачив.

— Що ж, за нашу майбутню успішну співпрацю, — промовив тост детектив, піднімаючи свою склянку.

Вістович був переконаний, що ніякої співпраці з цим типом у нього не буде. Жодної, а тим більше успішної. Втім, усе-таки випив. Алкоголь видався йому занадто теплим і від того неприємним на смак. Пляшку ніби відкоркували завчасно і так само заздалегідь розлили вміст у чарки.

— Доп'ю в купе, — з натягнутою посмішкою сказав він, підвівшись і поклавши на стіл гроші за свою вечерю. — На все добре, пане Салтіні.

Детектив відсалютував йому склянкою. Збоку могло здатися, що це двоє друзів після веселих посиденьок прощаються, домовившись зустрітися вранці на цьому ж місці за сніданком, а в обід знову випити разом.

Виходячи з ресторації, Вістович наштовхнувся на полковника Редля. Той також тримав у руках бокал, але вони розійшлися, не озвавшись один до одного навіть півсловом. Втім, як виявиться, вже за кілька годин, щойно поїзд перетне німецький кордон, ця мовчанка порушиться. Вони говоритимуть багато, гучно і з погрозами в голосі...

Поставивши бренді на стіл, комісар клацнув умикачем світильника. Якусь мить спостерігав, як всередині крихкого абажура поволі засвічувалася жарівка. Тоді зняв із себе маринарку і, лишившись у сорочці, закотив по лікті рукави й розв'язав краватку. Тоді підійшов до невеличкого вмивальника в кутку, набрав у пригорщу води й з приємністю плеснув собі в обличчя. Витерся рушником, трохи постояв, дивлячись на своє відображення у темному вікні. За цим відображенням час від часу мелькали скупі вогні якихось безіменних станцій і десь вгорі ясним нерухомим диском виднівся повний місяць. Вістовичу подумалось, що коли вимкнути світло всередині, то, мабуть, вдасться роздивитися нічні краєвиди. Дорогою з Берна до Страсбурга вони мають бути казковими. Навіть вночі і навіть якщо дивитися на них крізь вікно експресу до Ґаліції.

За пів години поїзд зупинився на кордоні. Перевірка минула доволі швидко. У купе до Вістовича зайшов зовсім молодий унтерлейтенант і попросив документи. З якоюсь байдужістю, зумовленою, мабуть, втомою, переглянув його австрійський паспорт, без жодних запитань повернув і побажав гарної дороги.

З німецького боку перевірка тривала на якихось двадцять хвилин довше. Після неї поїзд вирушив далі до Страсбурга, куди мав прибути о восьмій тридцять ранку.

Увесь цей час, впродовж якого експрес простояв між кантоном Базель-Штадт і німецьким Ельзасом*, комісар використав для того, аби вкотре заглибитися в шифр, що його він, їдучи в фіакрі передмістям Берна, переписав з листа Редля. За денного світла, щойно потяг відправився, Вістович скопіював увесь набір літер і цифр на нову сторінку. Зашифрований текст тепер мав зґрабніший вигляд, проте зрозумілішим від цього не став.

Втім, досить швидко комісар мусив закрити нотатник. Від швидкого руху й вагонної хитавиці написані на папері символи почали зливатися в одне суцільне мереживо, позбавляючи розум усякої можливості знайти ключ до цієї загадки чи принаймні зрозуміти, в якому логічному керунку його шукати. Вечірня втома далася взнаки, і Вістович сам не помітив, коли влігся на канапі й провалився в сон.

Розбудив його звук пострілу.

Якусь одну зовсім коротку мить комісар нерухомо лежав, дивлячись у стелю широко розплющеними очима,

* Після перемоги Пруссії над Францією у 1871 році внаслідок Франкфуртського мирного договору Ельзас відійшов до новоствореної Німецької імперії і залишався окупованим до 1919 року.

намагаючись зрозуміти, чи був постріл насправді, чи йому це приснилося.

Врешті, коли свідомість остаточно до нього повернулася, він схопився з місця. Тієї ж миті поїзд добряче хитнуло, і комісар усім тілом навалився на дверцята шафи. На щастя, вони виявилися достатньо міцними, аби витримати навіть чималу вагу Вістовича. Відновивши рівновагу, поліціянт вискочив зі свого купе й завмер у порожньому коридорі. Постріл пролунав ліворуч від нього й достатньо гучно. Найпевніше – одразу за стіною. Тобто в купе під номером дванадцять, в якому подорожує Салтіні. Невдовзі зі своїх відділів обережно почали визирати й інші пасажири, а в кінці коридору вигулькнула стривожена постать кондуктора.

Комісар натиснув на ручку дверей з римською цифрою XII. Купе виявилося незачиненим. Всередині було темно, а в ніздрі вдарив запах алкоголю і порохових газів. Вістович ступив кілька обережних кроків і ввімкнув світильник. Його скупе жовто-червоне світло лилося на стіл, де стояла напівпорожня пляшка бренді, далі на канапу і пасажира, що сидів на ній, звісивши голову на груди. З-під щелепи в нього розпливалася широка пляма, змінюючи колір дорогої сорочки з білого на темно-червоний. Світло від електричних жарівок заведено було називати мертвим, позбавленим того життя, що мають в собі денні сонячні промені. Таким же мертвим було й тіло детектива Ебербаха.

У правій руці чоловік все ще тримав револьвер. Це був той самий «*Zig-Zag*», про який вони згадували за вечерею. Видавалося, ніби детектив пустив собі кулю в голову, приставивши зброю знизу, під щелепою, паралельно до шиї.

— Що діється? — почув комісар чийсь голос за спиною.

Він озирнувся. Перед ним стояв худий довготелесий кондуктор, на пів голови вищий за Вістовича. Обличчя мав стривожене й заспане одночасно. Італієць, який чергував перед ним, очевидно, зійшов десь у Базелі або на самім кордоні. Комісар навіть встиг подумати про те, як той зрадіє, дізнавшись, що ця халепа сталася не на його зміні.

— З пасажиром у цьому купе дещо сталося, — промовив комісар.

— Сталося серйозне? — перепитав той.

— Настільки, що проситиму нікого сюди не впускати, — сказав Вістович голосніше, аби його почули решта. Ті, хто протираючи зі сну очі й сяк-так одягнувшись, також підходили й юрмилися в коридорі, намагаючись з'ясувати хто, в кого і чому стріляв.

— А ви хто? — з недовірою перепитав кондуктор.

— Я з поліції, — коротко повідомив Вістович.

Службовець кивнув і голосно промовив:

— Пані та панове, просимо вас повернутися на свої місця! Виник незначний інцидент, який жодним чином не вплине на нашу подорож. За три години, згідно з планом руху, ми зупинимося в Страсбурзі.

«Незначний інцидент» прозвучало для Вістовича трохи комічно, але на решту пасажирів це подіяло потрібним чином. Поволі, неохоче, увесь час ставлячи питання, на які ніхто не збирався відповідати, вони розбрелися по своїх купе, щоб доснити, кому вдасться, свої подорожні сни.

— У вас є перелік пасажирів? — запитав Вістович кондуктора, коли останній роззява зачинив за собою двері.

— Звісно, — відповів той.

— Принесіть його мені.

— Хочете викреслити бідолаху зі списку? — несподівано сказав кондуктор, кивнувши в бік трупа.

Своє службове чако він зняв з голови і тримав тепер у руках.

— А ви, бачу, полюбляєте мертвецький гумор, — глянувши на нього скоса, сказав комісар.

— Даруйте, — перепросив кондуктор. — У шістнадцять я потрапив на війну з французами, і відтоді, попри те що минуло багато років, трупи мене не лякають. Список зараз буде...

Заклавши чако на голову, він швидким кроком попрямував до свого службового місця. Комісар тим часом повернувся в купе самогубця. Увагу його привернув рукопис у брудноватій оправі, що стирчав із валізи Ебербаха. Так, ніби хтось збирався витягнути його й почитати перед сном або недбало поклав туди, вже прочитавши. «Читати стільки тексту — це, мабуть, останнє, чого б мені запраглося, якби я вирішив накласти на себе руки», — подумав комісар, швидко хапаючи рукопис. Потім, у два кроки опинившись перед своїми дверима, прочинив їх і кинув папери на стіл. Після цього знову опинився біля покійника.

Надійшов кондуктор зі списком у руках. Забравши в нього листок, комісар швидко пробігся поглядом по кривих літерах і цифрах. Серед них було і його прізвище, написане з помилкою, як «*Herr Wistrowytsch*». Раптом всередині неприємно вкололо: навпроти цього пана Вістровича було позначено купе No 12. Саме те, де зараз лежав мертвий Ебербах.

Звісно, нічого дивного в цьому не було, адже він сам запропонував лжеіталійцю помінятися місцем, аби той не перебирався і спав собі далі. Здавалось би, нічого дивного...

— Чи можу я залишити список собі? — запитав він у кондуктора.

— Якщо повернете, — відповів той.

— Поверну, — пообіцяв комісар і роззирнувся уважно по купе. — Чи знайдеться у вас ліхтар?

— Звичайно, — з готовністю промовив той, ніби йому й не набридло бігати. — Мене звати Франк, — додав він, — Франк Мюллер.

— Адам Вістович, — представився комісар у відповідь. — Ну ж бо, Франку. Швидко несіть те, що я попросив...

Той кивнув і знову помчав уздовж коридору. Комісар тим часом наблизився до трупа. Обережно притримуючи мертву голову за скроні, він звів її дещо догори. Електричне світло зблиснуло на чималій вогнепальній рані: розірваних клаптях шкіри й усе ще пульсуючій крові. Кілька хвилин поліціянт уважно придивлявся до цих моторошних субстанцій, потім так само обережно дозволив голові Ебербаха зайняти її попереднє положення.

Коли повернувся Франк, Вістович узяв у нього ліхтар і найперше освітив його світлом мертву руку з револьвером. Не зрушивши її ні на міліметр, довго вивчав положення пальців і шукав на них сліди пороху. Далі роздивився вагонну шибку. Особливо уважно в тому місці, навпроти якого відбувся постріл.

— Як відчиняється вікно? — несподівано запитав він у кондуктора.

— Вгорі є важіль, — промовив той, вказуючи пальцем на продовгувату металеву ручку, схожу на дверну, що стриміла над фрамугою.

Комісар направив світло на неї. Роздивився, а потім дістав з кишені хустинку, щоб не торкатися її голою рукою, й спробував відчинити вікно. Зробити це виявилося важко навіть для нього. Втім, Вістовича цікавило інше: він хотів знати, чи можна було б відчинити його ззовні, а потім знову зачинити. Схоже, що навряд...

З тим же ліхтарем у руках поліціянт обстежив підлогу й канапу. У шафі висіло кілька запасних костюмів і сорочок, елегантний плащ і тепле пальто. Вістович, з огляду на присутність кондуктора, вирішив не перевіряти вміст кишень. Зрештою, нічого особливого й не сподівався там відшукати.

Увагу його привернув алкоголь на столі.

— Випивка з нашого ресторану? — запитав комісар у Франка.

Той знизав плечима.

— Гадки не маю.

Вістович придивився до пляшки. Французький десятирічний бренді. Такий самий, що вони пили за вечерею. Очевидно, Ебербаху не вистачило однієї склянки, і він замовив собі цілу пляшку, вирішивши далі пиячити на самоті. При цьому начебто забувши замкнути двері... Вихлявши пів пляшки, він раптом вирішує вкоротити собі віку. Не зрозуміло чому, адже за лічені години до цього з азартом оповідав комісарові, що має справи в «темному Лемберзі». І врешті, перед тим як притулити до себе зброю для смертельного пострілу, Ебербах знову не замкнувся зсередини. «Що за чортівня? — думалося Вістовичу. — Чи не забагато суперечностей?»

Йому не було шкода вбитого, але його не полишала думка, що купе під номером дванадцять, де лежав зараз мертвий Ебербах, полковник Редль зарезервував для нього. І хтозна, чи то не Вістович мав би зараз лежати отак нерухомо, як лежить приватний детектив із Зальцбурга?

Комісар обернувся до кондуктора.

— Хто заходив до пана Салтіні після вечері? — запитав він.

Франк стенув плечима.

— Начебто ніхто.

— Що означає «начебто», пане Мюллере? — сердито перепитав поліціянт. — Хіба зі свого місця ви не бачите весь коридор?

— Бачу, — кивнув той.

— Тоді напружте вашу бісову пам'ять.

— Але я не пригадую... Я трохи дрімав.

— Можливо, кельнер? Адже Салтіні перед смертю замовив пляшку бренді.

— Рація! — аж підстрибнув Франк, хоч при його зрості він мав усі шанси вперіщитись головою в стелю. — Рація! Коли в ресторані закінчилася вечеря, до цього купе приходив кельнер із тацею в руках!

— О котрій годині? — перепитав комісар.

— Десь близько півночі.

Вістович глянув на годинник. Була п'ята ранку, постріл пролунав якихось двадцять хвилин тому. Виходить, між візитом офіціанта й смертю Ебербаха минуло чотири години й сорок хвилин.

— Офіціант одразу вийшов? — знову поставив питання поліціянт.

— Цього не пам'ятаю, я відволікся на щось.

— Який на вигляд кельнер?

— Середнього зросту, брюнет... Непримітної зовнішності, — з сумнівом у голосі проговорив той.

— Не буває «непримітної зовнішності», Франку. Затямте собі, — сказав комісар, проте більше не розпитував. — Замкніть це купе і відімкніть тільки для поліції у Страсбурзі, — наказав він йому, — або для мене, якщо знадобиться.

Мюллер кивнув.

Комісар кинувся до ресторації. Крім двох офіціантів, що готували столи для сніданку, там не виявилося нікого. Один із них був лисий, інший мав світле волосся, тож обоє не підпадали під опис Франка.

Кельнери відірвалися від роботи й з подивом глянули на пасажира.

— Вибачте, у нас ще зачинено, — проказав лисий, що серед цих двох був, очевидно, старшим.

— Мені потрібно знати, хто вчора відносив замовлення в купе під номером дванадцять, — проговорив поліціянт, і кельнери здригнулися від його жорсткого тону.

— З нас двох ніхто, — відповів старший.

— Гаразд. Тоді дізнайтеся, хто з ваших колег, — наполіг комісар. — Це було приблизно опівночі.

— Тут лише двоє офіціантів, — пояснив лисий, — і вони перед вами.

— Віднести замовлення міг бармен, але не опівночі, — додав блондин. — У цей час ресторацію вже зачинено.

Вістович сердито закусив губу. Виходить, кельнер, який приніс Ебербаху випивку, насправді міг бути вбивцею. Тільки чому постріл пролунав аж під ранок? А головне — як убивці вдалося зникнути так швидко? Адже комісар опинився перед дверима вбитого майже одразу?

Не озвавшись до кельнерів більше ані словом, поліціянт повернувся назад, до вагона, але подався не до свого місця, а до купе під номером шість. Тут, як він пам'ятав зі списку пасажирів, мав перебувати «*Herr Oberst Redl*».

Вістович постукав і, щойно полковник відчинив, рвучко зайшов досередини, відіпхнувши того від входу й не даючи можливості закрити двері йому перед носом. Редль, гепнувшись усім тілом на канапу, дивився на нього виряченими від подиву очима.

— Здивовані, що я живий? — запитав комісар, закочуючи правий рукав.

— Збираєтеся зійтися зі мною навкулачки? — промовив Редль. — Тоді дайте мені можливість підвестися.

— Щоб ти схопив свій револьвер? Е, ні! Спершу ти мені розкажеш, де зараз Грумм, — Вістович нетямився від люті.

— Грумм у Швейцарії. Він узяв конверт і...

Редль замовк. Спіймавши погляд поліціянта, зрозумів, що брехати не було сенсу.

— Гаразд, він у поїзді.

— Де? В якому купе? Його немає в переліку пасажирів.

— Він під іншим прізвищем, у вагоні другого класу.

— Прямує, як і ви, до Львова?

— Так.

— Навіщо?

Редль не відповідав.

— Я запитав, полковнику, — нагадав комісар.

— Цього я не скажу вам, комісаре, — він заговорив раптом твердо, мовби згадавши, яку посаду обіймає в Генштабі, — є таємниці, яких не видають за жодних обставин.

— Наказ убити мене віддали йому ви?

— Що? — здивувався Редль.

— У купе номер дванадцять лежить труп. У цьому купе мав їхати я. Причин бажати мені смерті у вас більш ніж достатньо, — пояснив комісар.

— Назвіть хоч одну.

— Не клейте дурня, полковнику... Саме цим і пояснюється ваша щедрість, коли в Берні ви подарували мені квиток у вагон першого класу. Я мав бути поруч. Тоді вбити значно легше.

Вістович зиркнув у бік гардеробу. Всередині висів плащ Редля, у кишені якого виднівся темно-коричневий край пістолетного руків'я. Поліціянт сягнув по нього і за секунду вже тримав перед собою красеня-браунінга, модель 1900 року. Переконавшись, що всередині є набої, промовив:

— Зброю я візьму собі. Поверну вам у Львові.

— Як ви смієте, чорт забирай! — закипів полковник і рушив до комісара, але Вістович одним різким поштовхом відправив його на попереднє місце.

— Грумм замість мене вбив іншого чоловіка. Типа неприємного, але непричетного до наших з ним і з вами порахунків, — сказав Вістович, повертаючись до дверей.

— А я чув, що той бідолаха наклав на себе руки, — промовив полковник.

Звичні спокій і нахабство, здавалося, до нього повернулися.

— Я іншої думки, полковнику. І неодмінно поділюся нею з поліцією в Страсбурзі. Наприклад, зверну увагу слідчих, що на ідеально білому манжеті сорочки покійника немає жодного сліду від пороху, або на те, що рана не обпалена гарячими пороховими газами, як це буває тоді, коли самогубець притуляє до себе зброю. Стріляли щонайменше з двох кроків.

— Це неможливо, оскільки пасажир був у купе сам, — заперечив Редль.

Він все ще намагався говорити спокійно, але помітно зблід.

— Маєте рацію, але кондуктор бачив, як у його купе заходив кельнер. Думаю, Салтіні в цей час там не було. Кельнером перебрався цей горлоріз Грумм. Побачивши на столі відкорковану пляшку бренді, яку пасажир незадовго перед тим сам приніс із ресторану, підсипав у неї снодійного.

— І що далі? — запитав Редль.

— Грумм вийшов, але повернувся вже після того, як ми перетнули кордон. Пристрелив сплячого з його револьвера, переплутавши в темряві його зі мною. Потім вклав зброю йому в руку.

Вістович повернувся, щоб відчинити двері.

— Гаразд. А як убивця потім вийшов? Адже переполох почався відразу? — сказав йому в спину Редль.

— Наразі не знаю, — відповів комісар, — нехай це з'ясовує страсбурзька поліція.

— Ви нічого не доведете й виглядатимете ідіотом. Тільки затримаєте поїзд, — сказав Редль. — А поліціянти зроблять усе, щоб записати це як самогубство. Кому, як не вам, знати, що розслідувати такі справи — це найгірше покарання для будь-якого слідчого. Я пропоную інше...

Вістович затримався й, озирнувшись, подивився на полковника.

— Пропоную перемир'я. До Лемберга. Ви не шукаєте Грумма, а він не шукає вас. Щодо мене, то також можете не турбуватись, адже тепер я беззбройний. Усі порахунки зведемо в Ґаліції... Нащо це робити чортзна-де, у чужій країні?

Кілька секунд обоє мовчали.

— То як? Згода? — перепитав полковник.

Вістович зітхнув. Слід було визнати, що Редль мав рацію.

— Убивця залишився всередині, так? — перепитав він перед тим, як вийти. — Був там весь час, доки я обстежував місце злочину?

— У гардеробі, за одягом, — холодно сказав полковник. — Б'юсь об заклад, ви зазирнули в шафу, але не мали часу відгорнути пальто й гарнітури, щоб роздивитися той невеликий простір як слід. Грумм цим скористався й увесь час перебував у вас під носом. Втім, якби ви натрапили на нього, не сумнівайтеся, він убив би й вас. Хоча б для того, щоб виправити свою дурнувату помилку. Приблизно тоді, коли ви кинулися до ресторації, я відімкнув двері купе і випустив його. На щастя, до цих замків підходить майже кожна відмичка.

Вістович відчинив двері.

— А загалом, — додав Редль, — аплодую вам, комісаре. Не сподівався на таку блискавичну реакцію.

— Завдання спрощується, коли знаєш, хто хоче твоєї смерті, — проказав той наостанок.

Повернувшись до себе, Вістович відчув несподіване полегшення. Зазвичай піти на угоду з полковником Редлем означало те саме, що домовитися зі змією, але цього разу він був переконаний, що начальник галицького *Evidenzbüro* дотримає слова. Попри те, комісар поклав перед собою трофейний браунінг і сів так, щоб увесь час бачити двері. Двері, за словами Редля, з ненадійним замком.

Відчуваючи, що спати сьогодні він вже не буде, поліціянт розгорнув записник і знову занурився в розгадування шифру. Переписав усі символи ще раз, намагаючись помітити повторюваність або якусь закономірність.

Комісару подумалося, що для цього запису мав би існувати ключ. Яка-небудь фраза або навіть слово, з допомогою якого кодують текст. Наприклад, пишуть його вгорі сторінки й від кожного слова проводять вертикальні стовбці. Потім повідомлення записують горизонтально й без пропусків, у кілька рядків... Власне, цифри й могли б означати, скажімо, номер рядка. Тоді як кожній літері з прихованого тексту відповідала б літера з ключа.

Але як дізнатися ключ? Адже ним може бути що завгодно. Від уривка з вірша Гете до випадкової фрази, позбавленої сенсу.

Зрозумівши, що тут він зайшов у глухий кут, Вістович спробував розбити текст на симетричні групи літер. Якщо і є якась закономірність серед цих символів, то вона мала б зрештою проявитися. Проте щойно йому здавалося, що відповідь от-от з'явиться, усі його логічні здогади й висновки розсипалися, наче карткові будинки.

Непомітно для нього за вікном почало світати. Перші ранкові промені зблиснули над виноградними пагорбами Ельзасу, між якими то тут, то там виринали дивовижно гарні шато й самотні руїни, що, втім, також притягували до себе погляд подорожніх.

Густі хвойні ліси змінювалися фермерськими полями, вкритими безмежним килимом соковитої і сміливої озимини, в якої вистачило сил і життєлюбності перетерпіти холодну пору, аби тепер заявити світові про свої права.

Кілька разів Вістович побачив береги й свіже плесо могутнього Райну. Ріка тягнулася і розтинала довколишній ландшафт, мовби начищена до блиску кавалерійська шабля, кинута поміж клаптів шовку та оксамиту.

До Страсбурга експрес прибув із запізненням на двадцять хвилин. Цього часу зазвичай достатньо, щоб пасажири встигли понервуватися, і замало, аби їхні плани полетіли під три чорти. Комісар бачив через вікно, як Франк Мюллер, кондуктор з його вагона, кілька хвилин перемовлявся про щось із поліціянтами на пероні. Звісно, мова йшла про самогубця з сусіднього місця. Поліціянти мали на собі прусську поліційну форму, хоча були, мабуть, французами. Присадкуватий капрал з люлькою в зубах і молодий червонощокий капітан слухали Мюллера зі знудженим виразом на обличчях. Їхні постаті виражали тільки втому і бажання якнайшвидше задокументувати покійника із поїзда, що так недоречно вигулькнув під кінець зміни, й передати його далі, в найближчий звідси судово-медичний заклад. Редль мав безсумнівну рацію. Будь-яке розслідування було б зараз марудним, довгим і не викликало б жодного ентузіазму в місцевих функціонаріїв.

Невдовзі після того, як Мюллер з поліціянтами закінчили свою розмову, на пероні з'явилися двоє санітарів з ношами. Вони зайшли в поїзд, і комісар чув, як ті перемовлялися упівголоса незнаною йому французькою, порядкуючи над тілом. Санітари кректали й лаялись, оскільки Ебербах, австрійський детектив, що вдавав із себе італійця, був за життя здоровилом. Таким самим здоровилом лишився він і після смерті.

З труднощами його винесли з поїзда. На пероні санітари трохи перепочили, емоційно при цьому пояснюючи щось капітану й капралу, а потім потягли свою ношу кудись на тутешній двірець. Вістович знав, що день-два поліція шукатиме родичів покійника, перебиратиме його речі, намагаючись знайти бодай якісь контакти, а потім, якщо не знайде, то Ебербаха поховають за кошт магістрату на якому-небудь місцевому цвинтарі, куди зазвичай потрапляють безіменні волоцюги, самогубці й злочинці, страчені в довколишніх в'язницях.

Потім Вістович спостерігав, як радісно з поїзда вийшла група ельзасців, вигукуючи щось своєю говіркою, і, незважаючи на ранішню пору, заходилася просто на валізах відкорковувати пляшку шампанського. Один із них театрально (хоч, може, й у щирому пориві) впав на коліна й поклонився, наче мурин у молитві, чималим літерам над входом до вокзального вестибюля. Літери були облущені, давно не знали свіжої фарби й складалися в слово «*Straßburg*».

Вістович засміявся, як, мабуть, і всі інші, хто спостерігав за цією сценою. Чоловік збирався вже й собі вийти на перон, аби ковтнути свіжого повітря, коли ж зауважив там молоду жінку в темно-синьому пальто й акуратному капелюшкові. На шиї вона мала шовкову хустинку, що трохи з'їхала вбік чи то від вітру, чи то від поспішної ходи. Слідом за нею йшов носій з валізою на спині.

Коли жінка зупинилася для короткої розмови з кондуктором, Вістович зміг нарешті розгледіти її обличчя.

Постать одразу здалася йому знайомою, а тепер зникли останні сумніви. Акуратні вилиці, тонкі рівні губи, уважний погляд великих очей. Під капелюшком, як він пам'ятав, ховалося темно-русяве волосся.

Її звали Маґдалена. Родом вона була з Позена, і вперше вони зустрілися саме там.

Це сталося минулої осені, коли Вістович втягнувся у ризиковану й карколомну справу, пов'язану із загадковими вбивствами прусських чиновників. Знайомство з нею закінчилося найкоротшим у його житті романом.

Розкривши свою «позенську» справу, комісар мусив повертатись до Лемберга. Попрощавшись із Маґдою, він добре розумів, що зустрітися знову в них шансів мало. Саме тому її поява на пероні так його приголомшила. Хоча йшлося, найпевніше, зовсім не про почуття, які навряд чи встигли тоді як слід розгорітися у них обох. Йшлося про те, що тут, в біса, в цьому експресі робить агентка A III b? Адже якби Маґда подорожувала у приватних справах, то навряд чи взяла би квиток у вагон першого класу. Як і він сам, зрештою.

Комісар глянув у список, який отримав від кондуктора. Вільними досі були купе під номером сім і чотирнадцять. Отже, Маґда зайде зараз у котресь із них. Коли через вікно він побачив, як Франк забрав у носія валізу, а потім вільною рукою допоміг їй піднятися до вагона, Вістович став прислухатися до їхніх кроків у коридорі. За кілька хвилин почулося, як вони пройшли повз його двері, а далі кондуктор запросив її зайняти викуплене місце. Значить, Маґдалена буде в чотирнадцятому... Зовсім близько від нього.

Комісар продовжив спостерігати за пероном. Цікаво, чи є тут ще хтось із Третього відділу? А якщо є, то куди вони, в дідька, їдуть? Чи не до Львова часом? Вістович усміхнувся й одразу ж відігнав цю думку. Найпевніше, A III b має якийсь інтерес у Відні або в Празі, куди, якщо вірити розкладу, експрес прибуває завтра о десятій ранку.

За десять хвилин на перон вийшов полковник Редль і, встромивши до рота сигару, попрямував до двірця. Але за ним Вістовичу спостерігати не хотілося. Він дістав з валізи свіжу сорочку, комірець і свою елеґантну темно-смарагдового кольору хустину, яку збирався зав'язати на шию замість краватки.

Змінивши сорочку, одягнув поверх неї світло-сіру камізельку, до якої пристебнув два ланцюжки: один для годинника, інший — для годинникового ключика. Потреби в другому не було, проте два ланцюжки створювали симетрію й додавали одягові поважності. Замість гарусової маринарки Вістович одягнув доброго піджака з великими внутрішніми кишенями. У них помістилися гаманець і відібраний у Редля браунінг. Наостанок чоловік витягнув зі свого багажу пляшечку кельнської води й делікатно скропив нею комір.

За хвилину комісар вийшов з купе й, прошмигнувши повз двері під номером XIV, перейшов до вагона-ресторації. Обличчя лисого й світловолосого кельнерів аж скисли при його появі, проте Вістович приязно їм усміхнувся і попросив приготувати подвійний сніданок для першого класу.

— Вам принести? — запопадливо перепитав старший офіціант.

— У чотирнадцяте купе, — відповів комісар, дістаючи з гаманця кілька грубих купюр. — І ще...

Вістович підкликав його до себе й промовив щось на вухо пошепки.

— Буде зроблено, *Herr Wistowytsch*, — змовницьким тоном пообіцяв кельнер і прийняв до рук гроші — його досвідчене око зауважило щедрі чайові.

Щойно поїзд вирушив зі Страсбурга, як той самий кельнер, тримаючи в руках важку тацю, обережно постукав у двері з цифрою XIV. На таці, крім ельзаських булочок, щойно куплених у місті, сиру, кави, свіжих фруктів і персикового варення, стояла відкоркована пляшка італійського «*Chianti*» й два бокали.

Маґда відчинила й оторопіла від здивування.

— Ви помилилися, — сказала вона й уже збиралася зачинити двері, але кельнер заперечив:

— Аж ніяк, пані. Мені наказано принести сніданок саме у ваше купе.

— І хто ж вам наказав?

— Я, Маґдо, — промовив з-за його спини Вістович.

Він став поруч з офіціантом і впевнено забрав тацю з його рук. Кельнер відкланявся й швидко пішов геть, залишаючи цих двох сам на сам.

— Вістович? — тепер замість здивування в її очах майнув острах. — Що ви тут робите?

— Подорожую, як і ви, — сказав львів'янин, відчуваючи, що цей переляканий і водночас офіційний тон його добряче зачепив. — Можна мені зайти? Стояти з цим усім незручно, мушу зізнатися.

— Я щойно сюди перебралася... — промовила Маґда, непевно озираючись на свою напіврозпаковану валізу. — Тому, щиро кажучи, поки не можу приймати гостей.

— Облиш, — впевнено сказав комісар і рішуче подався вперед. — Я ж не гість.

Жінка відступила, пропускаючи його досередини. Вона й справді встигла зняти пальто, рукавички й капелюшок, прилаштувавши всі ці речі в гардеробі. Одним рухом елегантної ніжки Маґда заштовхнула валізу під канапу.

Комісар поставив тацю на стіл і заходився наливати каву з кавника у два керамічні горнятка.

— Готовий побитися об заклад, ти ще не снідала сьогодні, — промовив він.

— Ні, — зізналася Маґдалена. — Але ж хіба пасує до сніданку вино? Навіть якщо це к'янті?

— К'янті, моя люба, пасує навіть замість сніданку, — незворушно відповів Вістович, — я міг би мати сумніви щодо хересу або, скажімо, рислінгу, але щодо к'янті — ніколи.

Маґда нарешті всміхнулася і, взявши каву, обережно відпила. Чоловік не зводив з неї очей, і обоє досі стояли, хоч це було й незручно, оскільки поїзд трясло.

— Куди ти прямуєш? — запитав нарешті комісар.

— До Лемберга.

— Це ж треба, — він здивувався цілком щиро.

Виходить, ніяка не Прага, і ніякий не Відень. Шпигунка з A III b має завдання в його рідному місті.

— Не розпитуй в мене нічого, будь ласка, — попросила жінка. — Я розумію, що тебе розпікає цікавість, проте не змушуй мене брехати.

— Гаразд, — зітхнув він, — скажи принаймні, чи їдеш туди сама, чи з тобою ще десяток агентів?

— Фішер і Клавдія також у поїзді, — відповіла Маґда, — з ними ще двоє чоловіків, не агентів.

— На пероні я бачив лише тебе. Вони в іншому вагоні?

Агентка кивнула.

— У тому, що з іншого боку ресторації.

На цих словах Маґда стиснула губи, аж вони побіліли, й відставила каву.

— Ти могла би бути зі мною відвертішою, — дорікнув їй Вістович, — врешті-решт дечим мені зобов'язана.

— А хіба я не достатньо сказала? — раптом випалила Маґда. — Ти тепер знаєш більше, ніж будь-хто сторонній.

— Що ви робитимете у Львові? — запитав комісар.

— Я ж просила, не розпитуй.

Жінка відвела очі до вікна, де виднілися малоприємні околиці Страсбурга. Інженери залізниць мають дивовижний талант прокладати колію найогиднішими дільницями навіть найчарівніших міст.

Вістович дивився на бліді щоки Маґдалени й натягнуту шкіру на шиї, таку делікатну й прозору, що під нею виднілися тонкі сині жилки. Був час, коли він припадав губами до цієї шкіри, відчуваючи, як під нею збуджено пульсує кров.

Він спробував узяти жінку за руку, але та сердито відмахнулася.

— Усе це недоречно, Адаме, — промовила Маґда. Вперше назвавши його на ім'я.

— Що саме?

— Твоя поява, залицяння, вино...

— Хіба ж я залицяюся?

Вона засміялася. Сміх прозвучав трохи нервово.

— Подивися на себе, — промовила Маґда, — огрядний немолодий Дон Жуан, що кілька хвилин тому поспіхом нарядився в ґарнітур, бо побачив перед собою ту, що може якось придатися. Яке щастя, правда?.. Удача сама йде до рук. Чому б зі мною не порозважатися, як з курвою, випитати все, що хочеш, а потім покинути? Як минулого разу?..

— Про що ти, Маґдо?.. — спантеличено видавив з себе Вістович.

— Забирайся під три чорти! — гнівно вигукнула вона й вказала на двері. — Я попрошу, аби все, що ти приніс, занесли назад.

— Не потрібно, — відказав він і, не зволікаючи більше ні миті, вийшов. — Вар'ятка, — сердито додав уже в коридорі, на ходу зриваючи з себе хустинку, що пахнула кельнською водою.

Втім, його роздратування потроху згасало, щойно він пригадав слова Маґди про Фішера й Клавдію. Що, в біса, мусило статися, аби всі вони в один час вирушили на окраїну Австро-Угорщини? І чи знають, цікаво, про те, що в них під носом вони з Редлем? Втім, якщо не знають, то от-от дізнаються. Найпевніше, Клавдія вже з'ясовує, хто подорожує в обох вагонах першого класу.

З іншого боку, що б не гнало прусських розвідників Третього відділу зараз до Львова, ті не обов'язково мають бути йому ворогами. Якраз навпаки. І Фішер, і Клавдія могли б стати його союзниками у протистоянні з Редлем. Звісно, якщо той не домовиться з ними раніше. Так чи інакше, лишалося чекати найпершої зручної можливості поговорити з майором Фішером.

Вдалося це зробити за обідом. Теодор Фішер сидів у товаристві худорлявого чоловіка з акуратною борідкою.

Незнайомець дивився стомленим відсутнім поглядом кудись перед собою, у той час як майор насолоджувався сигарою й неспішно щось йому говорив. Так ніби втішав свого співрозмовника або доводив, що життя — не тільки неприємності й труднощі, а відрізок часу, не позбавлений також і приємних речей.

Як не дивно, побачивши комісара, майор першим подав йому знак, запрошуючи приєднатися до їхнього товариства. Львів'янин кивнув у відповідь і попрямував до них.

— Пане Вістовичу! — Фішер підвівся йому назустріч і простягнув руку для привітання. — Радий вас бачити. Зізнаюся, неабияк втішився, дізнавшись, що ви також у цьому поїзді.

«Як же чудово в нього виходить брехати, — подумки зауважив комісар, — насправді ж йому хочеться, аби я вийшов і випадково залишився на якій-небудь одинокій станції подалі від цивілізації».

— Пане Фішере! — не менш радісно промовив львів'янин, тиснучи йому руку. — Яка несподіванка! Їдете до Відня? Чи до Праги?

Вістовичу здалося, що ці запитання прозвучали трохи фальшиво, адже він добре знав відповідь, проте вирішив не перейматися. Врешті-решт уся ця розмова була фальшивою, і жодне слово в ній не коштувало найменшого недоїдка з цієї самої ресторації, де вони перебували.

— Не вгадали, комісаре. Будете вражені, але я прямую до Лемберга, — сказав Фішер.

Вістович удав глибоке здивування.

— Як і пан Бобровський, — вказав він на чоловіка навпроти себе. — До речі, познайомтеся...

— Яків Олександрович Бобровський, — підвівшись з-за столу, сам представився той, вимовляючи кожне слово повільно й виразно, мовби для того, щоб комісар запам'ятав його ім'я на віки вічні й не смів ніколи переплутати з будь-яким іншим.

— Адам Вістович, — відповів комісар.

Зачувши слов'янське ім'я, Бобровський пожвавішав. Уважно подивившись на комісара, він запитав:

— Можливо, ми не мусимо говорити з вами німецькою? Ви знаєте російську?

— На жаль, ні.

— Чому? Хіба ви не з Галичини?

— У Галичині говорять польською, українською й німецькою. Але не російською.

В очах Якова світилося щире здивування, він, здавалося, досі був переконаний, що російською говорять усі слов'яни.

Вістович сказав правду: знайти навіть у Львові мовця російською було важко. Що вже й говорити про менші міста. Сам він міг, за потреби, порозумітися з росіянином і на службі навіть мусив читати ліві пропагандистські газети російською, проте зазвичай волів уникати таких лінгвістичних потуг.

На додаток запротестував Фішер:

— Е ні, пане Бобровський! Жодної мені тут російської! Чи ви хочете, аби я ні чорта не розумів?

— Даруйте, — знічено, як гімназист на уроці, відповів той.

— Ми ще нічого не замовляли, — сказав майор тепер уже Вістовичу, — тож ви нагодилися якраз вчасно. Пообідаймо разом, якщо не заперечуєте.

Комісар погодився. Підійшов світловолосий кельнер, що найперше приязно кивнув комісару, а далі приготувався записати їхні побажання. Усі троє замовили шніцель «Кордон блю» з картопляним гарніром і гострою приправою. До цього — по чарці міцного виноградного шнапсу.

Розмова спочатку поточилася, здавалось, на цілком посполиті теми. Хоч усі троє уважно слухали один одного, прагнучи не проґавити момент, коли співрозмовник вибовкає щось важливе. Коли принесли їжу, йшлося про міжнародну політику:

— Світ потроху охоплює параноя, — розрізаючи шніцель надвоє, аби переконатися, що той добре просмажений, зауважив майор. — Від Британії до Італії ледь не кожна газета пише, що мир у Європі тимчасовий. Ми живемо на діжці з порохом і чекаємо лише на іскру.

— Якщо так, то цією іскрою мала б бути Франція, — докинув комісар, — горді французи досі не змирилися з утратою Ельзасу.

— Можливо, — згодився Фішер. — До того ж Франція — єдина серед усіх республіка. Страчувати монархів там вміють, як ніде. Думаю, її слід остерігатися хоча б через це.

Розсміявшись над власним жартом, він ковтнув трохи шнапсу.

— Ви забуваєте про Сербію, — промовив Бобровський. — Точніше, про те, як ця країна вміє скидати тиранів.

Шніцель йому не смакував, і він повільно, наче змушуючи себе, їв гарнір.

— «Тиранів», — напівсерйозно перекривив його майор, — ох, це ваше лівацтво, добродію. Ніяк не збагну, звідки воно в російського вельможі.

— Але монархія в Сербії залишилася. Адже після травневого перевороту* трон посів Петар I**, — сказав Вістович.

— Який, що цікаво, у 70-му воював за французів, — додав Фішер, — у мадам історії, як бачимо, своєрідний гумор.

Яша стенув плечима.

— Петар — надзвичайно м'який король. Сербія при ньому розквітла.

— І зблизилася з Росією, — додав комісар.

— У цьому нічого дивного. Південні слов'яни — наші брати.

— Гаразд, тоді міркуємо далі, — майор підпалив свою згаслу сигару. — Сербія зближується з Росією, а отже, віддаляється від Австрії. Вам, панове, не здається, що Франц Йозеф врешті-решт захоче відновити свій вплив?

— Тобто, на вашу думку, «іскрою» стануть Балкани? — перепитав Вістович.

— Я лише розвинув думку пана Бобровського.

— Франц Йозеф захоче, якщо захочуть у Берліні, — відповів росіянин, — адже вся австрійська політика робиться там.

— Не перебільшуйте, — сказав майор.

---

* Військовий переворот, що стався в Сербії 29 травня 1903 року. Офіцери на чолі з капітаном Драгутином Дмітрієвичем жорстоко вбили короля Александра, останнього з династії Обреновичів, його дружину, її братів, а також прем'єр-міністра й міністра оборони. Цікаво, що Драгутин Дмітрієвич надалі очолив терористичну організацію «Чорна рука», причетну до вбивства австрійського ерцгерцога Франца Фердинанда 1914 року в Сараєво. Саме «Сараєвське вбивство» стало причиною Першої світової війни.

** Петар I Карагеоргієвич (1844–1921) — сербський король, а з 1918 року також король хорватів і словенців.

— Я хотів би перебільшувати, але хіба не ваш кайзер називав австрійського імператора «прусським генералом»?

Мовби відчувши, що говорить забагато, Бобровський опустив очі й знову взявся до своєї картоплі, до якої, як і до шніцеля, все більше втрачав інтерес.

Спостерігаючи за ними, комісар ніяк не міг зрозуміти, що, зрештою, змусило цих двох до кооперації. Адже вони, безумовно, вирушили в одному керунку, до Лемберга, в якійсь спільній справі.

— Чи знаєте ви, пане майоре, що полковник Редль також в цьому поїзді? — врешті запитав він. Йому хотілося розповісти й про Карела Грумма, але вирішив зробити це пізніше.

Фішер кивнув і видихнув дим кудись угору, як цирковий штукар видихає вогонь.

— Ви хотіли сказати «був у цьому поїзді», комісаре, — виправив він співрозмовника.

— Що ви маєте на увазі? — не зрозумів той.

— Те, що полковник вийшов у Страсбурзі.

— Он як?

Непідробне здивування Вістовича добряче потішило майора.

— Уявіть собі. Просто наш знайомий знайшов спосіб швидше дістатися до Лемберга, ніж ми, — пояснив Фішер. — Об одинадцятій звідти вирушив інший поїзд, який не робить так багато зупинок, як наш, і прибуває в Ґаліцію швидше. На кілька годин.

Обідати вони закінчили майже мовчки. Комісар відмовився від десерту, бо не надто полюбляв солодке, а випити ще шнапсу, як пропонував йому Фішер, не хотілося.

Зрештою, вони попрощались, і Вістович подався до свого місця у вагоні.

Знімаючи піджак, чоловік пригадував їхню розмову. На позір, звичайну. Таку ж могли провадити будь-де в Європі, щоб убити час або порушити незручну тишу в товаристві. Проте комісар зауважив пильність, з якою Фішер за ним спостерігав. Мовби намагаючись вловити не просто кожне слово, а й інтонацію, з якою воно промовлене, а надто — прихований смисл, що міг за ним ховатися. Майор не запитав комісара, що той робив у Швейцарії, знаючи, певно, що Вістович не скаже йому правди. Тому цю правду майор із A III b намагався відшукати сам.

Вістович, зрештою, не був проти поговорити з майором щиро. Настільки щиро, наскільки дозволив би йому здоровий глузд і обставини. Можна було б розповісти про імовірну співпрацю Редля з росіянами. Бо хоч полковник стверджував, що має справу з приватним шпигунським агентством, комісар у це не вірив. Однак, завадив росіянин, що був з ними. Хто він, цей Бобровський? Шпиг? Арештант? Компаньйон Фішера?

Наступні кілька годин комісар знову присвятив розгадуванню шифру. Цього разу він вирішив шукати ключ інакше. Спробував проаналізувати, які символи в цій головоломці трапляються найчастіше. Якщо тут використано алгоритм заміни, тобто за літерою шифру ховається літера повідомлення, то вони мали б означати голосні «а», «е» або «о». Крім того, мусили б знаходитися переважно після приголосних, найчастіше — на другому місці в складах... Комісар виписав їх в окремий рядок. Далі спробував розшукати в тексті сполучники, як-от «і», «у» та «в». Зрештою, Вістовичу навіть здалося, що справа посувається і де-не-де в шифрі почав угадуватися зміст.

Непомітно минуло кілька годин і дві станції. Сонце за вікном висіло вже зовсім низько над горизонтом, віщуючи завершення дня й близьку ніч. Ельзас лишився позаду, і тепер їхній експрес мчав поміж горами Шварцвальду, долаючи мости-віадуки й занурюючись у довгі тунелі. Потрапляючи в темряву, пасажири перелякано скрикували й намагалися намацати вмикач світильника. Звісно, стосувалося це тільки пасажирів першого класу, котрі мали в купе власне освітлення. Іншим же доводилось тільки терпляче очікувати, коли поїзд знову виїде з тунелю на світ Божий. У другому класі жарівки вмикалися не раніше восьмої години.

Несподівано в його двері хтось постукав. Вістович стрепенувся й витягнув з кишені браунінг. Відчинив, тримаючи зброю напоготові.

У коридорі стояла Маґда.

— Можна мені зайти? — запитала вона.

Комісар, не кажучи ні слова, відступив убік, одночасно ховаючи браунінг. Жінка зайшла досередини. В руках у неї виявився ресторанний кошичок, в якому зазвичай доставляють клієнтові їжу додому. З нього визирала та сама нерозпита пляшка «*Chianti*», знову закрита корком.

— Майже все з нашого сніданку згодиться на вечерю, — сказала Маґда, ставлячи кошичок на стіл.

Вістович все ще мовчав.

— Гаразд, якщо не хочеш мене бачити, я піду.

Він обережно її стримав.

— Давай нарешті поснідаємо, — запропонував чоловік, і Маґда не стримала усмішки.

За пів години все їхнє невеличке приміщення вже заливало червоним призахідним світлом.

Сир і фрукти зі сніданку чудово смакували до вина. Трохи зачерствілі ельзаські булочки мали, втім, досі апетитний вигляд, і варення з персиків пасувало до них не гірше, ніж пасувало б уранці.

Чоловік і жінка багато жартували й балакали про подорож. Обговорювали австрійську залізницю і тішилися, що живуть у часи, коли технічні можливості дозволяють людям за короткий час, усього за дві з половиною доби, переміститися з Берна до Лемберга. Тоді ще як на початку минулого, дев'ятнадцятого століття, це здавалося лише надміру сміливою мрією. Ці двоє ніби хотіли наговорити якнайбільше слів, щоб ті віддалили їх від неприємного ранку в Ельзасі, коли спочатку з поїзда винесли тіло самогубця, а потім Маґда прогнала Вістовича геть.

Коли теми для розмов і жартів закінчилися, жінка обережно запитала, що за рукопис лежить у нього під канапою. Комісар спершу здивувався, а потім зрозумів, що цілковито забув про папери, які поцупив з купе Ебербаха. Забув, хоч у ту мить вони здалися йому важливими, що він вирішив навіть приховати їх від страсбурзької поліції.

— Гадки не маю, що це, — сказав він, беручи рукопис до рук. — Текст італійською, тому прочитати я не можу.

— Дай сюди, — сказала Маґда.

— Ти знаєш італійську? — здивувався він.

Вона не відповіла й узялася читати. Добрих чверть години мовчала, аж Вістовичу набридло чекати, і він уже хотів запитати її, про що там ідеться.

— Це любовний роман, — засміялася вона. — І доволі сороміцький.

— Жартуєш?

— Ні, ось послухай: «Зазвичай мені вдавалося вгадати його бажання. Як саме йому хочеться взяти мене сьогодні... Чи прагне він спочатку мене попестити, а потім насолодитися моїми пестощами, чи без прелюдій, одразу оголитися й оголити мене. А далі, вибравши зручне положення, увійти у моє лоно...». Звідки це? — запитала Маґда.

Вістович вагався з відповіддю. Якщо розповісти їй правду, то, найпевніше, вона вважатиме його дурнем. Бо тільки дурень міг замість справді важливих паперів ухопити якусь порнографічну писанину, якою Ебербах, мабуть, збуджувався перед візитом до коханки. Або дружини. Комісар сподівався, що в рукописі знайде доказ проти вбивці, а натомість — мав лише сповідь невідомої авторки, яка вибирала любовну позицію зі своїм любасиком. Тому Вістович тільки стенув плечима, мовби забув звідки або це не має ані найменшого значення. Наповнив спорожнілі склянки вином і трохи відпив.

«Що ж до мене самої, то найбільше я любила, коли нам прагнулося трохи гри й солодкої розпусти, — читала далі Маґда. — Я не соромилася пестощів на французький манер, дозволяючи моїм вустам і язикові ковзати по його животу і навіть опускатися нижче. Я дозволяла собі вкривати поцілунками його твердь, мліючи від думки, що от-от вона опиниться в мені... Втім, спочатку просила його делікатно поніжити пальцями моє лоно. Мені хотілося такого ж збудження, яке вирувало в той момент у ньому...»

— Увесь рукопис про це? — запитав комісар, допиваючи вино зі своєї склянки.

Маґда перегорнула кілька сторінок.

— Не весь, — сказала вона. — Але ось що цікаво...

Жінка якусь хвилину мовчки вчитувалася.

— Події цієї любовної історії відбуваються в Лемберзі, — продовжила вона.

— Он як, — Вістович не знав, як реагувати на цю новину.

— Авторку звати Ельвіра Сапфо... Гм, думаю, це псевдонім... — досліджувала далі Маґда, повернувшись до перших сторінок. — Переклад зроблено з німецької в Цюриху 27 березня цього року. Ім'я перекладача також вказано: Антон Піллер. Чув про такого?

— Ні, — похитав головою комісар.

— Але найцікавіше тут — назва історії.

— Яка?

Жінка показала йому титульну сторінку.

— «Розпусний міністр», — провела вона пальчиком по великих літерах, виведених чорним атраментом, — і підзаголовок: «Скандальна молодість міністра поліції Фердинанда фон Шпрегорфа».

Вістовичу перехопило дихання.

— Отже... — промовив він, але не знайшов слів, щоб продовжити.

— Отже, тобі дістався компромат на імперського міністра, який переклали італійською. Думаю, хтось збирався це видати, — замість нього договорила Маґда.

— І в такий спосіб помститися за щось?

Тепер вже Маґда стенула плечима.

— Про це краще запитати в пані Ельвіри Сапфо. Цілком можливо, що вона львів'янка. Знайди її й запитай, навіщо їй це все здалося.

Жінка повернула йому рукопис.

— Мені насправді байдуже... Навіть якщо йдеться про міністра, — сказав комісар, відкладаючи папери вбік.

— І до мене тобі байдуже? — раптом запитала Маґда, підводячись зі свого місця.

Підійшовши до Вістовича, стала над ним і поклала руки йому на плечі.

— Аж ніяк, — відповів той. — Але я для тебе «огрядний і немолодий Дон Жуан»...

Маґда приклала палець йому до вуст, і коли той замовк, одним рухом вимкнула світильник. У сутінках звела руки догори.

— Зніми з мене сукню, — тихо мовила вона.

Чоловік підвівся й обережно виконав прохання. Долоні його ковзнули вздовж усього її тіла, від колін до плечей, впізнаючи його на дотик. Тільки тепер він зрозумів, що скучив за Маґдою, тому коли весь одяг уже було знято, не поспішав, а й далі насолоджувався її оголеною присутністю, запахом волосся, шкіри й передчуттям того, що от-от станеться.

Торкнувся пальцями її плаского живота, малюючи на ньому невидимі кола, як шаман, що здійснював ритуал. Потім пальці пірнули між її пружних стегон, і вона, ніби втративши рівновагу, сперлася на свого коханця, обхопивши руками його шию. Трохи подалася вперед, притулившись до нього персами. Поставила ноги ширше, на ширину плечей, мов гімнастка, що готувалася виконати вправу. Насправді ж Маґда хотіла, аби чоловіча долоня, що її пестила, мала більше простору.

— Я більше не можу, — простогнала вона за хвилину й потягнула коханця до себе. Одночасно піднесла коліно вгору, мов танцюючи з ним танґо.

Він входив у неї обережно, хоча кортіло зробити це сильно. Дослухався, як вона реагує. Коли проник повністю, на кілька секунд завмер, відчуваючи, як пульсує зсередини її тіло. Маґда вкривала поцілунками його шию, гладила плечі, вимагала продовжувати. Він, зрештою, хотів того самого, тому більше не зупинявся.

Переїжджаючи черговий міст безмежного Шварцвальду, коханці врешті вдовольнилися, скрикнувши, либонь, занадто голосно. Аж Маґда від сорому прикусила губу. Втім, їх навряд хто-небудь почув. На щастя, експрес торохтів у цю мить особливо гучно.

Маґдалена не повернулася до свого купе. Хоч, мабуть, слід було б — на випадок, якщо Клавдія чи Фішер матимуть до неї розмову. Вістович застелив постіль і дістав з полиці теплу ковдру. Вкрив Маґду та ліг поруч, хоч заснути не зумів.

Прокинулася вона о шостій, вже коли минули Прагу. Вістович встиг одягнутися й принести з ресторації сніданок.

— Що ж, цього разу наш романс затягнувся, — усміхнулася жінка. — Минулого разу в Позені ми попрощалися значно раніше.

Купе наповнилося запахом кави і свіжої богемської випічки, яку кельнери купили під час зупинки пів години тому.

— Маємо час до Лемберга, — відповів чоловік, обережно наповнюючи горнятка. — У Лемберзі ти знову зникнеш...

— Мабуть, — згодилася вона.

Жінка спочатку прикривалася ковдрою, але потім відкинула її. П'ючи каву, вона більше не ховала свої спокусливі груди.

Вістович спостерігав за нею, запаливши свою першу на сьогодні цигарку.

— Чи могла б ти допомогти мені з шифром? — раптом запитав він.

— З шифром? — здивовано перепитала Маґда.

— Так. Думаю, пані Шраґмюллер вчила вас криптографії.

— Гаразд, — погодилася жінка.

Він розгорнув блокнот і поклав його перед нею на столик. Маґда відставила горнятко й сперлася на лікоть, відкривши таким чином решту тіла. Кілька хвилин вдивлялася в символи. Далі переглянула марні спроби Вістович знайти розв'язок. Відкинула назад волосся, вправно закрутивши його на потилиці. Груди її при цьому підстрибнули й заколихалися. Потім знову схилилася над записами.

— Подай мені мій ридикюль, — попросила Маґда за якийсь час.

Вістович виконав прохання. Маґда витягнула з нього невеликий округлий футляр. Могло здатися, що всередині — компас або збільшувальне скло. Натомість жінка дістала звідти щось, що нагадувало радше кишеньковий сонячний годинник. На тонкій дерев'яній підставці розташовувався бронзовий диск, по краях якого були вирізані літери. Диск виявився подвійним: всередині нього оберталася така сама, але, звісна річ, меншого розміру кругла пластинка. На ній також був алфавіт. У початковому положенні внутрішні й зовнішні літери збігалися. Зовнішня «А» знаходилася навпроти внутрішньої, внутрішня «В» — навроти зовнішньої і так далі по колу. Втім, було зрозуміло, що з рухом внутрішнього диску ця симетрія зникає. Тоді, приміром, «A» опиняється навпроти «C», а «D» — навпроти «E». Усі інші літери також отримували свою нову «пару». Поверталася внутрішня пластина, очевидно, за допомогою ключа, оскільки в ній виднілася характерна шпарина.

— Ти чув щось про шифр Цезаря? — запитала Маґда.

Вістович невпевнено кивнув.

— Здається, так. Це коли одна літера замінюється іншою, і для запису утворюється новий алфавіт.

— Саме так.

— Але хіба це не занадто легко? — засумнівався комісар. — Адже врешті-решт можна перебрати всі можливі варіанти. Їх буде стільки, скільки літер в алфавіті. Тобто 26*.

— Так, якщо змістити алфавіт лише один раз...

З цими словами вона дістала з футляра маленького ключа і повернула диск на дві літери.

— Зміщення — 2, — промовила Маґда, — кожна літера «A» відповідає літері «C». Варіантів для шифру і справді тільки 26, і розгадати нескладно. Але зміщення пластин можна проводити перед кожним новим реченням або навіть перед кожною буквою. Кількість варіантів тоді зросте до тисяч.

Вістович нетямився з радощів.

— Гадаєш, текст зашифровано саме в такий спосіб? — запитав він.

— Я лише припускаю. Думаю, той, хто писав, приховуючи зміст, робив поворот диску перед кожним новим словом. Звісно, деякі цифри можуть означати власне цифри... Але спробуймо.

---

* Для українського алфавіту шифр Цезаря має 32 варіанти.

Наступної миті Вістович і Маґда з неабияким азартом, забувши про все на світі, взялися до роботи.

Агентка мала рацію. Менше ніж за годину на новому аркуші комісар записав прихований зміст:

«Повідомляю і гарантую, що вантаж прибуде в Лемберг 19 квітня. Склад на Підзамчі. Всі дані передано також Орлову.

З повагою,
Ніцетас

P.S. Номер мого рахунку в Швейцарії не змінився. Буду вдячний, якщо отримаю обіцяну винагороду не пізніше середини травня».

— Ну ось, — з неприхованим тріумфом і гордістю в голосі промовила Маґда. — Тепер ти знаєш усе, що знає відправник.

Вона почала вдягатися, і Вістович не міг відвести від неї очей. Хоч більше, ніж тіло, його заворожив її розум.

— Знаєш, про що йдеться у цьому тексті? — запитала жінка.

Комісар вирішив не приховувати.

— Думаю, Ніцетас — це псевдонім полковника Редля. У мене є підозри, що той провадить нечесну гру, — сказав він і коротко розповів про свою пригоду в Берні.

— Якщо наважишся на протистояння, то в тебе в руках серйозні карти, — підсумувала Маґда.

Вона майже вдяглася, проте обом хотілося ще близькості. І обоє відчували це навзаєм. Втім, часу в них уже не було.

— Чому ледь не весь A III b вирушив до Лемберга? — запитав комісар.

— Якщо я розповім тобі, мене повісять, — напівсерйозно сказала жінка.

— Облиш. Ніхто не дізнається.

— Не можу, Адаме.

Маґда дивилася в люстерко і сяк-так намагалася приборкати своє неслухняне волосся.

— Ну, гаразд. А хто цей Бобровський? Той тип, якого я бачив біля Фішера.

Цього разу Вістович вирішив дотиснути:

— Маґдо, я розповів тобі стільки, що *Evidenzbüro* мало б усі підстави зварити мене живцем у котлі, як за часів середньовіччя. Якщо Редль зрадник, то найперше я мав доповісти про це у Відень, а не розпатякувати прусській агентці...

Вона закусила губу. Схоже, «прусська агентка» з вуст чоловіка, з яким провела ніч, прозвучало для неї не надто приємно.

— Бобровський — це російський багатій і вельможа, який рік тому підтримав есерів. Мусив тікати до Пруссії... — промовила жінка. — Друзі в Бадені сховали його до психіатричної клініки під виглядом пацієнта.

— Що за друзі?

Маґда витримала паузу. Доволі довгу, але Вістович терпляче чекав.

— Ім'я одного з них у твоєму шифрі, — вона вказала на блокнот.

— Орлов?

— Так.

— І ти хотіла змовчати?

— Чорт забирай, Адаме, якби не я, ти б розгадував його до кінця життя! — в очах її загорівся гнів.

— Або віддав би криптографу, — сказав комісар. — Зрештою, зміст листа виявився корисним не лише мені, але й тобі.

— Орлов — емігрант, як і Бобровський. Але впливовіший.

— Щось цих емігрантів у вас забагато, — іронічно зауважив Вістович.

— Нічого дивного. За останній рік з Росії втекло більше людей, ніж за попереднє сторіччя. Але Орлову вдалося добре пристосуватися. У Пруссії в нього міцні зв'язки і з російською амбасадою, і з багатими росіянами.

— І з «охранкою»?

Маґда хитнула головою.

— Спочатку він щиро допомагав своєму другові, але потім Варшавський відділ* «переконав» його видати їм Бобровського. В Орлова на батьківщині лишилися родичі, тому натиснути було нескладно.

Вістович кивнув.

— А як про це дізналися ви?

— У нас є подвійна агентка. Коханка Бобровського, співачка...

Маґда сіпнулася, мовби від раптової мігрені.

— Боже, я тобі все вибовкала.

— Заспокойся, — Вістович з ніжністю торкнувся її руки. — Ти ж і дізналася чимало.

---

* Варшавський відділ — військовий округ збройних сил Російської імперії, що розташовувався у Варшаві (на той час місто було окуповане росіянами). При Варшавському окрузі містилось Розвідувальне бюро.

– Що це за Підзамче? – запитала Маґда за якийсь час.

– Дільниця у Львові, – пояснив комісар, – але тут, очевидно, йдеться про залізничні склади.

Кілька хвилин вони мовчали.

– Коли вийду звідси, у нас не повинно залишитися нічого спільного, – промовила врешті Маґда.

– Крім спогадів, – сказав Вістович.

– І навіть спогади треба стерти.

– Аж ніяк. Нехай вони залишаться. Часом, коли все летить під три чорти, спогади – це єдине, що повертає притомність. Не дає з'їхати з глузду. Вони мені знадобляться...

VI

Лемберг
14–18 квітня 1906 року

На станції «Лемберг» Вістович тільки мигцем побачив Маґду й Фішера. Зійшовши на перон, вони віддавали короткі розпорядження вокзальному носієві щодо свого багажу. Були схожі на німецьке подружжя, що з якихось причин вибралося до Галичини. Зрештою, цілком можливо, що саме за чоловіка й дружину вони себе тут видавали. Тоді, мабуть, іншим «подружжям» були Бобровський і Клавдія. Вістович криво посміхнувся від цього здогаду і рушив до стоянки фіакрів. Хотілося швидше дістатися додому.

Була Великодня субота, й візники підвищили ціну вдвічі. Клієнти обурювалися, втім, однаково платили, бо не мали вибору. Не йти ж додому пішки з багажем у руках. За інших обставин комісар дістав би поліційний жетон і, не добираючи надто пристойних слів, пообіцяв би хапугам усі жахи пекла. Аж врешті ті мусили б везти його задурно. Та сьогодні не хотілося.

Заплативши, скільки просили, Вістович сів у незручний міський екіпаж, котрий через Казимирівську*, повз недобудовані, обвиті риштовками стіни, що мали в майбутньому стати стінами костелу святої Єлизавети, попри костел святої Анни й далі повз «Бригідки»** виїхав спершу до Нового театру***, а відтак — на Вірменську. Візникові наказав зупинитися трохи раніше. Хотів прогулятися.

Днина була погожа. Сонце нагрівало бруківку й стіни кам'яниць, об які терлися ліниві коти. Вірменська була майже безлюдна, проте, як не дивно, гамірна. Гамір долинав з відчинених вікон разом із божественними запахами страв, що їх господині готували на Великдень. Від цих ароматів печені, варива й солодощів комісар ковтав слину, бо не встиг подбати про обід, а тим часом потроху зближався час вечері. На ратуші пробило п'яту по полудні.

У своєму помешканні Вістович відчув, як поряд з голодом усередині зароджується інше, значно сильніше й нещадніше відчуття. Це було відчуття провини. З'явилося воно, щойно комісар побачив, що в кожній з його кімнат панує ідеальна чистота. Тільки одна людина в цілому світі могла подбати про його житло. І, зрештою, тільки їй він би й довірив свої ключі.

Бейла з'явилася в житті Вістовича ще до того, як дружина комісара, акторка Анна Каліш, одного разу поспіхом

---

* Тепер — частина вулиці Городоцької.

** «Бригідки» — діюча донині в'язниця, що була заснована 1782 року на місці монастиря св. Бригіди. Звідси й назва.

*** Тепер — Львівський національний академічний театр опери та балету імені Соломії Крушельницької.

спакувала речі й нічним експресом утекла до Берліна. Життя з поліційним комісаром виявилось не для неї. До того ж берлінський Шаушпільгауз пропонував їй контракт, про який актриса з провінційного австрійського Лемберга могла тільки мріяти.

Після скандалів, які влаштовувала Анна, Вістович зазвичай мовчки виходив з дому. Але піти міг лише у двох керунках: або до кнайпи, звідки потім брів у перший-ліпший готель, або до помешкання Бейли поруч зі Стрийським парком. Туди він, щоправда, також часто приходив напідпитку.

Бейла не ставила зайвих питань, ніколи не дорікала і нічого від нього не вимагала, крім як прийняти ванну й трохи протверезіти, перш ніж опинитися з нею під однією ковдрою. Розуміла, як потрібна йому, і розуміла, що створює для цього чоловіка, можливо, єдиний у світі прихисток, де Вістович міг бути собою. Вночі з ним вона брала своє. Попри грубуватий вигляд, він несподівано виявився делікатним і вправним коханцем.

Ця жінка нічого не розпитувала у комісара, але нічого й не розповідала про себе. Вістович знав тільки, що Бейла, як і Самковський, була родом з Дрогобича. Помешкання у Львові, невеличка, проте зґрабна вілла, дісталося їй у спадок... Ось і все.

І хоч Бейла не сказала б йому ані слова, якби й дізналася про його ніч у поїзді з іншою жінкою, саме через це Вістовича нестерпно розпікала провина. А заодно й думка, чи не робить вона того самого? Чи не проводить ночі в обіймах іншого чоловіка? Адже іноді вона зникає на тиждень або й на місяць. Потім пояснює, що мусила відвідати родичів...

— Яких родичів? — допитувався комісар. — Хто в тебе є в Дрогобичі? Чи не в Дрогобичі?.. Чи, може, й не родичі?..

Питань вона не любила, тому мовчала у відповідь.

— Все одно ти моя, — сміявся тоді Вістович.

— Ми не речі, любий, — відповідала Бейла цілком серйозно й дивилася на нього своїми великими карими очима, — ми не можемо комусь належати. Свобода й спокій — це найбільші людські цінності. Не треба зазіхати на жодну з них, бо й друга тоді не значитиме нічого.

— Свобода й спокій, — повторив він тепер, ставлячи на підлогу валізу й знімаючи плаща. — Втративши спокій, мені тепер і справді до дупи моя свобода...

Не переодягаючись, зайшов до вітальні й відшукав у кредενсі почату пляшку «*Baczewski*». У кухні стояв кошичок зі свіжими булочками й тарілка з сиром. Бейла знала, що він повернеться сьогодні, й відправила служницю трохи поповнити його запаси. «Як доречно...» — подумав комісар і налив собі першу чарку. Хотілося залити це бісове відчуття провини, навіть якщо знадобиться більше, ніж одна пляшка.

— Ти негідник, Адаме... — пробурмотів він сам до себе за годину й, не роздягаючись, побрів до ліжка. — Найбільший, курва, негідник в усьому бісовому світі...

Вранці його розбудили дзвони на церковних вежах міста.

Щойно Вістович спробував підвестись, як йому здалося, що ці дзвони б'ють просто в його голові. Жорстоке похмілля підсилювало їх у тисячу разів, і вони відлунювали у скронях пекельним болем. До всього, страшенно мучила спрага.

Підвівшись нарешті, комісар поплентався до ванної, де, знайшовши мидницю, заповнену водою до країв, не роздумуючи, занурив у неї голову. Рідина виплеснулася і розтеклася по підлозі. За кілька секунд Вістович підняв голову й судомно хапнув повітря. Відчув, що йому трохи полегшало, втім, тепер до горла підступила нудота. Глибоко вдихнувши й видихнувши, чоловік промовив перше на сьогодні слово:

— Курва...

Обережно сперся на стіну і з ненавистю подивився у дзеркало. Звідти на нього витріщилася неголена спухла мармиза з розкуйовдженим волоссям. Під нею виднівся мокрий комір, що був пристебнутий до зім'ятої сорочки.

— Курва, — повторив комісар і відвернувся від свого відображення.

Він почовгав до вітальні, де з надією відшукав учорашню пляшку. Ухопив її й підняв до рівня очей. Всередині не було ані краплини, отже, похмелитися й трохи полегшити свої страждання йому не вдасться. На столі лежали недоїдки сиру й хліба, проте думки про їжу викликали хіба що відразу. «Треба вийти й перехилити десь чарку, — подумав комісар, — інакше до завтра не покращає...»

Вістович переодягнув сорочку й поверх неї одягнув камізельку. Марно спробував причесати волосся. Врешті перестав ним перейматися і просто насадив на голову капелюха. Одягнув плаща і, поклавши до кишені свій порожній портсигар, вийшов на вулицю.

Погода знову була сонячна й тепла. То тут, то там з'являлися святково вбрані містяни з великодніми кошиками в руках. Радісно перемовляючись, усі вони поспішали до своїх помешкань, аби узятися до святкового сніданку.

Комісар вийшов на Домініканську площу, а звідти, через коротку вулицю Божого Тіла — на площу Ринок. З палкою надією він подивився на двері кав'ярні «Атляс», проте вони були зачинені. Вістович зиркнув на годинник. Одинадцята ранку... Це означало тільки одне — кав'ярня вже сьогодні не відчиниться.

Облизавши губи, чоловік рушив далі на пошуки, та жоден заклад у цей святковий день не приймав відвідувачів.

— От паскудство... — видихнув комісар і подався Сербською, а далі звернув на Собеського*.

Втім, і тут кожна, навіть найбрудніша, кнайпа була зачинена. Та найгіршим було те, що й купити цигарок йому сьогодні не вдасться. Оскільки власники тютюнових генделиків також воліли у святковий день бути вдома.

Біля старого міського Арсеналу Вістович раптом побачив мале дівча років шести, що, підібгавши ноги, сиділо просто на холодній бруківці. Придивившись, комісар помітив, що дівчинка схлипувала.

Він наблизився повільно, аби її не злякати, проте в якусь мить дитина звела на нього очі, повні сліз і страху. З жахом Вістович помітив на її маленькому личку чималий синець. Мала схопилася з місця.

— Не бійся, — якомога лагідніше промовив комісар.

Дівчинка не рухалася, але все ще з недовірою дивилася на неохайного незнайомця. Руки тримала перед собою, перебираючи пальчиками тканину маленької сукні.

---

* Тепер — вулиця Братів Рогатинців.

— Як тебе звати? — запитав Вістович, все ще тримаючи дистанцію.

Вона не відповіла, тому комісар назвався першим:

— Мене звати Адам.

— Той, що був у Раю? — раптом запитала дівчинка, і в її очах сяйнула цікавість.

Вістович усміхнувся.

— Ні, я інший Адам, — сказав він. — А ти маєш ім'я?

Вона кивнула.

— Ляна.

— Гарно... А скажи, Ляно, — Вістович намагався тепер втамувати внутрішню злість, — хто тебе скривдив?

Він торкнувся пальцем свого обличчя, даючи зрозуміти, що має на увазі її синець. Дівчинка скривилася, ніби збиралася заплакати.

У цей самий час у будинку праворуч від них почувся погрозливий чоловічий крик, а вслід за ним — переляканий жіночий.

— Ти мешкаєш там? — запитав чоловік, вказавши поглядом на будинок.

Ляна кивнула.

— Не йди нікуди, гаразд? — попросив комісар, додаючи у свій тон стільки спокою й безтурботності, скільки тільки міг. — Обіцяєш?

Дівчинка пообіцяла.

— Я зараз усе владнаю! — з усмішкою промовив чоловік. — Зараз усе буде добре.

І, підморгнувши їй, Вістович подався до будинку, звідки чув крики.

Долинали вони крізь відчинені двері, з помешкання у пивниці. Вістович зайшов спочатку в тісний передпокій, звідти у невелику кімнату, посеред якої було накрито скромний великодній стіл. У кутку стояв широкоплечий здоровань у полотняній сорочці й засмальцьованому жилеті. Перед ним вклякла на колінах розтріпана жінка з червоним від побоїв обличчям.

Вістовича цей бугай помітив не одразу. Та коли перевів на нього погляд, то спершу занімів від здивування.

— Ти хто? — врешті загорланив він.

— Тихіше, — скривився комісар і торкнувся долонею розпеченого лоба.

Облишивши жінку, господар загрозливо наблизився до гостя.

— Ти хто й чого приперся? — повторив він запитання.

Вістович зняв капелюха і дбайливо поклав його на стілець. Потім спокійно закотив рукави.

Здоровилу урвався терпець. Гаркнувши щось іще, він кинувся вперед на прибулого. Тієї ж миті комісар спрямував йому назустріч два коротких удари: лівий і правий. Обидва точно в щелепу.

Нападник завмер, наче від здивування. Вістович бачив, як його очі закотилися кудись угору, потім голова повернулася набік, і він усією масою повалився на підлогу. Пролунав гуркіт, наче впала важка переповнена шафа.

Натомість його жертва звелася на рівні ноги. Жінка переводила розгублений погляд з лежачого на свого рятівника і навпаки, не знаючи, що сказати.

А Вістович тим часом жадібно подивився на їхній святковий стіл.

— Можна? — запитав він, вказавши рукою на карафку з горілкою. — Ви дозволите?..

І, не чекаючи відповіді, тремтячою від похмілля й несподіваного боксу рукою налив собі повну склянку. Одразу ж випив одним ковтком.

— Ляно! Ляночко... — раптом заголосила жінка й вибігла назовні.

Комісар знову взявся за карафку. Вже коли підносив до рота нову порцію, почув, що здоровило на підлозі зарухався.

Вістович відставив, випивку, вхопив того за сорочку й допоміг йому підвестися. Губи в нього були розтовчені й невпинно кривавили.

— Подивись на мене й запам'ятай, — промовив комісар йому в обличчя. — Скривдиш їх ще раз, переламаю всі кістки. Зрозумів?

Господар кивнув.

Вістович відчув, як у голові застугоніло так, мовби там працював паровий двигун. Щоб зігнати лють, щосили зацідив здорованю кулаком під ребра. І, коли той знову опинився на підлозі, випив удруге, загриз огірком, узяв капелюха й вийшов на вулицю.

— Мамо, це Адам! — почувся голос маленької Ляни.

Вістович ґалантно уклонився їй і побрів убік Валової.

Від випитого трохи полегшало. Комісар втягнув носом весняне повітря, наповнивши ним груди й усе своє розпечене нутро. Йому подумалося, що незайвим буде зайти в Дирекцію. Хоча б тому, що в його кабінеті могли залишитися цигарки. На біду, можна буде взяти одну-дві в чергових. Та й, зрештою, завтра йому на службу, слід наперед дізнатися, що нового сталося за час його відсутності.

Двоє поліціянтів на вахті при його появі схопилися, мов ошпарені, й виструнчилися. На столику поруч із телефонним апаратом та грубим потріпаним журналом, куди вони занотовували всіх і все, що потрапляло й вибувало з будівлі Дирекції, лежала розкладена газета. На ній шматочки паски, кілька писанок, шинка й металева креманка з потертим хріном.

— Христос Воскрес, пане комісаре! — вимовили вони в один голос.

Обоє дивилися на Вістовича трохи перестрашено, бо їсти на посту заборонялося. Сподівалися хіба, що комісар буде мати Бога в серці й на Великдень їх не каратиме.

— Воістину Воскрес! — відповів той.

Раптом погляд його впав на два карабіни, що стояли одразу поруч зі столом.

— Це що? — запитав він. — Чому зброя тут? Хто дозволив?

— Не дозволив, а наказав, пане комісаре, — уточнив один із чергових. — Директор Шехтель.

— Он як? Це ж чому?

— Вас не було в Лемберзі, тому й не знаєте останніх новин. Убито вже трьох наших...

Паровий двигун у голові комісара знову запрацював із шаленою силою.

— Убито трьох поліціянтів? — перепитав Вістович, мовби не зрозумів, про кого йшлося.

— Так, пане комісаре. 13 квітня — віцекапрала Шварца, 14-го — фельдфебеля Цайса, і вчора знайшли мертвим постерункового Вільху.

— Хто веде справу? — запитав комісар.

— Спочатку доручили пану Самковському, — сказав другий черговий. — Але потім його звільнили і слідство очолив сам директор.

— Самковського звільнили? — несподівано навіть для самого себе голосно вигукнув Вістович.

Чергові знову виструнчилися.

— Так є, пане комісаре! — знову в один голос відповіли вони.

Якийсь час Вістович мовчав, дивлячись кудись на сходи, що вели на другий поверх, де був його кабінет. Крізь пелену похмілля розум комісара намагався зрозуміти, де зараз можна дістати якнайбільше відомостей про ці вбивства. Матеріали, без сумніву, замкнені, а канцеляристів сьогодні на службі немає. Телефонувати Шехтелю? Також марно. Навіть ведучи таку справу, директор не схопиться з-за великоднього столу тільки для того, щоб поспілкуватися з Вістовичем. Що ж до Самковського, то невідомо, чи після звільнення він залишився у Львові. Швидше за все, повернувся на свята до рідного Дрогобича.

— Маєте найновіші газети? — запитав він у чергових.

— Так є, пане комісаре! Зараз!

— Тільки цієї мені не потрібно, — Вістович вказав пальцем на розгорнуту шпальту «*Kurjera Lwowskiego*», що правив їм за скатертину на столі.

Обоє у відповідь реготнули й витягнули з поштової шафи перев'язаний пакунок.

— Це за три попередні доби!

— Чудово. І ще дайте мені цигарок.

Чергові здивовано вибалушили на нього очі.

— Дайте мені цигарок, матолки два, бо зараз дістанете за те, що жерли на посту! — гаркнув на них Вістович.

Ті миттю подіставали з кишень кожен по кілька сигарет. Забравши їх і вклавши у портсигар, комісар подався врешті до кабінету.

Всередині найперше відчинив вікно й підійшов до столу Самковського. Як завжди, на стільниці панував ідеальний порядок: рівно складені папери, зв'язані папки, олівці підстругані однаково, як за міркою. На кріслі висів вовняний коц. Вовна його просмерділася тютюновим димом і місцями мала дірки. Втім, якщо залишилися папери і його улюблений коц, значить, Самковський ще не встиг передати справи й мусить повернутися після свят.

Комісар підійшов до свого столу, де, на відміну від робочого місця ад'юнкта, панував безлад, вмостився у своє крісло і, закуривши, взявся перечитувати газети. Поступово, шпальта за шпальтою, стаття за статтею, він більш-менш починав розуміти, де й за яких обставин відбулися всі три вбивства. Журналісти особливо наголошували на тому, що, вбиваючи поліціянтів, невідомий маніяк щоразу здійснює той самий ритуал. Після смерті вибирає трупам очі.

З неприхованою іронією кілька видань написали, що слідчого в цій справі, ад'юнкта Антоні Самковського, звільнено з поліції за неналежне виконання служби. І правильно, мовляв, нічого доручати такі справи жовтодзьобим дилетантам. Коли місто в передвеликодній час змушене жити в страху, то розслідування таких справ слід доручати справжнім майстрам, як-от директору поліційному Вільгельмові Шехтелю.

Вістович криво всміхнувся. Можливо, Шехтель колись і був добрим детективом, але кілька років на посаді директора перетворили його на звичайного бюрократичного щура, який понад усе дбає, аби на емеритуру піти з добрим статком. А тому хоче, щоб усі звіти до Відня писалися так, мовби у Львові немає жодного злочинця. Замість них лише ксьондзи й монахині в молитовних процесіях. Ніби немає шльондр і перемитників, ґвалтівників і збоченців, крадіїв і вбивць...

Через годину, занотувавши все необхідне в блокнот, Вістович спустився донизу. Сніданок у чергових закінчився, і вони тепер звично нудьгували на своєму посту. Він повернув їм газети й попрощався.

На вулиці рушив до трамвайної зупинки. Трамвай у цей день робив усього кілька рейсів, але один із них, згідно розкладу, був за п'ятнадцять хвилин. Це була електрична лінія «Z», що провадила на Замарстинів. Звідти Вістович збирався прогулятися на станцію Підзамче.

Дорога загалом зайняла в нього пів години. А завдяки прогулянці на свіжому повітрі майже безлюдним тереном похмілля його практично минуло. На станції не було ані душі. Тільки сторож ліниво глянув у його бік і далі втупився у свою газету. Комісар мовчки пройшов повз нього й попрямував уздовж товарних колій, де, як він знав, були старі склади. Дорога була тут широка, призначена для возів, що тягли звідси вантаж у місто, але курна і повна крем'яха, яким засипали ями. Йти ставало незручно й важко.

Попереду несподівано виникла чоловіча постать. Невідомий, як і Вістович, був одягнений у довгий плащ і капелюх. Вони йшли приблизно в одному темпі, аж врешті чоловік попереду почав сповільнюватись. Постать раптом видалася Вістовичу знайомою.

— Агов, там! — гукнув комісар.

Чоловік зупинився, але повертатися не поспішав. Вістович зупинився й інстинктивно потягнувся до браунінга в кишені. Того самого, що відібрав у Редля. Чоловік попереду нарешті став до нього обличчям. Одночасно зблиснули скельця окулярів і револьвер у руці.

— Самковський! — здивовано промовив комісар.

Той опустив зброю. Подив його був не менший.

— Що ви тут робите, Самковський? — швидко наблизившись до ад'юнкта, запитав Вістович.

Водночас він придивився до обличчя підлеглого. Воно було вимучене й неголене, так само, як і обличчя самого комісара.

— Важко сказати, що я тут роблю, шефе, — зітхнув Самковський, ховаючи зброю. — Але тут безлюдно, отже, я можу почуватися в безпеці.

Вістович подивився на нього одночасно з недовірою і співчуттям. Навколо справді було порожньо, якщо не враховувати кількох бродячих собак, які сновигали поміж коліями, старими загорожами і горами важкого іржавого залізяччя. Проте безпечним це місце точно не назвеш.

— У місті мені за кожним кутком ввижається Брюкнер, — мовби прочитавши його думки, пояснив Самковський, — це той маніяк, що вбиває поліціянтів.

— Мій давній знайомий, — промовив Вістович і сплюнув у пилюку.

Ад'юнкт кивнув.

— Я багато маю розповісти вам, шефе. Хоч, може, якась частина вам уже відома.

— Знаю, що вас звільнено, — промовив комісар.

— Це не найгірше, — криво посміхнувся ад'юнкт, — мене невдовзі чекає суд. І розраховувати на м'який вирок у мене немає жодних підстав.

Вони пішли поволі в бік міста, і комісар вислухав його розповідь про засідку на Погулянці й смерть Заремби від руки Берла Брюкнера.

— Смілива авантюра, — чи то похвалив, чи то покепкував з нього Вістович.

— Шкодую, що на таке зважився, — сказав Самковський. — Тепер кінець усьому. В мене більше ані грошей, ані...

Він замовк, проте Вістовичу здалося, ніби той хотів сказати «ані бажання жити».

— Послухайте, ад'юнкте, ви ж мешкаєте неподалік?

— Пів милі звідси, — відповів той.

— Може, хоч тут, на Підзамчі, відчинена яка-небудь кнайпа? Я б зараз душу продав за гальбу холодного пива.

— Можливо, «Тлуста риба». Це те саме місце, де я вперше зіткнувся з Брюкнером, — з сумнівом у голосі сказав Самковський, — але, щиро кажучи, мені не хочеться туди потикатися.

— Годі вам, — комісар узяв його за лікоть. — Тут ми на видноті, а це ще гірше. Ходімо, я маю до вас розмову.

«Тлуста риба» справді була відчинена, щоправда, всередині нікого, крім господаря, не було. Зайґельт розставляв на поличках над шинквасом якісь трунки в різноформних і різнокольорових пляшках. Озирнувся на відвідувачів і, за звичкою, розтягнув на обличчі привітну усмішку. Приязно привітався із Самковським, повідомивши, що радий бачити його знову. Той змовчав у відповідь.

— Прошу панства, маю до диспозиції тільки напої та холодну закуску, — промовив він. — Кухня нині не працює.

— Два пива, — коротко промовив комісар. — Хліб і полядвицю з гірчицею.

— Одну хвилину, — сказав Зайґельт і зник у коморі.

Поліціянти вмостилися за той самий стіл, де кілька днів тому Самковський розмовляв із Брюкнером. Вістович полегшено видихнув, відчувши тільки тепер, як стомився після своєї прогулянки.

— Гляньте, комісаре, — засміявся раптом ад'юнкт, — ось отвір від моєї кулі. Стіл навіть не замінили.

Він вказав рукою на продірявлену стільницю.

— Наскільки серйозно ви поранили Брюкнера? — запитав Вістович.

Самковський знизав плечима.

— Він зміг вискочити звідси на своїх двох, тож... Гадаю, моя куля лише незначно його зачепила.

— Ну, знаєте, важко підстрілений кабан часом ще довго тікає від мисливців...

Вістович витягнув і поклав на стіл портсигар, але той виявився порожнім. Цигарки, здобуті у чергових, він викурив, ще коли читав газети. Врятував Самковський, який поділився з шефом самокрутами.

— Цигарок більше не купуєте? — здивувався Вістович. — Схоже, у вас направду паскудні часи.

— Ще й які, — відвівши очі, зізнався ад'юнкт. — Але після того, як мене звільнять, настануть ще паскудніші. Думаю, після суду доведеться піти до в'язниці.

Вістовичу стало його жаль. Самковського він знав давно, той завжди був надійним помічником і, попри все, таки вправним слідчим.

— Коли мусите остаточно передати справи? — запитав він у нього.

— Післязавтра або й пізніше... Після свят Шехтелю буде не до мене.

— Але від служби вас відсторонено?

Ад'юнкт кивнув.

— Чудово, — комісар випустив струмінь темного гіркого диму. Від самокрута нестерпно зашкребло в горлі, аж Вістович мусив відкашлятися.

— Чудово? — здивовано перепитав Самковський. — Ви тішитесь?

— Хіба я сказав, що тішуся? Чудово, що наступні два дні зможете не бути на службі, а попрацювати на мене. Я вас наймаю.

З цими словами комісар дістав з гаманця три банкноти по п'ятдесят крон і підсунув їх ад'юнктові. Той здивовано витріщився.

— Сховайте гроші, — наказав йому комісар. — Мерщій.

Самковський підкорився.

— Півтори сотні? — перепитав він майже пошепки. — За що?

— Я хочу, щоб наступні дві або й дві з половиною доби ви спостерігали за старими складами, неподалік яких ми зустрілися. Невдовзі туди має прибути якийсь вантаж. Мені потрібно знати, хто іще напередодні буде цікавитися цим місцем. Хто буде там вештатись і приглядатись, — так само стишено сказав комісар. — Ніхто краще, ніж ви, цього не зробить, Самковський. Розумію, що самому буде важко, тому найміть надійного помічника. Нотуйте все, що вважатимете за потрібне й важливе... Покладаюся на вас.

Ад'юнкт кивнув.

Тим часом з'явився Зайґельт, несучи в одній руці одразу два кухлі з пивом, а в іншій — тарілку з м'ясом і хлібом.

— Прошу сердечно! Пиво коломийське «*Marcowe*» з броварні Вайса. Полядвиця з масарського складу Йозефа Лінттнера! Правдивий великодній лігумін!

Побажавши поліціянтам смачного, він повернувся на своє попереднє місце.

— У поліції Зайґельта допитали? — поцікавився Вістович після першого жадібного ковтка. Холодне пиво полилося нутром і здавалось йому божественною амброзією.

Самковський кивнув і теж хильнув пива. Після цього обидва з апетитом вгризли два шматки полядвиці й по скибці хліба, рясно намащеного гірчицею. Одразу за цим знову припали до гальб.

— І що він розповів? — допитувався Вістович.

— Що з Брюкнером не знайомий і гадки не має, де той може переховуватися, — знехотя сказав Самковський, беручи до рук наступний кавалок.

— Думаю, він бреше, — прошепотів комісар.

— Чому?

— Бо прямо зараз намагається підслухати нас зі своєї комірчини, — сказав він уже голосніше. — Агов, ти, сучий сину, виходь сюди! — схопившися з місця, гукнув він Зайґельту.

Той вийшов і став за шинквасом, мовчки кліпаючи очима.

— Маю кілька питань, — промовив комісар, — точніше одне, але важливе. Чи Берл Брюкнер навідувався сюди після того, як мій колега намагався його затримати?

— Мене вже допитували, і я все сказав... — заторохтів той.

— Зачиніть двері, Самковський, — промовив Вістович, беручи в руку чиюсь забуту тростину.

Комісар підійшов до шинквасу й щосили вгатив нею по пляшці заокеанського бурбону. Відмінний «*Heaven Hill*» розлетівся на друзки, а господар завив з розпачу.

— Чи навідувався сюди Брюкнер? — повторив комісар.

— Ні!

Ще одну пляшку довелося принести в жертву.

— Так, так! Він приходив! — закричав Зайґельт.

— Коли?

— Вчора.

— Сам?

Господар мовчав. Тоді Вістович, не вагаючись, вперіщив тростиною по товстезній пляшці французького бренді. Як не дивно, пляшка витримала, і обоє якусь мить здивовано її споглядали.

— Оце так скло, — пробурмотів комісар і замахнувся вдруге.

— Стійте! — зупинив його Зайґельт. — У мене тільки одна така пляшка...

Він дістав хустинку й витер чоло.

— Ну й Великдень, — простогнав господар. — Щоб ви всі здохли.

— З ким він тут був? — запитав комісар.

— З якимось своїм кумплем...

— Який той на вигляд?

— Міцно збудований, кремезний, одягнений пристойніше. Брюнет.

— Грумм... — сказав тихо Вістович. — І що, отак спокійнісінько теревенили за столиком? — запитав він вже голосніше. — Адже обидвох розшукує поліція!

— Вони прийшли після закриття. Близько півночі.

— Повтори.

— Я впустив їх до кнайпи, коли всі відвідувачі пішли! — істерично вигукнув Зайґельт. — Інакше мені б розтрощили голову так, як ви пляшки!

З цим Вістович був згоден.

— І про що ж вони говорили?

— Не знаю. Їх я не смів слухати.

За якийсь час Вістович виклав на стіл кілька крон.

— Це за пиво й закуску.

Господар на нього не дивився, спрямувавши погляд кудись на стіну. Поліціянти вийшли.

— Дарма ви з ним так, — сказав Самковський вже за дверима, — він непоганий чоловік. Іноді я міг навіть повечеряти в борг.

— Цей «непоганий чоловік» дивився, як Заремба ледь не розніс вам голову, а потім не зізнався поліції, що гостив у своїй кнайпі двох терористів. Запевняю вас, ад'юнкте, ті розбиті пляшки він заслужив, — промовив комісар.

Самковський змовчав, але було помітно, що він погодився зі сказаним.

— Виконайте моє доручення, — нагадав йому Вістович.

— Буде зроблено, шефе. Дякую за підтримку.

Комісар поплескав його по плечу.

— Важкі часи нас чекають, Самковський. Але бувало й гірше.

Вони попрощалися, і кожен з них, ідучи в свій бік, мав підстави сумніватися. Вістович — у тому, що сказав. Ад'юнкт — у тому, що почув. Паскудніших часів, ніж зараз, у них насправді не було.

Надвечір комісар дістався вілли на Понінського. Не сподівався, що Бейла прийме його сьогодні. Про свій візит він не попередив. Зрештою, її могло й не бути вдома. Але, як виявилося, вона була й навіть чекала на нього.

Служниця забрала в нього верхній одяг і провела до вітальні. Попросила зачекати й запропонувала чаю. Комісар не відмовився. Великим поціновувачем не був, але пам'ятав, що Бейла на цьому знається, тому гербата йому засмакує. Господиня дому особисто раз на місяць складала замовлення в крамниці колоніяльних товарів на Сикстуській*. Найбільше полюбляла китайський «Лапсанг» та квітковий індійський «Дарджилінг». А для заварювання мала безліч начиння, різного для кожного сорту, й свою служницю навчила всім цим користуватися.

Вістович знав, що в тій крамниці Бейла замовляє не тільки чай, але й прянощі, ароматичну олію, тканину для одягу й книжки, написані загадковою для нього мовою їдиш.

Господиня не спустилася до вітальні, а наказала служниці одразу покликати гостя нагору. Вістович відставив горнятко і неквапно піднявся сходами, дослухаючися до своїх кроків, мовби в кожному їхньому звукові був зміст, що його він намагався розгадати. Відчинив двері її кімнати.

Інтер'єр був добре знайомий: вікно з оксамитовими шторами, акуратний дамський столик з великим люстром над ним, книжкова шафа, до якої усі книги не вмістилися, тому декотрі стояли стосами на підлозі. Поруч з ними був електричний торшер, що трохи розсіював темряву, перетворюючи її на сутінки. Просторе ліжко, застелене лляним покривалом із непомітними візерунками по краях.

---

* Тепер — вулиця Дорошенка.

Між ліжком і столиком пролягав теплий килимок. З кутка виступала дерев'яна тумба з увімкненим патефоном. Приємний жіночий голос виконував «*Lamento della Ninfa*» Монтеверді. Вістович знав усіх улюблених композиторів Бейли: Скарлатті, Кореллі, Перселл... Вона обожнювала барокову музику.

Жінка стояла біля вікна. Постать її була майже невидима на тлі портьєри. Втім, Вістович здогадувався, що вбрана вона в легкий шлафрок, а своє довге чорне волосся зібрала у вузол на потилиці.

Якийсь час вони мовчки дослуховували арію Аріадни з патефона. Коли та закінчилася, Бейла нарешті озвалася:

— Запис із «Ла Скала»*. Сьогодні привезли на Сикстуську. Увесь день не могла наслухатися і от вирішила поставити цей запис тобі.

— Добре жити в часи, коли техніка дозволяє нам чути голоси з Мілана, — зауважив комісар, все ще стоячи на місці.

— Проходь. Сядь у крісло, — запросила Бейла.

Чоловік зробив, як вона сказала. Насправді Вістович любив їй підкорятися. Тим більше, сидячи в кріслі, тепер краще її бачив. Акуратні риси обличчя, довгу шию і делікатні плечі. Волосся й справді було у вузлі на потилиці. Їй так надзвичайно пасувало.

— Як твоя поїздка? — запитала вона.

— Краще б я лишився в Лембергзі, — зізнався комісар.

— І краще б зі мною, — додала жінка й підійшла до нього.

---

* «Ла Скала» — знаменитий оперний театр у Мілані.

Якийсь час вона дивилася на Вістовича згори вниз, ніби прочитуючи його, як дорожній щоденник. Йому нестерпно було під цим поглядом, і водночас він божеволів, відчуваючи її парфуми.

— Я матиму до тебе прохання, — сказав він раптом.

— Яке? — запитала вона, обережно торкаючись кінчиками пальців його скронь.

— Ти ж опікуєшся єврейськими дівчатками-сиротами, правда? Допомагаєш їм з наукою, аби потім вони мали професію.

— Опікуюсь, — зі здивуванням у голосі сказала Бейла. — А чому запитуєш?

— Бо хочу, аби ти допомогла одній дівчинці. Їй десь шість років, й виростає вона в паскудній сім'ї. Сумніваюся навіть, що ходить до школи. Правда, це не єврейська дитина. Але я міг би оплатити її навчання.

— Що-небудь придумаю, — пообіцяла Бейла і забрала руки з його скронь, аби зняти свій одяг.

— Сьогодні залишишся в мене, — почув він черговий наказ. — Бодай на службу підеш, поснідавши.

Він засміявся і притягнув її до себе.

Прокинувшись вранці, Вістович одразу зрозумів, що проспав. Вранішні сонячні промені були яскраві й упевнено пробивалися у спальню, минаючи портьєри. Найпевніше, була вже восьма або й пів до дев'ятої. Бейла дивилася на нього, лежачи на своїй половині ліжка й спершись на лікоть. Її акуратні груди були напівприкриті волоссям. Вістович любив ці груди. І просто обожнював пестити їх до безмежності довго, відчуваючи, як Бейла тремтить від усе нових і нових приливів насолоди.

— Шехтель з мене шкуру здере, — вимовив комісар, але без краплі жалю.

— Кесарю кесареве, а мені ось це, — відповіла Бейла, грайливо запускаючи руки під його ковдру.

— Що ти робиш зі мною, жінко? — сказав комісар, відчуваючи, що його ранкове збудження досягло неймовірних масштабів.

Втім, уже в наступну мить він замовк, спостерігаючи, як його коханка опинилася згори і зі звабливою грацією спрямувала його плоть поміж своїх стегон. Вістович більше не переймався спізненням. Навіть якби в цю мить настав кінець світу, йому було б начхати. Бо й серед руїн і згарища він би продовжував дослухатися до відчуттів, що дарувала йому ця жінка.

Сніданок, що чекав його на столику біля патефона, встиг захолонути.

— Коли ми побачимось знову? — запитав він її, ковтаючи каву просто із дзбанка.

— Коли я захочу, Адаме, — відповіла Бейла, сідаючи за свій столик. Вістовича при цьому вона бачила в люстрі. — Або коли ти справді того потребуватимеш.

— Я потребую тебе завжди, — сказав комісар.

Вона хитнула головою.

— Ця спальня — наш сховок. А ми одне для одного — відрада. Тож давай не перетворювати все це на буденність.

Вістович наблизився до неї і вдихнув її запах так, ніби вдихав тютюновий дим. Глибоко й з насолодою. Так, щоб можна було дотягнути до наступної зустрічі.

— Я провідаю тебе незабаром, — сказала Бейла наостанок, — іди...

До кабінету шефа комісар зайшов о пів на одинадцяту. Шехтель був заклопотаний, але спізнення Вістовича сприйняв спокійно. Зрештою, був другий день Великодніх свят, і він сам залюбки побув би ще вдома.

— А, Вістовичу... — промовив він, розгрібаючи якісь документи на столі. — Вітаю вас. Як минула ваша відпустка?

Комісар знав, що директору насправді начхати, як вона минула, тому відповів якоюсь шаблонною фразою і подякував за турботу.

— Були в Швейцарії? — поцікавився несподівано шеф, указуючи тому на стілець.

— Так... Мав там деякі справи, — спантеличено сказав Вістович.

— Мабуть, уже знаєте, яка чортівня в нас тут коїться.

Шехтель знервовано відкинув документи й сперся ліктями на стіл.

— Читав у газетах, пане директоре.

Комісар очікував, що Шехтель зараз оголосить, що доручає йому провадити слідство, але той мовчав. Витягнув з кишені зім'яту хустинку й голосно висякався. У директора на весну загострювався хронічний нежить.

— Паскудно все, Вістовичу, — прогугнявив він, — ваш підлеглий Самковський взявся за цю справу, я повірив йому, але, як виявилось, дуже дарма. Цей гівнюк усе зіпсував. До того ж через нього загинув важливий свідок. Наступного разу вибирайте собі в помічники когось розумнішого.

Комісар змовчав. Про Самковського він був кращої думки, ніж директор, проте вирішив не перечити. Шехтель не любив такого й зривався тоді на істерику.

— Ось усі документи, пов'язані з убивствами поліціянтів, — продовжив директор, підсуваючи йому зв'язану папку, — але тільки для ознайомлення.

— Що ви маєте на увазі? — не зрозумів Вістович.

Йому здавалося, що, вийшовши з кабінету, він одразу мав би розпочати пошуки вбивці.

— Те, що сказав, комісаре. Наразі вивчіть матеріали. Справу я вам не доручаю!

— Так, пане директоре, — Вістович взяв папку й підвівся з місця.

— Сядьте, — махнув йому Шехтель і одразу ж приклав долоню до чола. Схоже, окрім нежитю, його мучив ще біль у голові.

— Маю для вас ще одну новину, — продовжив Шехтель. — Ополудні до Лемберга прибуває міністр поліції Фердинанд фон Шпрегорф. А вже о п'ятій гоститиму його у своєму маєтку в Зимній Воді. Вам також бути обов'язково, Вістовичу.

Комісар мусив прикусити губу, щоб стримати усмішку. Це ж той самий міністр-казанова із рукопису, що йому читала в поїзді Маґда! На щастя, Шехтель у цей момент дивився кудись у вікно свого кабінету, тому не помітив такої реакції.

— Ви чули, комісаре? — перепитав директор за мить.

Він глянув на підлеглого, але той вже встиг посерйознішати.

— Так є, пане директоре.

— Підіть додому, скажімо, о третій і приготуйтеся як слід. Маю на увазі, вдягніться святково, як належить. У мене мусите бути за чверть до п'ятої. А доти вивчайте цю бісову справу...

Шехтель знаком показав, що розмову закінчено й підлеглий може собі йти.

Опинившись у своєму кабінеті, Вістович полегшено зітхнув і, перш ніж узятися до матеріалів, дістав з кишені пачку *«Muratti»*, куплених неподалік дому Бейли, й з насолодою закурив. Це була перша цигарка на сьогодні. Кілька хвилин, перш ніж зануритися у свій звичний кривавий вир, сповнений зла й насильства, він дозволив собі позгадувати ніч і ранок. Десь над шлунком запекло від туги за Бейлою. Та щойно цигарка закінчилася, зі спогадами також довелося прощатися. Вістович запалив наступну, але радше за звичкою, бо звик думати, вдихаючи й видихаючи дим.

Потім довелося таки заглибитись у справу. Серед усього він бачив кілька рапортів Самковського, які той написав після сутички в «Тлустій рибі», фото загиблих поліціянтів і звіти доктора Фельнера. Жертви вмирали миттєво, напад був несподіваним і застав кожного зненацька... Нападник був високого зросту і фізично дужий.

«Що ж, Самковський має рацію, убивця — без сумніву, Берл Брюкнер, — подумав Вістович. — Утік з етапу і тепер мститься львівській поліції. А понад усе йому хочеться дістатись нарешті до мене. До того, хто колись його впіймав. І якщо справді Карел Грумм зі Страсбурга вирушив сюди, то разом вони здатні влаштувати тут пекло...»

Одне, щоправда, видавалося Вістовичу дивним: на тілі жодного вбитого поліціянта не було інших насильницьких слідів, окрім ран від ножа. Фельнер стверджував, що убивця нападав несподівано, але Брюкнер був, як пам'ятав комісар, доволі громіздким. Підкрастися непомітно такому важко, залякати поліціянта при зброї не вдалося би навіть йому. Брюкнер мав би спочатку подолати опір своїх жертв. Схопити, вдарити, збити з ніг... Але жоден з убитих не мав на собі свіжих синців. Не йшли ж вони покірно до нього, наче вівці на забій. Знаний своєю хоробрістю віцекапрал Шварц, бувалий і перевірений не однією облавою фельдфебель Цайс, молодий енергійний постерунковий Вільха... Жоден з них не дав би себе заколоти просто так.

З такими роздумами комісар невдовзі вийшов зі свого кабінету й попрямував на Вірменську. Там швидко переодягнувся у святковий гарнітур, одягнув пальто й чорний мелонік. Ще за пів години Вістович прямував у фіакрі до Зимної Води.

Це було передмістя Львова, що називалося часто й на німецький манер – *Kaltwasser*. Свого часу сюди заселилися німецькі колоністи, запрошені австрійською владою, й донедавна переважали серед тутешнього населення. Нічого дивного, що для австріяка Шехтеля тут існувало цілком комфортне мовне середовище. Хоч зрештою і посеред Львова порозумітися німецькою було нескладно. Багато містян знали німецьку, більшість розуміли й навіть могли сяк-так відповісти.

Шехтель мав у Зимній Воді гарну двоповерхову садибу з велетенським садом і літніми будиночками. Пора їхня ще не надійшла, але для гостей, з огляду на теплу погоду, частунок все ж приготували просто неба. Тим більше абрикоси вже зацвіли, а на клумбах давно з'явилися тендітні первоцвіти.

Міністр вже прибув. Більшість запрошених на цей прийом гостей також: віденський намісник, директор

Львівської залізниці, декотрі крупні тутешні землевласники та провіденські депутати Галицького сейму.

У дерев'яній альтанці посеред саду розмістився струнний квартет. Двоє скрипалів, віолончеліст та альтист виконували Гайдна, вочевидь, на догоду віденському гостеві. Навпроти них було розставлено п'ять столиків із шахами, і запрошений славетний гросмейстер Ян Флібель давав сеанс одночасної гри.

Гостей, що прибували, зустрічав кельнер, пропонуючи їм келих шампана або вина на вибір. Вістович вибрав вино.

Невдовзі винесли гарячі наїдки: печену свинину, курчат у декількох різних соусах, шніцелі, крученики, м'ясні кнедлі, а до них декілька пляшок «*Baczewski Antique*» та трохи дешевшої «Англійської гіркої». Пані могли скуштувати львівських лікерів: бананових, вишневих чи персикових. Якщо ж ці трунки не смакували, то кожен охочий міг випити підігрітого вина чи пуншу з велетенських казанів, під якими палахкотіли гасові грілки, аби ці ароматні рідини не охололи.

Посеред саду стояло також кілька камінів, у яких садівники збиралися запалити дрова. Попри теплі дні, вечори ще були холодними. А теплих ковдр і алкоголю не вистачало, щоб зігрітися.

Вістович подивився у бік поважного гостя, намагаючись не думати одночасно про той рукопис, що досі лежав у його дорожній валізі. «Розпусний міністр» був чоловіком близько шістдесяти. Був середнього зросту, мав кайзерівські сиві вуса, рівний ніс і проникливий погляд. Ліву руку тримав за спиною, мов фехтувальник, праву перед собою. Між пальців затискав сигару, яку час від часу плавно підносив до рота. Так само плавно потім опускав. Іноді просив у когось підкурити її, наче своїх сірників не мав або просто не хотів добувати руку з-за спини.

Коли винесли портвейн і солодку випічку, Шехтель спіймав комісара за лікоть.

— Міністр хоче з вами поговорити, Вістовичу, — упівголоса, проте гаряче сказав директор.

При цьому він зміряв підлеглого уважним поглядом. Здавалося, хотів переконатися, що підлеглий має підходящий вигляд і не встиг набратися.

— Зі мною? — здивувався комісар. — Ви не плутаєте?

— Ні, чорт забирай, я не плутаю, — сердито відповів Шехтель. — Я, по-вашому, не розумію німецької? Фон Шпрегорф мені говорив, що матиме до вас розмову. Саме тому я наказав вам тут бути. Ходімо, я вас проведу до нього.

Чоловіки наблизилися до головної особи вечора, і поліційний директор стримано кашлянув у кулак, щоб привернути увагу.

— Пане міністре, дозвольте вам представити нашого найкращого слідчого — комісара Адама Вістовича, — урочисто вимовив він, коли міністр повернувся до них обличчям.

Фон Шпрегорф привітно усміхнувся.

— А-а-а, пане Вістовичу! Радий познайомитися, — поворушив він своїми вусами. — Чув про вас багато хорошого. Зокрема й від шеф-інспектора віденської поліції. Він і досі пам'ятає, як ви упіймали того маніяка на прізвисько Упир. А негідник же наганяв страх на пів імперії!..

Промовивши це, міністр переклав сигару до рота й простягнув комісару звільнену руку. Вістович потиснув її, одночасно дякуючи за приємну характеристику.

— Для мене велика честь особисто з вами познайомитись, пане міністре, — додав він і одразу помітив на собі схвальний погляд шефа.

— Я знаю, що контррозвідка також має на вас плани, — продовжив фон Шпрегорф, — але ми вас не віддамо. Правда ж, директоре?

Міністр засміявся і, щоб не загубити через це свою сигару, знову взяв її у праву руку.

— У жодному разі, пане міністре! — сказав Шехтель.

Фон Шпрегорф раптом посерйознішав.

— У мене до вас невелика справа, пане Вістовичу... — сказав він і замовк на хвилину, мовби обдумуючи, з чого почати.

Затягнувся димом і перевів погляд на директора.

— Вільгельме, друже, чи знайдеться у вас ще одна пляшка такого ж бренді, що ми з вами розпили за обідом? — запитав він у Шехтеля.

— Звісно, — кивнув той, — у мене цілий запас для таких випадків. Беру гуртом на заводі Бачевського.

— От і чудово. То, може, принесете? Я б іще випив.

Директор потемнів на обличчі, але слухняно подався виконувати побажання міністра.

— Так-от, пане комісаре, — сказав фон Шпрегорф, коли господар відійшов досить далеко, — справа стосується моєї репутації. Тому найперше мусите мені дати слово, що ні зараз, ні потім про неї не дізнається ніхто інший.

Сказавши це, він із вимогою в очах подивився на співрозмовника.

— Ясна річ, пане міністре. Обіцяю, — відповів комісар.

— Чудово. Тоді перейдемо до суті: понад тридцять років тому мене, тоді ще простого капітана, відрядили сюди, до Ґаліції. Як інженер за фахом я допомагав укріплювати Цитадель і оснащувати її на випадок війни. Втім, це не надто важливо... Важливіше, що якось на Гетьманських Валах я познайомився з милою особою двадцяти з чимось років на ім'я Ельвіра Сафронська. Ми зустрілися вдруге, потім втретє, аж доки в нас не розгорівся роман. Нічого прекраснішого зі мною не ставалося ні до, ні після цього, пане Вістовичу. Зізнаюся вам як чоловік чоловіку... — тут міністр зробив паузу і рвучко затягнувся димом. — Була, щоправда, одна деталь, яка перетворювала наші стосунки на злочин: Ельвіра була заміжня. Чоловіком її також був військовий, майор Казимир Сафронський. Достойний офіцер і чесна людина, яку ми змушені були обдурювати.

Ми з Ельвірою втратили розум, думали тільки одне про одного, і світ наш простягався не далі взаємних обіймів. Сподіваюсь, ви пробачите цю недолугу поетичність...

Вістович кивнув. Він вже не сприймав міністра як героя з відвертого рукопису, але потроху почав здогадуватися, про що піде мова далі.

Фон Шпрегорф за мить продовжив розповідь:

— Невдовзі збіг термін мого відрядження, і я повинен був збиратися назад до Відня. Сказати, що ми були в розпачі, — нічого не сказати. Ельвіра благала мене покинути службу і втекти з нею подалі з Лемберга, а може, й з Австрії, проте я вирішив, що це буде дурницею. Що чекало би нас, двох самотніх втікачів у якому-небудь незнайомому місті без грошей, без друзів, без нікого, хто міг би підтримати нас бодай кілька місяців?

Я їй відмовив. У день мого від'їзду, перед тим як сісти в поїзд, я купив газети в дорогу. Кілька з них повідомляли про смерть майора Сафронського від отруєння арсеном.

Поліція звинуватила Ельвіру, стверджуючи, що вона підсипала отруту йому в чай.

Знаю, тоді я мав би виявити мужність. Вийти з вагона і повернутися до неї. Підтримати її в цьому пеклі, але я так не зробив. Просто згорнув газети і спостерігав у вікно, як поїзд все більше й більше віддаляється від станції Лемберг.

Суд над Ельвірою тривав майже рік. Про нього писали віденські газети, тому я був у курсі подій. Їй пощастило із захисником. До того ж обвинувачення так і не змогло чітко довести, що майора отруїла саме його дружина. Ельвіра уникла смертної кари, проте отримала десять років жіночої в'язниці. Умови утримання були доволі м'якими, проте, ясна річ, це зламало їй життя.

Увесь цей час я відчував на собі вину. Мені снилися кошмари, я ламав голову над тим, чи справді Ельвіра зважилася через мене на вбивство, але навіть отримавши свою першу високу поліційну посаду, не спробував зв'язатися з нею. Хоч слід було. Бодай для того, аби попросити вибачення.

А тепер до суті справи... Ельвіра знайшла спосіб мені помститися. Вона мовби навмисне чекала, доки я піднімуся на саму верхівку кар'єри. Бо ж що вагоміша моя посада, тим болючіше я відчую удар.

Взявши собі псевдонім Ельвіра Сапфо, ця жінка написала огидний порнографічний роман, в якому відвела мені роль головного героя, ще й називаючи мене моїм справжнім іменем. Ви не повірите, але цей твір під назвою «Розпусний міністр» поширився з такою швидкістю, що у Відні він опинився вже за два тижні після того, як його опублікували в Лемберзі. Мої люди вдалися до рішучих дій: з книжкових крамниць і складів були вилучені всі примірники, декотрих книгарів поліціянти заарештували й протримали в буцегарнях кілька днів, аби вони затямили, що ця книжка не принесе їм добра. Друкарні й видавництва, що випустили цей непотріб у світ, отримали гігантські штрафи. Словом, ми зробили все, щоб німецькомовний читач ніколи не взяв цю книжку до рук. Ні у Відні, ні у Лемберзі, ні у Зальцбурзі, ні в іншому місті...

Однак авторка не заспокоїлася. Жодного примірника вже не знайти, але слава про цю книжку поширилася поміж шанувальниками такого брудного чтива. І що гірше — проникла за кордон. Мої агенти повідомили, що Ельвіра продала права на переклад італійською, і невдовзі «Розпусний міністр» має вийти у Венеції. Я знову мусив удатися до рішучих дій і найняв детектива... За планом він повинен був зв'язатися з її швейцарським перекладачем і, вдаючи з себе редактора чи власника італійського видавництва, отримати оригінал перекладу. А також, за можливості, виманити й рукопис цього бісового роману...

Міністр замовк.

— І що сталося далі? — обережно запитав Вістович, хоча продовження історії добре знав.

— Гадки не маю, — фон Шпрегорф знизав плечима. — Той детектив більше зі мною не зв'язувався. Сучий син, мабуть, мене обдурив, хоча я й отримав від нього телеграму, в якій він повідомив, що переклад у нього...

— А ось і я, мої панове! — почувся збоку голос директора.

Шехтель в одній руці тримав пляшку темно-бурштинового кольору, а в іншій, вертикально, мов суцільну скляну квітку, три порожні чарки.

— Потримайте-но, Вістовичу, — звернувся він до підлеглого, простягнувши йому склянки.

— Так-от, моє прохання, пане комісаре, — продовжив міністр, коли Шехтель кожному налив порцію випивки, — знайдіть цю Ельвіру Сапфо.

Чоловіки випили. Бренді від Бачевського справді смакувало чудово.

— Знайти... А потім? — запитав Вістович.

— Переконайте віддати рукопис, якщо він у неї. Якщо не вийде, то я зустрінуся з нею сам... Маєте три дні. Рівно стільки я ще перебуватиму в Лемберзі.

Вістович замислився на якийсь час. Три дні... Часу небагато, але, маючи в рукаві деякі козирі, які він, сам того не знаючи, отримав по дорозі з Берна, можна виконати це доручення навіть за коротший час.

— Розумію, що термін, відведений на пошуки, малий, але й ви, комісаре, знаєте свою справу, як ніхто інший. Ви зробите послугу міністру поліції, тож можете бути певні, що й він зуміє вам віддячити, — додав фон Шпрегорф.

— Гаразд, але я маю одну умову, — сказав Вістович.

— Комісаре, як ви можете? — спалахнув Шехтель. — Що ви дозволяєте собі?

Однак міністр знаком показав йому, що все гаразд.

— Кажіть, — звернувся він до Вістовича.

— Нещодавно звільнено мого помічника, ад'юнкта Самковського, — промовив комісар і тієї ж миті побачив, як обличчя Шехтеля налилося кров'ю. — Я хотів би, щоб він повернувся на службу.

— У чому винен цей ад'юнкт? — запитав у директора фон Шпрегорф.

— Він вчинив злочинну службову недбалість, — процідив той крізь зуби, — через нього загинув дуже важливий свідок.

Міністр зробив ковток бренді і якусь мить подумав.

— Ви наполягаєте, пане Вістовичу? — перепитав він.

— Так, до того ж я хотів би, щоб справу проти нього закрили.

Фон Шпрегорф ковтнув ще алкоголю.

— Це все? — мовив він коротко.

— Так, пане міністре.

— Пане директоре, прошу взяти це до виконання, — наказав він Шехтелю.

— Буде зроблено, — промовив той здавленим голосом. — Тільки на жодні підвищення, доки я керую львівською поліцією, Самковський нехай не розраховує...

— Я зупинився в готелі «Метрополь», — не звертаючи більше уваги на Шехтеля, сказав комісару фон Шпрегорф. — Від сьогодні можете зв'язуватись зі мною в будь-який час доби. Я попереджу рецепцію.

Вістович кивнув.

— Хай щастить вам, комісаре, — побажав міністр наостанок. — Точніше, нам.

Після цього, мов утративши до Вістовича будь-який інтерес, фон Шпрегорф у супроводі господаря подався слухати музикантів, які помітили, що той наближається, і почали новий твір з неабияким завзяттям і піднесенням.

Комісар зрозумів, що більше йому тут робити нічого, і, вирішивши не прощатися з Шехтелем, рушив до виходу. Свою порцію бренді він допив уже біля фіакра. Кілька місцевих візників завбачливо тримали свої екіпажі поблизу, знаючи, що невдовзі матимуть заробіток, розвозячи підхмелілих гостей по домівках.

— На Вірменську, — голосно сказав комісар, сідаючи в один із таких фіакрів.

— До середмістя буде дорожче, — відповів незворушно візник.

— Я тобі дам, курва, дорожче! — гримнув на нього Вістович. Вдруге поспіль зіткнувшись з перевізницькою жадібністю, не мав наміру терпіти. — Отримаєш звичну плату, а як ні — поїдеш задурно!

— Та я хіба що... Як пан собі зичить... — пробурмотів той і хлеснув свою клячу батогом.

Наступного дня Вістович прийшов на службу раніше, ніж зазвичай. Вже о пів на восьму він, тримаючи під пахвою кілька свіжих газет, піднімався сходами до свого кабінету. Йому хотілося прийти раніше, аніж в Дирекції з'явиться Шехтель, однак не вдалося. Більше того, директор підстеріг його, щойно комісар опинився на другому поверсі. Вигляд Шехтель мав невиспаний і похмільний.

— Доброго ранку, Вістовичу, — привітався він з підлеглим.

— Доброго ранку, пане директоре, — відповів той, повертаючи ключ у дверях кабінету.

Коли він прочинив їх, Шехтель зайшов усередину слідом за комісаром. Якусь мить спостерігав, як той кладе газети собі на стіл, знімає капелюха й плаща, а потім чіпляє їх на порожній вішак.

— Вчора добре дісталися додому? — з удаваною турботою запитав шеф.

— Цілком добре, пане директоре. Дякую вам за гостину.

— Пробачте, що не зміг з вами попрощатися. Мусив опікуватися міністром.

— Ясна річ. Не переймайтесь.

Шехтель всадив до рота цигарку, і комісар підніс йому вогонь зі своєї «*Ronson*».

— Гарна річ, — похвалив директор запальничку.

— Сувенір із Берна, — відповів Вістович, також закурюючи.

Якусь хвилину чоловіки мовчки затягувалися димом.

— Що думаєте про справу, яку вам доручив міністр? — запитав нарешті директор.

— Дещо незвично буде таким займатися в той час, як у місті маніяк вбиває поліціянтів, — зізнався комісар, — але що ж...

— Погоджуюся, — кивнув Шехтель. — Проте, якщо фон Шпрегорф у подяку за цю послугу стане другом львівської поліції і нашим з вами безпосередньо, в подальшому це принесе чимало користі. Зокрема й місту.

— Розумію.

Вістович неквапно перекладав цигарки з пачки до портсигара. Діставати їх потім звідти було для нього звичніше.

— Фельнер, до речі, знайшов між згинами пальців одного із загиблих кілька ниток. Бідолаха, очевидно, перед смертю вхопився за одяг убивці, — зазначив директор, — зараз це не має жодного значення, оскільки ми й так знаємо ім'я маніяка, але на суді обвинувачення матиме ще один доказ. Якщо знайдемо в цього Брюкнера пальто чи плаща такого ж кольору, як і нитки, то повісять цього сучого сина значно швидше.

– Буду тільки радий, – сказав комісар, – у нього на мене давній зуб.

– Так, пригадую.

Шехтель підійшов до столу й загасив у попільничці недопалок.

– А ви з чого збираєтеся розпочати пошуки тієї... Саломеї... Чи як її там?

– Сапфо, – виправив його Вістович, – Ельвіри Сапфо.

– Один біс, – відмахнувся директор. – То з чого?

– Ще не думав, – сказав комісар. – Можливо, слід ще раз перевірити друкарні, що надрукували її книжку? У когось там міг залишитися з нею зв'язок.

– Сумніваюся, – промовив Шехтель. – Ви ж чули міністра, ми все зробили для того, аби жодна друкарня не хотіла мати з нею справу. Після наших візитів друкарі й видавці відреклися від цієї авторки. Ніхто вам ні в чому не зізнається.

– І все-таки, я спробую, – наполіг Вістович.

– Як хочете, комісаре. Але пам'ятайте, що у вас лише три дні.

– Я не забуду, пане директоре.

Більше не кажучи ні слова, Шехтель вийшов з кабінету. Щойно двері за ним зачинилися, Вістович усміхнувся. Ясна річ, ходити по друкарнях – марно. Він, зрештою, і не збирався... За пів години комісар вийшов з Дирекції й попрямував на Марійську площу*, звідки через Пасаж Міколяша** дістався вулиці Сенкевича***, а звідти попрямував

* Тепер – площа Міцкевича.

** Пасаж Міколяша – торговий критий пасаж, що існував у Львові з 1901 до 1939 року. Зруйнований під час німецького бомбардування.

*** Тепер – вулиця Вороного.

на Словацького. Тут Вістович зайшов до триповерхової будівлі ц. к. Дирекції пошти.

Галас, шум і тріскотіння телеграфних апаратів огортали кожного, хто сюди заходив. Вістович не без труднощів відшукав відділ, який займався міжнародними відправленнями. На щастя, тут було не так людно, як у всіх інших. Чекаючи, доки підійде його черга, комісар дістав з нагрудної кишені блокнот і ще раз перевірив запис, зроблений ще в експресі: «Переклад зроблено в Цюриху 27 березня 1906 року. Перекладач — Антон Піллер». Ця нотатка нагадала йому про Маґду, і приємні спогади про її пристрасть обпекли чоловіка зсередини. Бейла так і не дізналася про неї. Точніше, він не розповів їй... Звісно, це зовсім не означало, що Бейла бодай частково про все не здогадалася.

— Уважно вас слухаю, шановний пане, — ввічливо звернувся до нього службовець пошти по той бік вікна.

Вістович, не кажучи ні слова, простягнув йому свою поліційну легітимацію.

— Так... — трохи розгублено промовив службовець. — Чим можу допомогти?

— Хочу перевірити всі відправки зі Львова до Цюриха за останні три місяці, — сказав комісар.

— Зайдіть сюди, — промовив той, вказуючи на невеличкі двері до своєї конторки й одночасно вивішуючи табличку «Зачинено».

Отримавши грубезну книгу відправлень, Вістович разом зі службовцем взялися до роботи. За годину комісар відшукав потрібний запис: «2 лютого 1906 року. Лемберг — Цюрих. Отримувач: Антон Піллер. Берґенґассе, 14. Відправник: Ельвіра Сафронська, Личаківська, 21».

— *Das ist alles, Herr Minister*[*], — тихо промовив комісар, знову опинившися на вулиці. — Далі — справа лише одного візиту.

Зі Словацького чоловік перейшов на Сикстуську і, дочекавшися трамвая, дістався ним на Личаківську. Вийшов на одну зупинку раніше, біля костелу кларисок, де Личаківська тільки починалася. Позаду виднілися Бернардинська Вежа і Глинянська Брама, що залишилася від середньовічних укріплень міста. Далі починалися новітні будинки, зведені вже за Габсбургів. Личаківська видавалася незвично широкою і модерною. То тут, то там майоріли яскраві вивіски численних ательє та крамниць з модним одягом. У будинку під номером 6 містилося славетне архітектурне бюро Івана Левинського, а трохи далі — відомий на весь Львів фотосалон пана Александера Буха.

До будинку під номером 21 Вістович дістався за якихось п'ять хвилин. Щоб дізнатися, яке з помешкань належить Ельвірі Сафронській, комісар придивився до прізвищ на поштовій скриньці. Авторка «Розпусного міністра» мешкала в квартирі на першому поверсі.

Двері довго не відчиняли. Вістович вирішив уже, що доведеться повернутися сюди зі слюсарем, який розкрутить дверний замок, але врешті зсередини почувся жіночий голос:

— Хто там?

— Пані Сафронська? — запитав комісар.

— Що вам треба? — замість відповіді промовила жінка.

— Я з поліції, пані Сафронська. Будьте ласкаві, відчиніть.

---

* Ось і все, пане міністре (*нім.*).

Нависла пауза. Потім клацнув замок і двері прочинилися, проте лише на стільки, на скільки дозволяв ланцюг між стіною і внутрішньою ручкою. У дверному отворі з'явилося худе виснажене жіноче обличчя. Настороженій вираз робив вікові зморшки ще різкішими.

— Покажіть документи, — сказала господиня.

Вістович виконав її прохання. Примруживши погляд, вона довго розглядала його легітимацію, то наближаючи, то віддаляючи її від очей.

— Гаразд, пане комісаре, заходьте.

Вона зняла з дверей ланцюга й пропустила гостя досередини. Темний коридор провадив до невеликої вітальні, яка, можливо, здавалася б просторішою, якби не коричневі, місцями вицвілі шпалери, завдяки яким цей простір став схожим на усипальницю. Меблі, старомодні й трухляві, також, схоже, доживали віку. Найбадьорішим у цьому сонному царстві був, мабуть, чималий маятниковий годинник під стіною, що розмірено відбивав тягучий час. Крізь щілини у шторах до кімнати проникало світло й свіже повітря. Вікно, мабуть, було відчинене.

— Сідайте, добродію, — господиня вказала Вістовичу на крісло.

Він сів обережно, наче боявся, що в будь-яку мить воно може під ним розсипатись.

— Вибачте, що не пропоную чаю, — промовила пані Сафронська. — На сьогодні я відпустила служницю, а сама не дам ради. Кепсько почуваюся.

— Дякую, не переймайтеся, — відповів комісар. — Я навряд чи надовго...

Годинник гучно пробив одинадцяту, змусивши Вістовича сіпнутись усім тілом від несподіванки.

Господиня лагідно всміхнулася.

— Даруйте, я мала б попередити, — сказала вона.

У кожному її слові й рухові відчувалася глибока шляхетність і вишуканість, мовби пані Сафронська володіла яким-небудь родовим маєтком, а не занедбаною квартирою.

Вона було невисокою і тендітною. Одяг мала неновий, місцями акуратно підрихтований. Погляд сірих очей був теплий і жвавий. На собі мала деякі прикраси, втім, навіть неозброєним оком було видно, що вони несправжні. Оригінали, мабуть, були продані й замінені дешевими копіями.

— То що привело вас сюди, пане комісаре? — запитала жінка. — Адже ви, либонь, перший гість у цьому домі за багато років.

— Я тут за розпорядженням міністра Шпрегорфа. Він доручив мені відшукати Ельвіру Сапфо, — відповів комісар.

Господиня міцно стисла бліді губи.

— Отже, це він назвав вам моє справжнє прізвище?

— Саме так.

— І що... що потрібно від мене цьому достойнику? — жінка говорила з ледь помітним хвилюванням і тремтінням у голосі.

— Він просить вас віддати йому оригінал вашого... роману й відмовитися від продажу прав за кордон.

Вона засміялась.

— Просить? Але якщо поліція вже тут, у моєму помешканні, то хіба я маю вибір?

Вістович зітхнув.

— Дорога пані, я — це не вся поліція. І перебуваю тут майже приватно... — сказав він.

— Що це означає?

— Що можу діяти на свій розсуд. Якщо ви віддасте мені рукопис, то, присягаюся, жодна душа не дізнається вашої адреси. Тільки раджу прибрати напис із вашим справжнім прізвищем на поштовій скриньці.

Жінка зазирнула йому в очі й кілька секунд дивилася в них, мовби хотіла розгледіти там якийсь прихований смисл його слів.

— Тобто Фердинанд... Пан міністр не шукав зі мною зустрічі? — раптом запитала вона.

— Навпаки. З його слів я зрозумів, що він хоче з вами зустрітися.

— Тільки щоб я перестала видавати свій роман?

Вістович набрав у легені повітря для відповіді, але господиня його зупинила.

— Нічого не кажіть...

Вони замовкли, й добру хвилину в кімнаті чулося тільки цокання годинника.

— Я продала права тільки на переклад італійською, — порушила тишу господиня. — Боюся, робота у видавництві вже почалася й книжка невдовзі побачить світ.

— На жаль, ні, — промовив Вістович. — Чи на щастя.

— Що ви маєте на увазі?

— Єдиний переклад італійською — в мене. Я знайшов його випадково в купе експресу, що прямував до Ґаліції, — пояснив комісар.

— У поїзді? — здивувалась Ельвіра. — Як він туди потрапив? І що з паном Піллером? Моїм перекладачем?

— Маю всі підстави стверджувати, що пан Піллер загинув.

— Боже мій, — жінка притулила руки до обличчя. — Боже мій... Це Шпрегорф винен?

Комісар стенув плечима.

— Навряд. Не думаю, що міністр доручав убити вашого перекладача. Йому залежало тільки на тому, щоб отримати його роботу.

— Якби я знала, що це спричинить чиюсь смерть, то ніколи б навіть не взялася писати, — зі сльозами промовила Ельвіра.

— Оригінал вашого рукопису в Цюриху? — обережно запитав комісар.

Вона кивнула.

— Ви відправили Піллеру єдиний примірник?

— Так... Тож, як бачите, нічим не можу бути вам корисною. Підіть і заспокойте свого міністра. Гру закінчено.

Вістович звівся на ноги, але виходити не поспішав.

— Чи не могли б ви розповісти мені про смерть чоловіка? — промовив він, хоч розраховував радше на відмову.

Ельвіра звела на нього переляканий і здивований водночас погляд.

— Я все розповіла багато-багато років тому! — майже викрикнула жінка. — Розповіла поліціянтові, що розслідував справу. Я незаслужено відсиділа у в'язниці. Чого ви ще хочете?

Руки, обличчя й усе тіло її дрібно затряслися. Комісар зрозумів, що подальша розмова з нею марна. Та все ж одне питання він мусив поставити:

— Як звали слідчого, що розслідував смерть майора Сафронського?

— Кронфельд, — видусила вона з себе. — Оберкомісар Франц Кронфельд... Пробачте, пане Вістовичу, я мушу попросити вас піти.

— Звичайно, — чоловік попрямував до виходу, — на все добре.

Не дочекавшись відповіді, поліціянт вийшов за двері й почув, як невдовзі господиня замикає їх зсередини. Вістович вийшов знову на Личаківську і повільним кроком вирушив у бік площі Митної.

Що ж, доручення міністра він виконав, і навіть зробив це завчасно. Залишалися ще два дні, які можна було б використати, щоб удовольнити цікавість. Вістович згадував коротку розмову з Ельвірою, і йому складно було уявити її вбивцею. За роки роботи в поліції він навчився вирізняти людей, котрі здатні позбавити життя інших. Оця жінка, що самотньо живе на Личаківській, видавалась йому іншою. І якщо вона все-таки отруїла свого чоловіка, піддавшись любовному одурманенню, то йому страшенно цікаво було б знати обставини, за яких це сталося.

Справи тридцятирічної давності ще мали б досі зберігатися в Дирекції, тож відшукати матеріали про вбивство майора Сафронського він міг би ще сьогодні.

Поспіхом пообідавши у кнайпі неподалік Бернардинів, комісар повернувся на Академічну і, не заходячи до свого кабінету, рушив одразу до секретаря поліційної канцелярії, в якого мусив отримати дозвіл на роботу з архівом. Той не заперечував, лише наполіг, щоб Вістович не виносив матеріали за межі відділу. Ознайомитися з ними він міг в архівній бібліотеці.

Отримавши чималу папку з позначкою «1876 рік», він зручно вмостився за стіл і розгорнув документи. Одразу потрапив на очі заключний рапорт оберкомісара Кронфельда з нерозбірливими примітками й підписом тодішнього поліційного директора. За ним — нескінченні протоколи допитів Ельвіри Сафронської. Покази свідків і кілька портретів дійових осіб цієї драми.

— А, Вістовичу! — почув він раптом за спиною бадьорий голос.

Заглиблений у читання комісар підскочив на стільці від несподіванки. Озирнувся. Позаду нього стояв доктор Фельнер і від душі реготав.

— Даруйте... Ох, чорт забирай... Даруйте мені, комісаре, — тамуючи свій скрипучий, мов старі двері, сміх, промовляв той. — Але бачили б ви себе збоку!

— Ідіть до біса, докторе, — відмахнувся Вістович, відчуваючи, правда, що й сам починає сміятися.

Той віддихався і врешті заспокоївся.

— А що за справа перед вами? — поцікавився раптом Фельнер.

— Стара як світ. Про отруєння одного майора...

— Отруєння? Чим? — перепитав Фельнер. І в його погляді загорівся вогник професійної цікавості.

Вістович зазирнув у папери.

— Згідно рапорту, арсеном.

— Можна мені глянути?

Комісар завагався.

— Та годі вам, Вістовичу, в моїй голові більше таємниць, ніж у цьому архіві. Показуйте, що там у вас.

Він перехилився через плече комісара, одночасно насаджуючи на носа окуляри.

— Так, ага... Казимир Сафронський. Смерть внаслідок отруєння... Особа вбивці встановлена... Послухайте, Вістовичу, — раптом посерйознішав доктор.

Фельнер зняв окуляри з носа й задумливо почав гризти дужку оправи.

— Послухайте... — повторив він. — Я пам'ятаю цю справу.

— Ви пам'ятаєте справу тридцятирічної давнини? — з недовірою перепитав комісар.

— До вашого відома, комісаре, я цікавлюся не тільки трупами у своїй мертвецькій, — зауважив Фельнер, — я також мешкаю у Львові. Свого часу цей випадок наробив галасу. Ви можете перечитати газети того часу. Журналісти зчинили справжню бурю, а суспільство розділилося навпіл: одні гаряче підтримували вдову майора, інші вимагали для неї смертної кари...

— Чому? Було недостатньо доказів?

— Наскільки пригадую, арсен і справді знайшли в цукерниці на їхній кухні. Але не в залишках гербати, яку випив тоді Сафронський. І від якої начебто помер, — пояснив доктор.

— А розтин? Адже отруту можна виявити в тілі покійника, якщо вона туди потрапила.

— Можна, Вістовичу. Але це були інші часи. Знайти фахівця, що виконав би пробу Марша*, тридцять років тому було не так просто. Минув би не один тиждень. Ми не могли стільки часу зберігати тіло й віддали його родичам на поховання.

Фельнер знітився, мовби відчував вину за недосконалість тодішньої криміналістики.

— А чому вас зацікавила ця справа? — запитав він у Вістовича.

— Поки не можу вам розповісти, докторе. Але цілком імовірно, що до цієї теми ми ще повернемось.

---

* Проба Марша — хімічний метод для виявлення арсену та арсенієвих сполук, що застосовувався у криміналістиці.

— Тоді, думаю, вам корисніше буде поспілкуватися з оберкомісаром Кронфельдом, — відповів той. — З тим детективом, що вів цю справу 1876 року. Зараз він вже на емеритурі.

— Маєте рацію, — згодився Вістович. — Знаєте, як його знайти?

Фельнер кивнув.

— Він мешкає неподалік від мене в кам'яниці на Потоцького*. Якщо хочете, я запишу вам адресу.

— Так, будь ласка.

Вістович розгорнув і простягнув йому свій блокнот.

Коли вони попрощалися, була майже шоста. Комісар вийшов з канцелярії і, трохи подумавши, попрямував у бік вулиці Потоцького. Він ще не знав, чи навідає сьогодні колишнього оберкомісара, але хотілося пройтися, тож чому б заодно й не перевірити адресу, яку записав Фельнер.

Як і вранці, Вістович минув Марійську площу, але оскільки Пасаж Міколяша вже було зачинено, рушив вулицею Коперника вгору до костелу Марії Магдалини. Тут зупинився й трохи віддихався. Вулиця Потоцького збігала далі вниз. По обидва боки давні кам'яниці чергувалися з новими. Деякі старі будинки вже були напівзруйновані, а нові — недобудовані.

Перепочивши, Вістович рушив донизу й за кілька хвилин зупинився біля кам'яниці під номером 11. Саме *тут*, як свідчив доктор, проживав Кронфельд. Кам'яниця була старою, але ще міцно трималася фундаменту. Двері, проте, було зачинено зсередини, а вікна на двох поверхах затягнуто шторами.

---

* Тепер — вулиця Генерала Чупринки.

Комісар відчув, як його охоплює інтерес. Старому поліціянтові зараз вже за шістдесят. Отже, потрапивши в його дім, він міг би певним чином зазирнути й у своє майбутнє.

Кам'яницю оминав невеликий провулок, і Вістович рушив ним, сподіваючись, що з протилежного боку до будинку є інший вхід. Ішов обережно, поглядаючи собі під ноги. Пройшовши лише десяток кроків, чоловік відчув, як серце його забилося гучно, ніби ковальський молот. Він напружив слух і прислухався до навколишніх звуків. Далеко десь задзеленчав трамвай, п'яний голос надривався нерозбірливим і безладним співом, до цього додалися його повільні кроки й важке дихання.

«Треба закурити, — подумалось йому, — і трохи заспокоїтися».

Комісар потягнувся до кишені, де був портсигар і запальничка. Клацнув нею і втягнув до легенів перший ковток диму. Край цигарки зашкварчав. Тієї ж миті десь угорі залопотіла крилами зграя міського вороння, і Вістович звів очі, якусь мить відстежуючи темні точки на тлі свинцевого вечірнього неба.

«Краще повернутися додому, — майнула в нього думка, — прихопити по дорозі пляшку чогось міцного, знайти недочитані книжки й провести з ними весь вечір. Нерви сьогодні гівняні...»

За спиною почулися квапливі важкі кроки. Рвучко повернувшись, Вістович просто перед собою побачив багряне від злості бородате обличчя й лезо ножа в здоровенній руці.

— От я тебе й знайшов, скурвисину, — зашипів Брюкнер і замахнувся для удару.

Комісар навіть встиг подумати, що ця бісова інтуїція ще жодного разу його не підвела. І щоразу, коли він до неї не дослухався, то неодмінно потрапляв у халепу. І от зараз, відчувши, як пришвидшилось його серце, міг би принаймні дістати з кишені свого браунінга. Але ж ні, замість пістолета він витягнув портсигар! Погляд його вловив криве лезо ножа, що от-от мало би ввіткнутись йому в шию чи груди, і шкіра в цих місцях, ніби передчуваючи рану, страшенно занила. Все це тривало соту частину секунди, одночасно з тим, як свідомість комісара гарячково вишукувала найкращий варіант самозахисту в цій ситуації. Зрештою, Вістович зробив те, що дуже добре вмів: лівою спробував перехопити озброєну руку нападника, правою ж щосили зацідив йому в писок. Цей правий боковий витримав би не кожен боксер в усій Ґаліції, але Берл, вищий і кремезніший за Вістовича, здавалося, його навіть не відчув. Вхопити нападника за ліву кисть поліціянтові також не вдалося. Ніж тільки трохи змінив траєкторію удару і пройшовся комісару по плечу, розрізавши тканину плаща й маринарки під ним. Вістович сіпнувся назад, але, перечепившись, гепнувся на землю.

— Радо б із тобою побоксував, — єхидно вищирився Брюкнер, — але часу катма.

З цими словами він навалився на комісара всією вагою й заніс над ним ножа для нового удару. Вістовичу сперло дихання й потемніло в очах. Він ще витиснув із себе слово «падлюка», назвавши так наостанок Брюкнера, й приготувався до найгіршого, коли почувся звук, що нагадував удар по важкому сталевому дзвону. Берл здригнувся й, облишивши комісара, спробував підвестись, але знову отримав удар. Брюкнер звалився набік.

Тоді Вістович, мов у тумані, побачив над собою постать, озброєну металевою рурою.

Схоже, Господь посилав йому поміч, отже, слід і самому не марнувати часу. Потягнувшись до кишені плаща, комісар нарешті вихопив звідти зброю і, не встаючи, спрямував її туди, де був Брюкнер.

— Ані руш! — видихнув Вістович, спостерігши, що той поступово приходив до тями й навіть намагався звестися на ноги.

Тієї ж миті в грудях комісара страшенно запекло. Так, мовби своєю вагою нападник роздавив йому нутрощі. Берл кинувся навтьоки, і Вістович натиснув на спуст. Гримнув постріл, втім, комісар із прикрістю побачив, що не влучив. Він вистрілив ще раз, але нападник вже зник за рогом будинку.

— Гукайте поліцію, — ледве дихаючи, вигукнув Вістович. — Телефонуйте в Дирекцію!.. Це той... той маніяк...

Постать, відкинувши своє знаряддя, нахилилася над ним, приглядаючись до його пораненого плеча.

— Гаразд, гаразд. Заспокойтеся, — почув над собою комісар.

Незнайомець був чоловіком уже поважного віку з посивілим волоссям і бородою.

— Хто ви? — запитав Вістович.

— Мене звати Франц Кронфельд. Я також колись служив у поліції... Ви поранені, тому найперше я покличу лікаря.

VII

Лемберг
18–19 квітня 1906 року

Ліза Хільке, більше знана, щоправда, як мадам Шене, щойно завершила свій перший номер у львівському клубі «Мінотавр». Це була жартівлива композиція Франца Легара «*Ja, das Studium der Weiber ist schwer*»*, яку вона виконувала на свій манер. Співала навмисне низьким голосом, зображаючи чоловіка, у той самий час, мовби ненароком, додаючи у свої рухи еротизму:

«*Nimmt uns Männer verteufelt auch her*», — і співачка «випадково» погладила виразне декольте.

---

* Ліза виконує фрагмент з оперети «Весела вдова» угорського та австрійського композитора Франца Легара (1870–1948):
Так, вивчити жінку непросто,
Взяти нас чоловіків, хай йому чорт,
Жоден не знає ні тіла, ні душі,
Жінки, жінки, жінки, жінки, жінки. — (*із нім.*)

«Niemals kennt man an Seele und leib», — тут вона удавано сердито ляснула себе по стегнах, але руки на них затримались, і кінчики пальців пробіглися від колін до живота.

«Man das Weib, Weib, Weib, Weib, Weib», — мадам Шене розпачливо вхопилася за голову, хоч насправді знову демонструючи публіці напіввідкриті груди, що піднялися від цього руху трохи вище.

До наступного виходу лишалося двадцять хвилин, і Ліза, сівши в гримерці за свій столик, спочатку поправила макіяж, а потім запалила тонку єгипетську сигаретку. Якийсь час уважно розглядала себе в дзеркало. Попри те що попередню ніч у поїзді не змогла заснути, вигляд у неї був свіжий. Шкіра на обличчі пружна, жодних «мішків» під очима, губи палахкотіли. Звісно, частково це — завдяки обережній дозі кокаїну, яку вона прийняла годину тому, але й природної чарівності їй не бракувало. Тому й спокусити будь-якого чоловіка для неї було заіграшки.

Взяти хоча б того кумедного молодого лікаря з клініки для вар'ятів. Щойно він знайшов у своєму пальті записку від неї, одразу ж, не розмірковуючи, прибіг на побачення. Винайняв номер у дорогому баденському готелі, замовив найкращого шампанського, купив кокаїну. Довго розповідав, як важко йому з дружиною Ґретою, що, вірогідно, йому зраджує, бо з ним останнім часом кохається стиснувши зуби, ніби через силу.

— Не вірогідно, дурнику, а таки зраджує, — сказала вона йому і втягнула до носа білий, ретельно подрібнений порошок.

— Звідки ти знаєш? — перепитав Краут. Порція кокаїну лежала й перед ним, але він з цим не поспішав.

Мадам Шене блаженно відкинула назад голову й кілька секунд дослухалася до приємного запаморочливого ефекту, викликаного наркотиком.

— Ми з нею одного віку, — сказала вона, знову глянувши на нього, — з твоїх слів я можу судити про її зовнішність і темперамент. Секс їй потрібен і потрібен часто. Якщо з тобою вона робить це неохоче, то комусь іншому, значить, віддається з усією пристрастю.

Краут побілів, а губи його затремтіли.

— Вибач, що кажу це, але краще тобі знати правду, — промовила співачка й потягнулася за шампанським.

— І що... що мені робити? — запитав Фелікс.

— Те, що й вона, — усміхнулася жінка й неквапно відпила. — Не відмовляйся від щастя.

Краут нахилився над столом і також прийняв кокаїн. Якусь хвилину чекав на ефект, але його не було, ніби замість наркотика він втягнув у себе дрібку борошна. Тоді він нервово ковтнув шампанського й схопився з місця, зриваючи з себе піджак, а потім сорочку. Ліза якусь мить спостерігала за ним, а потім відставила бокал.

— Зі мною будь, будь ласка, ніжнішим, ніж зі своїм одягом, — сказала мадам Шене. — Не люблю грубощів...

Вона ще гарцювала на ньому, відчуваючи, що от-от настане мить сатисфакції, коли двері прочинились і на порозі кімнати постали Фішер і ювелір Вайсманн.

— Хай вам чорт! Невже так важко дати мені закінчити? — сердито вигукнула Ліза, прикриваючи руками збуджені груди.

Їй самій нечасто вдавалося отримати насолоду від чоловіка, а сьогодні, здавалося, була саме та унікальна мить.

— Вибач, крихітко, — усміхнувся Фішер, зачиняючи за собою двері. — Наступного разу будемо делікатніші, обіцяю.

Мадам Шене зіскочила з коханця й подалася до ванної. Краут сперся на лікті й втупився невидючим поглядом кудись перед собою.

— Ти, здається, переборщила з кокаїном, — додав майор і з огидою накрив Фелікса покривалом. — Схожий тепер більше на своїх пацієнтів, ніж на лікаря. Втратив будь-який глузд.

— Хіба це важливо? — сказала жінка, виходячи з ванної. Її спокусливе тіло тепер прикривав шовковий халат. — Він розповів мені все, що потрібно.

— Тоді розповідай мені, — посерйознішав майор.

— В їхній лікарні є пацієнт-росіянин. Його називають Яшею, але не думаю, що це його справжнє ім'я.

— Звісно, що несправжнє, — пирснув сміхом Вайсманн, — Яків Бобровський став Яшею... Це ж треба...

— Продовжуй, — перебив того Фішер.

— Поза лікарнею ним опікується Орлов, — додала Шене. — Наскільки мені відомо, завтра граф повинен його звідти забрати.

— Отже, треба встигнути раніше, — промовив майор. — Викрасти цього Яшу під виглядом утечі, наприклад.

Ліза розвела руками, мовляв: «Це вже не мій клопіт».

— Скажіть, мадам, де особисті речі цього добродія? — запитав Вайсманн, кивнувши в бік асистента Краута, що досі безпомічно борсався під покривалом.

— На канапі, — відповіла вона.

Ювелір подякував і, ступивши два кроки, узяв до рук піджак Фелікса. Методично обшукав його й витягнув звідти згорток з купюрами.

— Лишіть гроші за номер, — кинула мадам Шене й знову зникла у ванній.

— Не турбуйтесь, моя пані, я при своєму глузді, — відповів чоловік і продовжив обшукувати одяг Краута.

— Ага, ось! Я мав рацію: він таки носив це все з собою, — тріумфально вигукнув він за хвилину, дістаючи з-під підкладки згорнутий папір.

— Що це? — запитав Фішер.

— Моє боргове зобов'язання, — відповів той, — я не збираюся йому платити. Досить того, що з моїх п'яти тисяч і так чимало потрачено.

З цими словами він зважив у руці пачку банкнот, мовби намагаючись зрозуміти, яка сума там залишилась.

— Лізо, якщо граф Орлов найближчим часом вирушить кудись у подорож, мусиш поїхати з ним, — сказав їй через двері Фішер. — Скажи, що хочеш влаштувати собі невеликі гастролі.

— Так, майоре, — відповіла мадам Шене.

Орлов і справді повідомив, що збирається до Ґаліції. Як і було наказано, його коханка Ліза Хільке поїхала з ним.

У двері гримерки хтось обережно постукав.

— Прошу, — з деяким роздратуванням у голосі гукнула вона.

Всередину зайшов молодий кельнер.

— Пробачте, пані Шене. З вами хоче зустрітися один чоловік, — сказав він німецькою з твердим і виразним слов'янським «р».

— Жодної зустрічі до останнього виступу, — нервово відповіла співачка.

— Він наполягає...

Кельнер поклав перед нею візитівку.

Прочитавши ім'я, мадам Шене важко зітхнула й загасила сигарету.

— Перекажіть — за десять хвилин.

Кельнер вийшов.

Співачка вирішила не перевдягатися, а лише накинути на себе плаща. Так її відверта концертна сукня не притягатиме зайвих поглядів, а перед новим виходом не доведеться знову вдягатися.

За осібним столиком біля виходу сидів граф Орлов. Мадам Шене наблизилася до нього й збиралася сісти навпроти, але він її стримав.

— Немає часу, солоденька, — сказав він, — треба їхати.

— Їхати? — вимовила вона. — Куди? В мене зараз вихід!

— Значить, перенесуть. А точніше, скасують.

Він підвівся.

— Ходімо.

— Але на мені ця сукня. Можу я хоча би перевдягнутися?

— Вона тобі дуже до лиця. Я бачив твій виступ. Поїхали.

Мадам Шене криво всміхнулась. Якщо він справді бачив її виступ, то, мабуть, несподівано відчув приплив чоловічої сили й тепер тягне до себе в готель, доки відчуває, що може.

— Гаразд, — відповіла вона з деякою втомою в голосі, — поїхали.

Не сказавши ні слова кельнеру, вони вийшли з «Мінотавра» й опинилися на нічній порожній Сербській. Лізу пронизав холод.

— Де машина? — запитала вона, тремтячи всім тілом.

Орлов махнув рукою в бік «Остіна», що стояв за кілька кроків, біля повороту на Руську. З авто вийшов водій і відчинив перед нею двері. Мадам Шене сіла позаду водія. За мить поруч вмостився Орлов. Водій, не питаючи, куди їхати, завів двигун, і машина, перетнувши нічну площу Ринок, вистрибнула через вулицю Кілінського* на Гетьманські Вали**, де, минувши Міський театр, невдовзі виїхала за межі міста.

Ліза тривожно визирнула у вікно автомобіля.

— Де це ми? — запитала вона.

— Я не львів'янин, тож гадки не маю, — холодно відповів Орлов, — знає наш водій. Він тутешній. Еге ж, полковнику?

Редль, що був за кермом, змовчав.

— Куди ми їдемо? — з тривогою в голосі запитала жінка.

— Замовкни, Лізо! — гримнув росіянин.

З пів години вони їхали мовчки. Холод пронизав Лізу до самих кісток, і вона вже не чула нічого, крім цокотіння власних зубів. Авто врешті зупинилося.

— Виходь, — наказав їй Орлов і сам виліз назовні.

Майже не контролюючи рухів і марно намагаючись закутатись у свій тоненький плащ, Шене підкорилася. Водій вийшов також.

Місце виявилося цілком безлюдним. Навколо не було жодного вогника. Звідкілясь із темряви долинав тільки плюскіт води й шурхіт очерету. Вологе нічне повітря забивало собою легені, наче мокре ганчір'я.

---

* Тепер — вулиця Памва Беринди.

** Тепер — проспект Свободи.

— Тепер говори, — сказав Орлов.

— Що... я маю... говорити? — тихо перепитала вона.

— А відколи ти працюєш на прусський Третій відділ?

— Не розумію... про що т-ти...

— Ти не розумієш? — закричав раптом граф. — Бісова ти наркоманко! Про те, що я відвідував пацієнта в психіатричній клініці в Бадені, знала тільки ти! Про те, що я мав його звідти забрати, знала тільки ти! І тут раптом він тікає просто в мене з-під носа!

— Це збіг... Клянуся, я тут ні до чого.

— І те, що пруссаки раптом опинилися тут, у Львові, це також збіг? — Орлов перестав кричати, задихаючись від злості. — Твій шеф з A III b недопрацював. Конфіденти пана полковника Редля сьогодні помітили його і Бобровського... Ти мене одурила. Одурила! — закричав Орлов і зімкнув руки на її шиї.

— Заспокойтеся, графе, — спробував зупинити його Редль. — Лишіть її.

Однак це не допомогло. Душитель його не чув.

— Припиніть, чорт забирай! — вигукнув він тоді й спробував звільнити бідолаху з його рук.

Втім, це було марно. Той вчепився в її делікатне горло сталевою хваткою. Коли його все ж вдалося відштовхнути, жінка нерухомо звалилася додолу. Редль нахилився до неї й спробував намацати пульс. За кілька хвилин підвівся й з ненавистю подивився на Орлова.

— Ти її вбив, сучий сину, — видихнув полковник.

Той не відповів, а тільки важко дихав. Врешті злодійкувато озирнувся довкола.

— Таке трапляється, — сказав він. — Врешті-решт вона була зрадницею.

Полковник потягнувся до револьвера. Йому хотілося пристрілити виродка, вгатити в нього цілий барабан, але замість цього він лише мовчки спостерігав, як той волочить тіло до річки й опускає його у воду.

Зрештою, Орлов повернувся до авто й сперся на капот.

— Здала нас пруссакам, — знову сказав він. — Подумайте лишень... Яша зник у мене з-під носа. І врешті прусська розвідка опиняється разом з нами тут. Адже ви самі говорили, що в цьому місті, ймовірно, сам Фішер.

— З мене досить, — коротко мовив Редль і відчинив дверцята авто.

— Куди це ви зібралися?

— Ось що, пане графе, — сказав полковник. — Я погодився відслідкувати маршрут вантажу, але не давав згоди брати участь у вбивстві. Я запропонував свої послуги приватному шпигунському бюро, але не персонально вам, не «охранці». Тож ідіть ви під три чорти!

— Хочете ви цього чи ні, але бюро, про яке ви згадали, належить насправді нам. Тобто ви, дорогий полковнику, весь час були російським агентом, — відповів Орлов.

— Ви на території Австрії, — з погрозою сказав той, — і в моїх силах заткнути вам пельку.

— А ви спробуйте. Вам доведеться мене заарештувати, а під арештом я матиму вдосталь часу, аби розповісти все вашим колегам-військовим. Їм буде цікаво послухати, як начальник галицького *Evidenzbüro* співпрацює з потенційним ворогом.

Редль знову потягнувся до зброї.

— Так, можете мене пристрелити, — іронічно сказав Орлов. — Це, звісно, вихід. От тільки замість одного трупа будете мати два.

Кілька хвилин вони мовчали, зі злобою дивлячись на темні силуети один одного.

— Поїхали, — сказав урешті граф, — завтра до Лемберга прибуде вантаж. Візьмете свою частку і про все забудете. І про неї також...

Він кивнув у бік мертвої Шене, тіло якої майже повністю занурилось у воду.

Вранці наступного дня у зовсім іншій частині міста комісар Вістович, відвідавши спочатку лікаря, що мусив оглянути й перев'язати йому рану на плечі, під'їхав кілька зупинок трамваєм до костелу Марії Маґдалини, а звідти пройшовся пішки до кам'яниці під номером 11 на вулиці Потоцького. Обійшов її тим самим провулком, де ледь не загинув напередодні, зчепившись з Брюкнером. Підійшов до непоказних дверей, які зазвичай у таких будинках використовували слуги, аби дістатися на кухню чи в погріб, проте в помешканні колишнього оберкомісара Кронфельда ці двері були головним входом.

Вістович постукав і терпляче дочекався, доки з іншого боку йому відчинять. Немолодий високий камердинер у потертій лівреї ввічливо запитав, що потрібно вранішньому гостеві.

— Хотів би побачити господаря, — відповів комісар.

— Голосніше! — крикнув слуга, повертаючись до нього правим вухом.

— Мені потрібен пан Кронфельд! — вигукнув гість, і перелякана облізла кішка, що досі спостерігала за ним настороженими очима, шугнула кудись у сусідні зарості глоду.

— Будьте ласкаві вашу картку, — попросив камердинер і простягнув до Вістовича відкриту долоню.

— Звісно... — комісар дістав візитівку й подав старому.

— Проходьте до вітальні. Я повідомлю пана Кронфельда про ваш прихід, — сказав він, пропускаючи гостя всередину.

За дверима виявилося двоє сходів. Одні вели вниз, очевидно, справді до пивниці, інші — нагору. Цими другими слуга запросив піднятися на другий поверх, де провів гостя до просторого приміщення, облаштованого на старомодний манер, а сам пішов кликати господаря. Ця вітальня нагадала Вістовичу помешкання Ельвіри Сафронської на Личаківській, щоправда, було воно не таким занедбаним. Темно-зелені шпалери, вкриті рослинним візерунком, щільно прилягали до стін. Скло в креденсі й на стільницях акуратних журнальних столиків було ретельно протерте. На одному з них містилася шахівниця з незакінченою партією. Вістович мимоволі наблизився й оцінив шахову ситуацію. Білі мали безперечну перевагу над чорними, в них було більше фігур і вигідніша ситуація на дошці. Втім, і становище чорних не видавалося безнадійним. За уважної гри ті могли б розраховувати на нічию.

— Цікавитеся шахами, пане Вістовичу? — почувся голос господаря.

Його худорлява постать з'явилася на порозі вітальні. Кронфельд був одягнений у темно-вишневу бонжурку, під якою виднілася біла сорочка без краватки. У руках мав запалену бріарову люльку. Все виглядало на те, що в таку ранню пору гостей він не чекав.

— Граю іноді, — відповів на його питання комісар. — А хто ваш суперник?

— Мій камердинер, — мовив Кронфельд, знаком запрошуючи гостя сісти. — Чоловік, що зустрів вас сьогодні.

— Ви, мабуть, грали за білих? — поцікавився Адам Вістович.

— Ні, за чорних, — усміхнувся господар. — Як бачите, Алоїз дуже добрий шахіст. Колись він був моїм помічником. Разом ми розв'язали багато складних задач. І не тільки шахових... А ще мій слуга має одну беззаперечну чесноту: він майже глухий, і в його присутності я можу розмірковувати над своїм ходом уголос.

Услід за сказаним колишній поліціянт від душі розсміявся.

— Як ваша рана? — запитав Кронфельд і приклався до люльки. Хмаринка запашного диму на якусь мить заховала від співрозмовника його обличчя.

— Усе гаразд. Як виявилося, нічого серйозного, — відповів Вістович.

— Вам пощастило, що мали на собі плаща й маринарку з грубої тканини, — зауважив Кронфельд, — мене колись також врятував мій одяг у схожій ситуації.

— Пощастило мені тому, що нагодилися ви, — сказав комісар, — власне, я прийшов, щоб подякувати.

— Пусте. Мені, знаєте, нудно на емеритурі, тому радий, що вдалося трохи розважитися... Ви знаєте нападника?

— Так, — відповів комісар, — ба більше, заочно горлоріза знає все місто. Його підозрюють у недавніх вбивствах поліціянтів.

Обличчя Кронфельда, рясно вкрите зморшками, раптом сіпнулось і на якусь мить застигло, ставши схожим на ритуальну маску.

— Так, я читав у газетах, — промовив оберкомісар. — Отже, це він? Тоді шкода, що я не проломив йому голову... Сучий син.

Вістович усе чекав, коли Кронфельд запитає, що він сам робив учора під його будинком, проте господар не квапився.

— Хочу передати вам вітання від доктора Фельнера, — мовив комісар, підходячи трохи ближче до справи.

— А-а-а, від Ебергарда? — зрадів Кронфельд. — Дякую! Передавайте навзаєм, хоч ми бачимося час від часу в одній ресторації тут поблизу. Любимо з ним однаковий сорт чилійського вина. В усьому Лемберзі його можна знайти тільки там.

— Пан Фельнер порадив мені звернутися до вас в одній справі, — продовжив Вістович.

— Справді? О, ласкавий Боже! Небеса послали мені вас, щоб я не вмер з нудьги, комісаре, — зрадів господар, — що ж, розповідайте.

— Власне, це я хотів би почути від вас розповідь, — промовив комісар, також закурюючи. — Мене цікавить убивство такого собі майора Казимира Сафронського, що сталося 1876 року. Чи пригадуєте цей випадок?

— Дайте подумати... Гм, тридцять років тому — це вам не вчора... — сказав Кронфельд і подивився кудись у кут своєї вітальні, мовби там були записані його спогади. — А як його вбили? Цього майора? — уточнив він.

— Отруїли арсеном.

— Ах, так! — оберкомісар ляснув себе по коліні. — Згадав! У мене тоді не виникло сумнівів, що це зробила його дружина. Майор помер за сніданком, випивши чаю, в якому замість цукру була отрута.

— Доктор Фельнер стверджує, однак, що арсену в чашці не знайшли, — зауважив Вістович.

— На бога, пане Вістовичу. Тридцять років тому криміналісти робили більше помилок, ніж учні на уроках латини. Пробу з тіла загиблого також не взяли, бо тут, у Лемберзі, не було ані потрібного устаткування, ані фахівців.

— Отже, доказом вини пані Ельвіри була тільки отрута в цукерниці?

— А хіба цього мало? — здивувався Кронфельд. — Ви, приміром, тримаєте в себе на кухні арсен, пане комісаре? Скажімо, для того, щоб додавати його в свої страви для смаку?

— Ні, звісно.

— Ну от. Крім них двох того ранку вдома нікого не було. Напередодні ніхто не заходив. Тож шукати вбивцю деінде було б дивно, — підсумував оберкомісар.

— А що було відомо про їхні стосунки? Маю на увазі Ельвіри з покійним Сафронським?

— У тому й річ. Розповідали, що майор був деспотом. Це й стало її головним мотивом. В останні місяці свого життя він влаштовував їй справжнє домашнє пекло. Казали, страшенно її ревнував.

— Спадку вдова не отримала?

— Ані копійки. Після чоловіка лишилися тільки борги, про які вона не здогадувалася. Причому велетенські.

Вони трохи помовчали, зосередившись на курінні.

— А чому вас зацікавила ця справа? — запитав Кронфельд.

— Випадково натрапив на неї в архіві, — збрехав комісар.

— Он як... І що ж? Думаєте, майор сам наклав на себе руки? Через борги?

— А вам це не спадало на думку? — питанням на питання відповів комісар.

Співрозмовник стиснув зубами люльку так сильно, що його безкровні губи стали блідішими за крейду.

— Ви розумієте, що коли це правда, то я пущу собі кулю в лоба? — промовив він хриплим голосом.

— Ви не зробите цього, бо переконані у своїй правоті, — сказав Вістович. — І в мене, зрештою, немає жодних сумнівів у тому, що слідство було проведено як належить.

— А як щодо вашої справи? Я маю на увазі ці нахабні вбивства поліціянтів? — запитав Кронфельд після нової паузи.

— Це поки що не моє розслідування, — сказав комісар, — офіційно я ним не займаюся.

— Гаразд. Але що про це думаєте?

— Я вже казав, ми знаємо, хто вбивця. Лишилося його спіймати.

Вістович підвівся, щоб іти.

— У мої часи поліція не мала стільки технічних можливостей, як зараз. Ми не знали нічого про відбитки пальців, а ідеї Бертільйона* лише входили у практику, — несподівано сказав Кронфельд. — У роки моєї служби кожен злочин сприймався як виклик особисто детективу. Детектив приймав його і ставав до поєдинку, сподіваючись лише на свій інтелект і вправність. Мені гірко дивитися, як здрібніли

---

* Альфонс Бертільйон (1853–1914) — французький криміналіст, що впровадив метод ідентифікації злочинців за антропометричними особливостями.

сучасні слідчі. Серед них більше немає ані мисливців, ані азартних гравців... Прошу, не сприйміть це близько до серця, пане Вістовичу. Я не маю на увазі конкретно вас. Просто давно не читав у газетах, як вправно львівський детектив заманив маніяка в пастку. Виграв партію за білих, якщо говорити мовою нашої з вами улюбленої гри.

Він підвівся й простягнув гостеві руку на прощання.

— Справжні маніяки, зрештою, також перевелися, — пожартував господар наостанок. — Ви тільки гляньте на цього вашого нападника. Такий стариган, як я, прогнав його шматком металевої рури.

— На все добре, пане Кронфельде, — попрощався Вістович. — Слугу не кличте. Вихід я знайду.

— Ви забули? Він глухий мов тетеря. Я б його й не докликався, — почув комісар уже за спиною.

У Дирекцію він повернувся не в гуморі. Зверхність колишнього оберкомісара добряче його вколола. І найгіршим було те, що відповісти Кронфельду, як хотілося, Вістович не міг. Старий поліціянт врятував йому життя. Причому відважно кинувшись на вдвічі більшого за себе Брюкнера. Так, мовби й справді функціонарії тих часів звикли брати найнебезпечніших злочинців голіруч або застосовуючи те, що трапиться під руку. Без сумніву, якби замість металевої рури цей чоловік мав при собі виделку, то і цим інструментом зумів би дати раду.

Біля вахти чергового комісар зіткнувся з капітаном військово-поліційної служби. Високий жилавий офіцер із хвацько підкрученими вусами, побачивши його, зупинився і, за звичкою, осмикнув свій темно-зелений мундир. На його поясі дзенькнув металевий ринґраф, на якому було витиснуто особистий номер. Поруч з ринґрафом висіла поліційна шабля, а з іншої сторони – кобура з револьвером.

– А, пане Вістовичу, – промовив офіцер.

– Вітаю, капітане, – комісар торкнувся пальцями краю капелюха. – Маєте новини?

– Ви про того маніяка? На жаль, нічого втішного.

– Тоді заздрю вашому спокою, – сердито мовив Вістович.

– Ми поставили на вуха всі експозитури поліції в місті. І ретельно прочесали все довкола тієї кам'яниці на Потоцького.

– Не сумніваюся у вашій ретельності.

Комісар, сам не розуміючи причин свого грубіянства, вже збирався пройти повз, коли капітан єхидно зауважив:

– Я міг би сказати, що й вам слід вправніше стріляти...

Втім, слідчий пропустив це повз вуха.

– Якби ви вчора не промахнулися, то, можливо, сьогодні не сталося б ще одного вбивства, – додав капітан вже йому вслід.

Вістович відчув, як по його тілу пробігли крижані мурахи.

– Ще одне? – перепитав він, наче недочувши.

Офіцер кивнув.

– Капрала Фільца знайшли мертвим на Замарстинові. Усе те саме: удар ножем точно в горло і виколоті очі.

Сказавши це, капітан надів на голову поліційне чако і вийшов з Дирекції. Вістович піднявся сходами, але замість свого кабінету попрямував до кабінету Шехтеля. Постукав у двері й, дочекавшись запрошення, зайшов.

На директора було шкода дивитися: зім'ятий гарнітур, непрана сорочка, сяк-так зав'язана краватка, спухлі від безсоння очі й скуйовджена чуприна. Схоже, він ночував на службі.

— А, комісаре... Чув, що ви ледь не вбили цього виродка Брюкнера. Боже, ви були за крок від того, щоб позбавити нас цієї виразки в дупі, — промовив Шехтель замість привітання. — Вам треба краще стріляти, Вістовичу, їй-Богу.

— Хочу зазначити, що стріляв я з доволі незручного положення і до того ж був на той момент поранений, — сказав комісар.

Чути таке зауваження вдруге було вже занадто.

Шехтель махнув рукою.

— Гаразд, не зважайте. Не хотів вас образити. Сьогодні сталося ще одне вбивство. Ви знаєте? Схоже, цей психопат, зіткнувшись з вами, потім вимістив усю злість на першому-ліпшому поліціянтові, якого надибав...

Директор підвівся й підійшов до вікна.

— Ви вже завершили ту ідіотську справу з рукописом? — запитав він.

— Ще ні.

— Курва! Вістовичу, то завершуйте! — вибухнув Шехтель. — Завершуйте до бісової матері й беріться разом зі мною за цього маніяка! Інакше він нас усіх переріже, як телят на бійні.

— Власне, щоб завершити, мені потрібен від вас один документ.

— Який ще документ до ясної холери?

— Дозвіл на ексгумацію.

Шехтель оторопів.

— Що? Збираєтесь ритися в могилах?

— Аби поставити крапку у справі отруєння майора Сафронського, мені потрібно, щоб Фельнер виконав деякі хімічні дослідження.

— Не пригадую, щоб міністр просив вас наново розслідувати цю справу, комісаре. Вам наказано було просто знайти той сраний рукопис і його авторку!

Вістович змовчав.

— Ви мене чуєте, комісаре? Чи я розмовляю сам із собою, курва?! — директор перейшов на крик.

— Пане директоре, з відведеного терміну в мене залишився тільки один день. Тож не пізніше, ніж завтра я почну допомагати з цими вбивствами. Але сьогодні прошу допомогти мені, — якомога спокійніше сказав Вістович.

Якусь хвилину Шехтель дивився на нього своїми запаленими очима, а потім рвучко підійшов до столу й, зігнувшись над ним, виписав комісару необхідний документ.

— Дідько з вами, — гаркнув він, ставлячи підпис.

Потім знову відвернувся до вікна, не дивлячись більше на підлеглого.

Вийшовши з його кабінету, Вістович найперше зателефонував Фельнеру на Пекарську і повідомив, аби той готувався досліджувати кістки убитого Сафронського.

— Що ви маєте на увазі під «дослідженням», комісаре? — запитав той, перекрикаючи свисти й хрипіння в слухавці.

— Дізнайтеся, чи є в кістках арсен.

— Впевнений, що нема, — відповів Фельнер.

— Чому?

— Навряд чи доза отрути була такою великою, щоб осісти в кістках.

— І все ж спробуйте. Ексгумація відбудеться ще сьогодні.

— Я вас ненавиджу, Вістовичу, — зітхнув той. — Але гаразд... І, до речі, нехай ніхто з поліції не пхається на цвинтар. Ваші бовдури можуть навіть мертвому нашкодити. Все зробить Бюро судової медицини. Врешті-решт ця справа досі моя...

Вони попрощались, і комісар, втішений, що Фельнер позбавив його організаційної тяганини, хутко вийшов з Дирекції й подався до трамвайної зупинки. Як і кілька днів тому, йому знову потрібен був маршрут «Z». Вже на вулиці його наздогнав черговий, вручивши запечатаний конверт.

— Від кого? — запитав комісар.

Той стенув плечима.

— Просунули під двері, — сказав він і повернувся на свій пост.

Записку Вістович прочитав уже в трамваї, прямуючи до Підзамчого. Текст був лаконічний і без підпису: «*Сьогодні о 7-й вечора. Вугільний склад на Замарстинові. Отримаєш свого маніяка*».

Комісар одразу зрозумів, про який склад ідеться. Залізниця Карла Людвіґа*, до того, як її поглинув транспортний державний монополіст, зберігала там вугілля для своїх локомотивів. Місце давно пустувало, оскільки нова компанія перепланувала маршрути сполучень, і локомотиви тепер доцільніше було завантажувати вугіллям в інших місцях.

---

* Галицька залізниця імені Карла Людвіґа (нім. *Galizische Carl Ludwig-Bahn*) — приватна залізниця, збудована в період 1856–1861 років. 1891 року перейшла у власність Австрійської державної залізниці.

Важко було збагнути, хто міг написати йому цю записку. Вістович не займався цією справою. Отже, або автор помилився, або вирішив з ним зіграти в якусь дурнувату гру. Зрештою, поліція дуже часто отримувала схожі анонімні листи. Декотрі були абсурдними й мали на меті розіграти слідчих, але частина з них іноді виявлялася корисною. Тому ігнорувати їх заборонялося.

Діставшись Підзамчого, комісар швидким кроком дійшов до помешкання Самковського. Це була невелика квартира в офіцині з кривими потрісканими стінами і ненадійними дверима. Ад'юнкт, утім, дорожив нею, бо оплату господиня брала більш ніж помірну. Постоялець відчинив комісару, поставши перед ним заспаний і неголений.

— Хто стежить замість вас за тим місцем, що я просив? — найперше запитав Вістович.

— Мій брат Ігнацій, — відповів той хриплим від сну голосом.

— Хіба він не в Дрогобичі?

— Приїхав мене відвідати, — пояснив Самковський, пропускаючи шефа всередину. — Мріє колись піти в поліцію, то що ж... Нехай звикає.

Житло ад'юнкта всередині було таким же понурим, як і ззовні. Брудна підлога, ненадійні старезні меблі й вицвілі стіни.

— Ніколи не думали переїхати? — поцікавився комісар, обережно сідаючи на скрипучий табурет.

— Якщо підвищать, то подумаю, — відповів Самковський, вмиваючись над старою мидницею.

— Прийшов лист із Дирекції, — витираючи обличчя рушником, додав ад'юнкт. — Повідомляється, що мене відновили на службі...

Голос його трохи здригнувся, і Вістович зрозумів, що так прозвучала вдячність.

— Підвищення якраз не обіцяють, — зазначив він, — але ви знаєте Шехтеля. Поверещить трохи й охолоне.

Самковський кивнув, надягнув окуляри й витягнув з шухляди списаний згори донизу аркуш паперу.

— Ось усе за дві доби, шефе, — сказав він. — Крім того, я дізнався у сторожа, які вантажі прибудуть сьогодні вночі на вантажний склад: о восьмій вечора зерно, о пів до одинадцятої — деревина з Ворохти і близько дванадцятої — бориславська сіль.

— Цікаво, що з цього потрібно Редлю? — вихопилось у Вістовича.

— Ви про полковника? — перепитав ад'юнкт. — Я помітив його кілька разів. Гляньте в список...

— Так, бачу. «Обійшов склад уздовж колії. Перевірив усі ворота... Озирався. Поводився обережно».

— За три години до нього був ще кремезний пан і дві дами, — додав ад'юнкт, намазуючи обличчя піною й беручи до рук бритву.

— Фішер, Клавдія і Маґда... — промовив комісар. — Виглядає на те, що цей вантаж однаково потрібен і тим, і тим.

— Виходить, ви всіх знаєте? — Самковський кривлявся перед дзеркалом, намагаючись якнайкраще зголити щетину, й від того слова його звучали дещо спотворено.

— Мені знадобиться сьогодні ваша допомога, — замість відповіді промовив комісар.

— Звісно, шефе, — з готовністю відповів той.

— О сьомій мусимо бути з вами на вугільному складі Карла-Людвіґа. Візьміть револьвер.

— Це той закинутий гадючник?

Вістович кивнув.

— Побачимо, які там повзають гади.

Ввечері обидва прибули на місце вчасно. Вістович мав при собі дві яскраві нафтові лампи з чималими лінзами, що в десяток разів підсилювали світло й спрямовували пучок променів у одному напрямку. Одну лампу він передав Самковському, іншу вирішив залишити собі.

— Зброя при вас? — поцікавився він.

— Так, — відповів ад'юнкт.

— Чудово, можете вже знімати з запобіжника.

Сказавши це, він дістав сірники й запалив лампи. Самковський тим часом витягнув з кишені поліційного «Ґассера» й перевірив уміст барабана, хоч, без сумніву, вже не раз це зробив перед тим, як вийти з дому. У Вістовича лишався браунінг, здобутий у поїзді.

Сонце ще не сіло, й надворі було доволі світло, але порожня вуглярня моторошно чорніла перед ними напівпрочиненими воротами, ніби пащею. Виставивши перед собою лампи та зброю, чоловіки обережно зайшли всередину. Світло ковзнуло по вологій долівці і відсирілих балках, що, здавалося, з останніх сил тримали стару покрівлю.

— Є тут хтось? — голосно вимовив комісар, дослухаючись, як його голос зникає у глибокій чорноті.

Кілька хвилин поліціянти обмацували променями ліхтарів простір довкола себе, а тоді Самковський опустив револьвер.

— Здається, вас розіграли, комісаре, — промовив він.

— Схоже на те, — сердито сказав Вістович.

Вони вже збиралися йти до виходу, коли в темряві почувся якийсь приглушений стогін. Два промені знову почали нишпорити по вуглярні.

Врешті комісар висвітлив ліворуч від себе зв'язаного чоловіка, що лежав на землі обличчям униз. Рота йому було заткано. Поліціянти обережно рушили до нього. Тим часом у глибині приміщення почулося клацання важкого вмикача, і потужний електричний промінь висвітлив їх широким сліпучим конусом. Вістович і Самковський мусили зажмурити очі й навіть затулити їх рукою.

— Дякую за пунктуальність, панове, — звернувся до них голос із темряви, що видався комісару знайомим. — Понад усе не люблю спізнень.

Вістовичу врешті вдалося сяк-так дивитися перед собою. Він поставив на землю свій непотрібний ліхтар і обома руками тримав тепер зброю, цілячись кудись у джерело світла. Те саме зробив і Самковський. Втім, від думки, що вони тепер зручна мішень, обох кидало в піт.

— Опустіть зброю, — спокійно продовжив голос. — Ви ж бачите, що користі з неї жодної.

Вістович нарешті упізнав того, хто говорив.

— Грумм? — промовив він. — Карел Грумм?

— Саме так, пане комісаре. І, якщо чесно, то почуваюся трохи ображеним, що ви не впізнали мене одразу.

— Отой зв'язаний — це Брюкнер, — пошепки сказав Вістовичу Самковський.

— Ваша правда, добродію, — підтвердив Грумм, — можете не шепотіти. Як і обіцяв, дарую вам вашого маніяка.

— Ти прийшов сам, Грумме? — запитав у нього комісар.

— Ні, тут іще полковник Редль.

— Отже, двоє моїх убивць, що сплутали мене в поїзді з іншим, — хмикнув Вістович.

— Зізнаюсь, я навіть зрадів, коли побачив, що вистрілив не в того, — промовив Грумм уже зовсім зблизька. Вони з Редлем також зайшли у світловий конус і стали навпроти поліціянтів. — Такий би розум пропав, — додав він.

— Що тобі потрібно? — Вістович дивився в огидну пику співрозмовника і відчував незборимe бажання врізати по ній ще раз, як це зробив у Берні.

— Ти зіпсував мені всі плани, — промовив Грумм, — я не збирався повертатися до цього сраного Лемберга. Редль повідомив мені маршрут вантажу, і я просто мусив передати цю інформацію у Варшаву.

— Росіянам?

— Не має значення.

— То чому ж ти все-таки тут?

— Бо був переконаний, що ти розшифрував ту записку. І я маю рацію, правда ж?

Комісар не відповів. Він перевів погляд на зв'язаного Брюкнера, що, повернувши голову, спопеляв його поглядом, сповненим ненависті. Від цього погляду в нього занило поранене плече.

— Відколи ти тримаєш його тут? — запитав комісар у Грумма.

— Відучора. Ми схопили його майже відразу після нападу на тебе. Він, бач, прийшов до мене пересидіти якийсь час, доки поліція прочісує місто, — відповів той.

Вістович і Самковський перезирнулись. Ад'юнкт також пригадав, що останнього поліціянта, капрала Фільца, було вбито якраз у цей час. Тобто коли Берл цього зробити не міг.

— І ти так просто його нам віддаєш? — запитав комісар.

— Ні, пане Вістовичу. Не просто віддаємо, — відповів за нього Редль. — Є одна суттєва умова.

Простір між ними був наелектризований. Здавалось, от-от у повітрі з'являться іскри.

— Яка умова? — запитав Вістович.

— Ви, безперечно, знаєте про надважливий вантаж, який очікується на Підзамчому. Наші конкуренти, пруська розвідка, також ним зацікавлені. Більше того, володіють тією ж інформацією, що й ми, — промовив полковник, роблячи паузи між реченнями, мовби для того, щоб співрозмовник собі краще затямив сказане. — Думаю, це сталося тому, Вістовичу, що розшифроване повідомлення бачив хтось із їхніх агентів. Наприклад, та гарненька чорнявка, яка разом із мадам Шраґмюллер проживає в готелі «Ванда» на Баторія...

Нависла коротка пауза.

— Переходьте до суті, полковнику, — сказав комісар.

— Сьогодні близько півночі туди прибуде вагон із бориславською сіллю, — промовив Редль. — Самі розумієте, що всередині не сіль, а дещо інше.

— Власне, що саме, я не знаю, — заперечив Вістович.

— Для вас так буде краще, — промовив Редль. — Цей вагон зустрічатиму я і мої колеги. Також туди прибуде Фішер та інші агенти Третього відділу, ваше завдання — заарештувати прусаків.

— На якій підставі?

— Не смішіть, Вістовичу! Невже комісар поліції не знайде приводу? Тільки візьміть із собою з десяток поліціянтів. Так просто вони вам не здадуться.

— А собі забирайте Брюкнера, — додав Грумм. — Впевнений, відзавтра ви з вашим колегою будете на перших шпальтах газет. Уявляю заголовки: «Маніяка спіймано!», «Відважний комісар та його помічник схопили злочинця, винного в смерті чотирьох поліціянтів!»...

— То що? Згода? — перебив його полковник і спрямував на Вістовича пильний проникливий погляд.

Якийсь час комісар лише дивився у відповідь, але врешті кивнув.

— Згода.

— От і гаразд. До зустрічі за кілька годин.

Грумм і Редль відступили за межі світлового конуса.

Не без труднощів доправивши Брюкнера до в'язниці на Баторія, Самковський і Вістович рушили в Дирекцію, де в своєму кабінеті кілька хвилин мовчки віддихувалися.

— Чи слід подзвонити Шехтелю? — запитав нарешті ад'юнкт. — Впевнений, він зрадіє, що Брюкнер тепер у нас.

— Не має значення, у нас він чи ні, — з деяким розчаруванням у голосі промовив комісар. — Брюкнер — не той, на кого полює поліція.

— Так, але директору це принесе тимчасове полегшення.

— Усім від цього тимчасово буде легше... Втім, маніяка все одно доведеться упіймати. Причому нам з вами, Самковський. Але...

Комісар виразно глянув на шафу позаду ад'юнкта.

— Але це турбота завтрашнього дня, — продовжив він.

Самковський простежив його погляд, а тоді підійшов до своєї шафи й, витягнувши з кишені невеликого ключа, відімкнув її. Далі відгорнув кілька стопок паперу й дістав звідти невідкорковану пляшку «*Bernardine Imperial*» від Бачевського.

— Знав, що у вас є запаси! — Вістович плеснув у долоні.

— Я збирався випити її з вами на прощання перед остаточним звільненням, — сказав Самковський, — але радий пригостити вас на знак подяки.

— Сердешний хлопче, а міг би знайти собі гарну роботу з притомним шефом! — мовив комісар, дістаючи дві чарки.

Ад'юнкт наповнив кожну з них рівно на третину. Більше вони дозволити собі не могли.

— Якщо все буде гаразд, то вранці доп'ємо з кавою, — промовив комісар.

— А як ні, то колеги доп'ють за нас.

— Еге ж, ці сучі діти тільки зрадіють!

Комісар і його підлеглий засміялись і випили кожен свою порцію. Настінний годинник пробив десяту вечора.

За двадцять хвилин до півночі два поліційних фургони зупинилися біля станції Підзамче. З одного вийшло четверо поліціянтів, озброєних карабінами, з іншого — їхній капрал у супроводі Вістовича і Самковського. Звісно, зібрати «десяток поліціянтів», як просив Редль, було неможливо, проте на кожного з цих п'ятьох комісар міг покластися, як на самого себе.

Вістович дістав з кишені складений учетверо план станції. Розгорнув його й передав капралу.

— Отже, пане Муравський, — звернувся він до нього, — ваше завдання — контролювати склад з усіх сторін. Займіть зручні позиції на відстані не ближче, ніж сто метрів. Зближатись до будівлі почніть тоді, коли під'їде локомотив із вантажним вагоном. Далі стежте за ситуацією. Кого слід брати на приціл, я вам описав.

— Все, як домовилися, комісаре, — бадьоро відповів капрал.

— Дякую, що погодились, — додав Вістович.

— Пусте, — відмахнувся той, — наші нічні зміни зазвичай нудні й довгі. А так хоч трохи розважимось. І зігріємось, бо зимно.

— То до роботи, панове, — звернувся комісар вже до всіх, і поліціянти швидко покидали додолу цигарки та позатоптували їх підошвами. За мить вони розділилися і, познімавши з плечей зброю, зникли в темряві.

— Що ж, Самковський, а ми з вами ходімо просто в пащеку монстра, — сказав він підлеглому.

І чоловіки неквапно рушили в бік велетенських воріт, до яких у темряві тягнулася хвиляста колія.

Простір всередині був яскраво освітлений чотирма прожекторами, що стояли в кожному кутку. Посеред складу височіла громіздка постать Фішера й ще чотирьох чоловіків. Одного з них Вістович впізнав одразу — це був росіянин Бобровський, з яким вони познайомились у поїзді. Окремо від усіх трималися дві жінки: Клавдія Шраґмюллер і Маґда.

— Пане Вістовичу! — з удаваною радістю гукнув йому назустріч Фішер. — Вам не спиться цієї чудесної весняної ночі?

— Як можна спати, якщо по твоєму місті бозна-хто вештається, — відповів комісар.

— Бачите, мої пані й панове! Я ж казав, що львів'яни гостинні, — сказав майор, звертаючись до колег.

Ті дружно засміялися. Всі, окрім Маґди. Вістович намагався не зустрічатися з нею поглядом, але все ж не стримався й на секунду жадібно вдивився у її бліде обличчя, трохи відтінене капелюшком.

Звісно, Редль правий. Розшифрувавши йому ту записку, вона слово в слово переказала все Фішеру. Саме тому всі вони зараз тут і, безумовно, тримають у кишенях зброю, націлену на них із Самковським. Зрештою, передбачити саме такий поворот подій було неважко.

Ворота з протилежного боку несподівано прочинились, і всередину зайшли ще три постаті. Коли світло впало на них, комісар впізнав Редля і Грумма. Третього, що був одягнений найелеґантніше й тримав у зубах сигару, він бачив уперше. Хоч і здогадувався, що це той самий Орлов, про якого йшлося у листі. Пруссаки відступили вбік, аби не опинитися до прибулих спиною.

— Ну от, тепер усі зібралися, — іронічно сказав полковник. — Бачите, пане Орлов. А ви хвилювалися щодо цього.

— Орлов? — хмикнув Фішер. — То ви, полковнику, тепер на боці охранки?

— Пан Редль на боці справедливості, — різко відповів граф.

— Точніше, на боці того, хто більше платить, — відповів майор.

— Це з'ясує австрійський Генштаб. Я неодмінно їм відрапортую.

— Хто писатиме рапорти — ще невідомо, — зауважив Редль.

— Ваша правда, живими звідси вийдуть не всі, — погодився Фішер і, глянувши на поліціянтів, запитав:

— А на чиєму боці ви, пане комісаре?

— На боці міста. Згідно моїх посадових інструкцій.

— Лемберг належить Австрії, — зауважив Редль.

— Лемберг належить мені, полковнику. А я належу місту.

У ту ж мить колія, що перетинала склад, застугоніла, й із того самого боку, звідки прийшли Редль, Орлов і Грумм, почулося наближення локомотива. За кілька хвилин велетенський паротяг з написом «*Wiener Neustädter Lokomotivfabrik*», що означав виробника, заїхав досередини, втягнувши за собою один-єдиний вантажний вагон. З паротяга визирнув переляканий машиніст, але побачивши, як усі присутні, мов за сигналом, вихопили зброю, знову сховався в кабіні.

— Вантаж належить російському підданому, Якову Бобровському! — вигукнув Орлов, цілячись у Фішера з нагана. — А отже, належить Російській імперії.

— І яким чином ви збираєтесь вивезти його звідси? — поцікавився той.

— Ми не так далеко від кордону, майоре. Години за дві цей паротяг домчить до Бродів. А всі супровідні документи давно готові.

— Ви мрійник, пане граф, якщо думаєте, що локомотив виїде з цього складу, — промовив Фішер.

— Впевнений, що виїде.

— Це ж чому?

— Зараз побачите... Полковнику, — звернувся він до Редля, не відводячи погляду від супротивника, — дайте команду солдатам.

— *Abteilung! Zielen!*[*] — вигукнув той.

---

* Відділення! Цілься! (*нім.*)

У ту ж мить над бортами вагона з'явилися люфи десятка гвинтівок і голови піхотинців у польових кепі.

— Ну от, — вдоволено сказав Орлов. — І оскільки солдати тримають вас на прицілі, то стуліть пельку, Фішере, і здайтеся поліціянтам. А вантаж попрямує в Росію.

— Мушу дещо уточнити, пане графе, — раптом сказав Редль.

Орлов здивовано глянув на нього.

— Що саме? — запитав він.

— Солдати, якими я командую, цілять ся зовсім не у Фішера і не в його людей.

— А в кого, чорт забирай?

— У вас і в пана Грумма.

Орлов оторопів. Щоки його затряслися від злості, а над нижньою губою з'явилися зуби, мов у звіра.

— Ах ти австрійська собако, — прошипів він, — подвійний зраднику! Думаєш, так врятуєш свою шкуру? Всі дані про співпрацю з нами завтра ж будуть оприлюднені!

Наган в його руках раптом вистрілив, і Редль звалився на долівку. Услід за ним стріляти почав Грумм, цілячись у Фішера. Втім, той вчасно повалився на землю, й куля його не зачепила. Продовжуючи відстрілюватись, Орлов і Грумм кинулися до воріт. Кілька разів натиснула на спуст Клавдія, проте світло прожектора било їй просто в очі, тому жінка також не влучила. Що ж до піхотинців, то, не отримавши жодної команди, вони й далі продовжували нерухомо за всім спостерігати.

— Чорт забирай, Вістовичу! Затримайте цих падлюк! — лежачи на підлозі, заволав Фішер.

Втім, і комісар, і Самковський зберігали спокій.

— Не переймайтеся, майоре. Далеко вони не втечуть, — відповів йому Вістович.

І справді, зовні почулися звуки пострілів і гучні прокльони російською.

— Капрал Муравський вже про все подбав, — мовив ад'юнкт і рушив до воріт.

Якийсь час усі присутні схилилися над Редлем. Тому пощастило — рана виявилася легкою, хоч і болючою. Солдатам було наказано негайно доставити полковника до лікарні.

Коли вони вийшли, обережно несучи пораненого офіцера, в приміщенні запанувала тиша. У цій тиші з кабіни вибрався нарешті машиніст і поспіхом вибіг за ворота.

— Пане Вайсманне, — озвався врешті майор, звертаючись до нерухомої постаті в кутку, — чи могли б ви перевірити вантаж у вагоні?

— Звісно, — відповів ювелір і з дивовижною спритністю заліз нагору.

Кілька хвилин він шурхотів усередині, залишаючись невидимим для решти, а потім його розчервоніле обличчя знову з'явилося над бортом вагона.

— Все тут! — схвильовано вигукнув він, а потім підняв руку, в якій тримав чималий золотий злиток. — Багатство Бобровського тут!

— Не галасуйте, пане Вайсманне, — заспокоїв його майор. — Усе треба зробити спокійно і з холодною головою.

— Ваша правда, пане Фішере, — погодився ювелір, хоча тремтіння у голосі в нього не зникло. — Будьте ласкаві, подайте сюди мій саквояж.

Майор виконав прохання, і Вайсманн дістав з нього рахівницю й чималий бухгалтерський журнал.

— Зробити що? — запитав комісар.

— Бачте, Вістовичу, пан Яків Бобровський, власник скарбу, в обмін на свою безпеку, прусський паспорт і нове життя доручив нам розпорядитися його багатством на свій розсуд. Точніше так, аби воно послужило усім на благо.

— Це ж як?

— Зараз побачите...

Фішер роззирнувся. За кілька метрів від них стояли Клавдія і Маґда. Самковський ще не повернувся. Більше тут нікого не було.

— Яких ви зазнали витрат, пане комісаре? Маю на увазі, допомагаючи сьогодні Третьому відділу? — запитав майор.

— Четверо поліціянтів і капрал, що ними командував, ризикували життям, арештовуючи Орлова й Грумма. Вони заслуговують на компенсацію.

— Отже... — промовив угорі Вайсманн, пересуваючи кісточки рахівниці. — По п'ятсот крон поліціянтам і сімсот капралу. Слухаю далі.

— Мій помічник, ад'юнкт Самковський, також заслуговує на винагороду.

— Тисяча крон пану Самковському.

— Це все.

— А вам, комісаре? — запитав його Фішер.

— Коли-небудь у Берліні я потребуватиму допомоги, — сказав після паузи Вістович. — Отоді й нагадаю про борг. Від прусських грошей у мене поки що самі неприємності...

Майор хмикнув, але ствердно кивнув.

— Куди ви відправите решту цього скарбу? — поцікавився комісар.

— Третину повернемо Бобровському, — відповів Фішер. — А все інше піде в Росію, як і хотів Орлов.

— Ви жартуєте?

— Ні, комісаре. Хіба до жартів, коли у вагоні золота й коштовностей майже на сімдесят мільйонів марок? Орлов хотів, щоб гроші прибрав до рук петербурзький Генштаб. Ми ж вкладемо їх у російську революцію. Ось тут, — він вказав на вагон, — гонорари усіх їхніх гапонів та ульянових, що, як інженерна вибухівка, підривають Росію зсередини.

— Сімдесят мільйонів? — не повірив Вістович. — Це ж гігантська сума!

Фішер скривив посмішку.

— Саме стільки, пане Вістовичу, коштують кілька годин ведення війни. І завдання нашої розвідки — щоб Росія її програла. Ще до початку, до першого пострілу. Повірте, вся Європа зітхне з полегшенням...

VIII

Лемберг
20 квітня 1906 року

У ресторації Вільгельма Вебера на вулиці Ґродзицьких* зазвичай збиралися поціновувачі добрих райнських вин. Сюди їх кожні два місяці постачали прямісінько з Пфальцу разом із добірними сортами німецького сиру. Влітку ж, у спекотні дні, кожен охочий міг замовити собі глек прохолодного *Apfelwein***, доставленого з Гессена у велетенських дубових діжках, які, втім, порожніли менше ніж за тиждень.

Вістович зайшов досередини й вмостився за вільний столик біля вікна. Звідси виднівся ріг вулиці, що далі переходила у площу Стрілецьку***. З цією площею

---

* Тепер — вулиця Друкарська.

** *Apfelwein* (*нім.*) — яблучне вино.

*** Тепер — площа Данила Галицького.

у комісара були пов'язані чи не найгірші спогади за всю його поліційну кар'єру. Приблизно в цю саму весняну пору чотири роки тому там відбувся мітинг робітників, який очолили галицькі соціалісти. Звісна річ, на площу стягнули ледь не всю львівську поліцію, якій доручили стежити за порядком і, не вагаючись, арештовувати тих, що закликатимуть до радикальних дій. Крім того, неподалік, на Старому Ринку, стояла рота піхотинців ц. і к. полку «Барон фон Георґі»*, яка, за необхідності, мусила допомогти поліціянтам.

Втім, очільник мітингарів Семен Вітик**, сам заспокоював гарячі голови і вже за дві години наказав усім розійтися. Вістович зітхнув із полегшенням. Попри те що це була найбільша демонстрація галицьких робітників за останній рік, тут вперше не прозвучало жодного заклику до повалення буржуазно-поліційної влади, а присутні, хоча й дискутували голосно й гаряче, втім, робили це без жодного злостивого азарту й ненависті в очах. «Можливо, вплинула добра весняна погода, — подумалося комісару, — а може, ці ліваки й справді не такі кровожерливі, якими здавалися раніше».

Раптом зі сторони монастиря бенедиктинок почулися голосні вигуки. Потім розбилося скло — чи то віконне, чи то пляшкове. Вістович, що разом із Самковським та ще п'ятьма поліціянтами стояли неподалік,

---

* «Барон фон Георгі» — цісарський і королівський галицький піхотний полк. У час оповіді дислокувався в Галичині, частково під Львовом.

** Семен Вітик (1876–1937) — громадський і політичний діяч. Засновник Української соціал-демократичної партії Галичини. Пізніше — член КП(б)У.

на вулиці Костельній*, одразу кинулись туди. Як виявилося, хтось із гурту робітників, проходячи повз піхотинців на Старому Ринку, не зміг минути їх спокійно й зачепив тих образливим словом. Дійшло до штовханини, і солдати відтіснили їх назад на площу. Поліціянти наспіли якраз у той момент, коли мітингарі почали жбурляти в піхотинців каміння, а ті відповіли залпом гвинтівок. Бійки, стрілянина й арешти тривали до кінця дня. Під вечір нарахували п'ятьох убитих і кілька десятків поранених. Причому жоден солдат чи поліціянт не постраждав. На цьому факті особливо наголошували наступного дня усі ліві газети, а через місяць — адвокати жертв у суді. Вирок видався м'яким навіть поліціянтам, які, ясна річ, свідчили на користь військових. Капітана, що командував піхотинцями, відправили на неспокійні Балкани, а солдатів покарали двома тижнями гауптвахти.

Вістович відігнав від себе неприємні спогади й подивився на годинник. Майже четверта по полудню. Невдовзі сюди мали прийти Самковський і доктор Фельнер, що, власне, й призначив їм тут зустріч.

Наблизився кельнер і люб'язно запитав гостя, чого той бажає. Комісар замовив п'ятирічний *Spätburgunder***. Якщо він вже в ресторації Вебера, то варто пити вино, яке у Львові знайдеш тільки тут.

Йому раптом подумалося, що десь о цій порі з Головного двірця відправляється той самий експрес, яким він повернувся кілька днів тому зі Швейцарії. Навряд чи

---

* Тепер — вулиця Гонти.

** *Spätburgunder* (*нім.*) — сорт райнського червоного вина.

Фішер, Клавдія, Маґда, Вайсманн і той росіянин Бобровський вирішили затриматися в Лемберзі надовше. Найпевніше, всі вони зараз на пероні й чекають прибуття поїзда.

Вчора, коли закінчилася вся та чортівня на Підзамчому, він намагався упіймати погляд Маґди, але вона вперто вдавала, що бачить Вістовича ледь не вперше. Можливо, так краще було для неї та її кар'єри в A III b. Є, зрештою, щось солодко-авантюрне в тому, щоб бачитися з нею отак випадково й за жорстких обставин, а при сторонніх вдавати незнайомців. Чимось це нагадувало картярську гру, де щаслива карта лежить поруч із тією, через яку можна втратити все.

У ресторацію зайшов Самковський і роззирнувся, шукаючи Вістовича. Комісар махнув йому рукою.

— Повірити не можу, — видихнув ад'юнкт після привітання. Очі його світились від радощів.

— Що сталося, Самковський? — запитав його шеф, хоч насправді розумів, що сталося.

— Тисяча крон, — стишивши голос, сказав ад'юнкт. — Щойно отримав повідомлення з пошти...

«Добре, що Фішер дотримав слова», — подумав Вістович.

За кілька хвилин з'явився доктор. Кельнери зустріли його широкими усмішками, знаючи того, вочевидь, вже не перший рік. Замовивши на ходу, він приєднався до колег за столом.

— Ви бачили, яка знадвору прегарна весняна погода, комісаре? — запитав доктор, вказавши пальцем на вікно.

Вістович кивнув.

— Так, потепліло.

— Потепліло настільки, що навіть я охочіше попрацював би у своєму саду, копирсаючись у землі, ніж перебирав би кістки давно померлого майора.

Фельнер говорив удавано ображеними тоном. Усі, звичайно, розуміли, що навіть якби не було відкопаних на Янівському цвинтарі останків Казимира Сафронського, доктор все одно перебував би зараз на службі.

— Аналіз ви також провели? — комісар відчув, як всередині нього зароджується легке хвилювання.

— Так, Вістовичу. І жодного арсену в кістках я не знайшов. Хоча підкреслюю, навіть якщо Сафронського й отруїли, не обов'язково ця сполука мала б осісти в кістковій тканині, — промовив доктор. — Тобто, якщо бути відвертим, комісаре, ексгумацію ми провели дарма. Не знаю, як ви це поясните Шехтелю.

— Недарма, — відповів комісар.

— Як скажете, — Фельнер розвів руками. — Так чи інакше, бажаю вам успіху.

Невдовзі підійшов кельнер із вином для доктора і Самковського. Чоловіки піднесли келихи й мовчки випили.

— До речі, — продовжив Фельнер, — вітаю вас, мої панове, з тим, що той зарізяка Брюкнер тепер за ґратами.

— Тільки жаль, що він — не наш маніяк, — розчаровано зазначив Самковський, — інакше ми б зараз пили святкового шампана.

— Я вже казав директору, що знайшов між пальцями одного з убитих кілька ниток, — мовив доктор. — Отож, замість копирсатися в саду...

— Дідько, Фельнере! Та вже дайте спокій з тим садом, — перебив комісар.

— Ви заздрите, Вістовичу, бо живете в кам'яниці, де можете вирощувати хіба що плісняву на стінах, — не здавався доктор. — Так-от, мої панове, нитки ці походять з доволі дорогого гарнітура, пошитого рік-півтора тому. Колір темно-синій. Можливо, це вам допоможе.

Комісар кивнув.

— Дякую, докторе.

Далі він закурив і звернувся вже до всіх:

— Друзі, чи не проти ви замовити цілу пляшку тутешнього відмінного вина й перебратися на Пекарську?

Фельнер поперхнувся від несподіванки.

— Куди-куди? — перепитав він.

— До вас у мертвецьку.

— Хай вам чорт, комісаре! Я щойно звідти. Повірте, тут значно приємніше!

— Обіцяю, після цієї поїздки ми розвіємо будь-які сумніви щодо смерті майора Сафронського.

— Але ж які тут сумніви, комісаре? Арсен...

Втім, Вістович його не слухав. Він підійшов до кельнерів, попросив ще пляшку і, розрахувавшись, рушив до виходу. Фельнеру й Самковському не лишалося нічого іншого, як іти за ним.

— Що ви взяли? — запитав доктор вже у фіакрі, який прямував на Пекарську.

— Рислінг, — відповів комісар і простягнув йому куплене вино.

— Хоч якась приємність, — зітхнув Фельнер і пригледівся до етикетки.

Фіакр зупинився навпроти Бюро судової медицини, і Самковський раптом пригадав, коли був тут востаннє. Тоді вся ця моторошна сіра будівля була для нього наповнена відчуттям присутності чорнявої асистентки доктора. Тепер, знову ідучи тим самим довгим вологим коридором, він мимоволі втягував носом повітря, ніби намагаючись у підгнилому повітрі вловити запах її парфуму.

— Тут лише ми? — вирвалось у нього запитання.

Фельнер глянув на нього поверх окулярів.

— Є кілька трупів у сусідньому приміщенні, — відповів доктор.

— Як добре, що вони не п'ють. Усе нам залишиться, — додав комісар.

Чоловіки розлили вино у три склянки й кілька хвилин його смакували.

— А Зося? — знову запитав ад'юнкт.

Фельнер почервонів як рак.

— Відпустив її сьогодні раніше. Одразу, як дав раду тим кісткам, — пробурмотів доктор.

— До речі, про кістки, — сказав комісар, відставляючи склянку. — Перейдімо до справи.

— Як скажете, — з полегшенням у голосі мовив Фельнер. — Ходімо в лабораторію...

Останки лежали на металевому столі, викладені у природному порядку.

— Для аналізу нам би знадобився усього один фрагмент, але ви, комісаре, попросили чомусь добути увесь скелет, — зауважив доктор, вмикаючи електричне світло.

— Насправді, я сподівався не лише на пробу Марша. Зараз поясню... — сказав Вістович. — Самковський, ви прихопили те, що я просив?

— Так, шефе.

Ад'юнкт відкрив свого затертого портфеля й дістав звідти папку з позначкою «Рік 1876».

— Якимось дивом, докторе, у справі Сафронського немає жодних анатомічних приміток. Не вказано, наприклад, чи мав цей чоловік переломи. Не зазначено його зріст і вагу. Словом, немає всього, що дозволило б перевірити, чи перед нами саме скелет жертви, — промовив Вістович. — Маєте рацію, стільки матеріалу й справді не знадобилося.

— Послухайте, комісаре, я тоді був лише асистентом і зазвичай щодня мав десяток трупів, — обурився Фельнер, — крім того, тридцять років тому усі канони були іншими.

— Я зовсім вас не звинувачую, докторе, — примирливо сказав Вістович, — я лише констатую факт...

Він розгорнув папку й обережно витягнув звідти фотопластинку з портретом офіцера.

— На щастя, світлину, на якій ми добре бачимо обличчя майора, у справу все-таки додали. Зверніть увагу на його широкий лоб. Зазвичай це ознака глибокого інтелекту, — продовжив комісар. — Також виразною особливістю я б назвав відстань між очима. Вони в майора були широко посаджені... А тепер давайте порівняємо фото з черепом.

З цими словами Вістович поклав портрет на стіл. Самковський і Фельнер якийсь час мовчали. Ад'юнкт озвався першим:

— Лоб у померлого вузький. Відстань між очима... у пропорції значно менша, ніж на портреті.

— Вилиці також різної форми, — додав комісар. — Висновок один: перед нами зовсім не скелет майора Сафронського. Вам, пане Фельнере, підсунули стороннього мертвяка.

— А де ж майор? — промовив доктор. — Куди подівся справжній труп?

Його обличчям котився піт, мов у студента, що провалив іспит.

— Нікуди, докторе.

— Що ви цим хочете сказати?

— Що Сафронський, найпевніше, щасливо дожив до наших днів.

Слова комісара, сказані упівголоса, прогриміли, мов грім. Самковський і Фельнер зблідли так, ніби скелет на столі раптом почав рухатись.

— Тобто його смерть була інсценізацією? — перепитав ад'юнкт.

— Я в цьому переконаний.

— Але хто розіграв цю комедію?

— Він сам. Як розповів мені оберкомісар Кронфельд, той, що вів цю справу, в майора були велетенські борги. Тож лишалося або зникнути, або гнити у в'язниці. У випадку смерті боржника закон стає поблажливішим до його родичів, що переймають боргові зобов'язання. Цим Сафронський і скористався. Його вдова, схоже, продала всі коштовності й дорогі меблі, які мала, розрахувавшись таким чином з усіма кредитними спілками. Хоч, може, й не сповна, і борги цього живого мерця досі висять над нею, мов Дамоклів меч...

— Якщо майор і справді не помер, то де він зараз? — промовив доктор.

— А ось це і я хотів би знати, — сказав Вістович.

Була вже шоста, й чоловіки, не допивши свого вина, розійшлися. Вістович вирішив не брати фіакра. Хотілося пройтися майже безлюдною вулицею до середмістя, щоб думки краще повкладалися в голові. Його роздуми перервав гучний дзвін на вежі Бернардинського монастиря.

Вірних скликали на вечірню месу. Мовби здивувавшись тому, як швидко він опинився в цій частині міста, комісар роззирнувся й пришвидшив крок. Перетнув Валову й через Галицьку швидко вийшов на Ринок. За кілька хвилин комісар уже був у своєму помешканні на Вірменській.

Всередині він довго не затримався. Знайшов рукопис, який у поїзді йому читала Маґда, поклав його у портфель і, замкнувши двері, знову вийшов на вулицю. Спогади про цю жінку знову нестерпно обпекли, тому думка, що сьогодні він позбудеться нарешті цих паперів, по-своєму тішила.

На рецепції готелю «Метрополь» він попросив повідомити про свій візит постояльця на прізвище фон Шпрегорф, а сам вмостився за столиком у вестибюлі й попросив кельнера принести йому гербати, яблучного штруделя і чарку коньяку. Комісару здавалося, що міністр буде спускатися довго, зрештою, невідомо, чи він у цей час перебуває в номері, можливо, його ще шукатимуть, а тому часу, аби так-сяк перебити голод, у нього буде достатньо. Втім, як не прикро, але вже за десять хвилин Вістович почув за своїм лівим плечем його тріскучий голос:

— *Bon Appétit*, пане комісаре!

Поліціянт був змушений поспіхом прожувати кавалок штруделя й ковтнути його, ледь при цьому не вдавившись. Постоялець і гість потиснули руки. Тоді фон Шпрегорф знаком попросив кельнера принести йому такий же коньяк, що мав перед собою Вістович.

— Тут можна вільно говорити? — запитав комісар.

Міністр кивнув.

— За десять хвилин прийде піаніст, тож будьте певні, нас ніхто не підслухає. Рецепціоніст і кельнер тут порядні й не підслуховують. За три дні я в цьому переконався.

— Сьогодні останній день з відведеного мені терміну, тож я мушу відзвітуватись перед вами, — почав Вістович. — Новини у мене для вас переважно хороші.

— Зізнаюся, я вже думав, що у вас нічого не вийшло, — усміхнувшись, сказав міністр, — радий, що помилився.

Вони закурили й дочекалися, доки офіціант принесе фон Шпрегорфу замовлення.

— Почну з того, що єдиний примірник рукопису італійською в мене. І я готовий передати його вам, — сказав комісар і витягнув папери з портфеля.

— Жартуєте? — зрадів міністр. — Повірити не можу... А як щодо оригіналу?

— Оригінал в єдиному екземплярі зберігається в Цюриху. У мене є адреса.

— Чудово! — похвалив фон Шпрегорф. — Шкода тільки, що Цюрих так далеко... Ви бачились із Сапфо?

Комісар кивнув.

— І як вона?

— Не сказав би, що добре. Живе без особливої розкоші.

Фон Шпрегорф відвів погляд і спрямував його у свій коньяк. Тим часом у вестибюлі почулися звуки рояля. Піаніст і справді почав роботу рівно о сьомій.

— Третій день його слухаю, — сказав міністр. — Блискучий виконавець і до того ж з прекрасним репертуаром.

— Є ще одна річ, яку ви мусите знати, — продовжив Вістович, не підтримавши його теми. — Чоловік пані Сафронської, найпевніше, живий.

Фон Шрегорф вирячився так, що очі його, здавалось, от-от опиняться на лобі.

— Що ви таке кажете?

— У мене є докази, з якими я принагідно вас ознайомлю.

— Авжеж, чорт забирай!

— Майор інсценував свою смерть, щоб позбутися боргів, у які заліз по самі вуха. Обставини сприяли: ходили чутки про ваш роман із його дружиною. Отже, всі підозри впали одразу на Ельвіру. Мовляв, осліплена коханням, спровадила на той світ чоловіка... Сафронський таким чином помстився їй і позбувся кредиторів. Одним каменем поцілив двох птахів.

— І де він тепер?

— Цього я ще не знаю. Але в мене є підстави підозрювати, що помститися він хотів не лише їй, але й вам і всій поліції, яку ви представляєте. Доки ви, пане міністре, були у Відні, помста видавалася неможливою. Аж ось повідомляється про ваш візит до Лемберга.

— Хочете сказати, що недавні вбивства поліціянтів — це його рук справа і мені слід остерігатися? — перепитав фон Шпрегорф.

— Радше вам слід якнайшвидше покинути наше місто, — уточнив Вістович, — така моя порада. Бо надто дивно вже дії маніяка фактично збіглися в часі з вашим тут перебуванням.

— Я збирався виїхати вранці.

— Правильне рішення.

— Але тепер залишусь надовше. Якщо йому потрібен я, то міністр поліції не тікатиме.

Фон Шпрегорф підвівся. Вістович також.

— Шукайте його, — сказав міністр. — Якщо буде потрібна моя допомога, зв'яжіться зі мною через тутешню рецепцію.

Залишивши на столі гроші за випивку, він рушив до сходів і піднявся ними нагору. Тепер комісар міг спокійно доїсти свій штрудель. Щоправда, той смакував йому вже значно менше.

За чверть години Вістович неохоче поплентався додому. З одного боку, втома пробирала його до самих кісток й хотілося виспатись як слід, а з іншого — помешкання в цю пору було сирим і порожнім.

Саме тому вечірній візит Бейли став для нього спасінням від самотньої нудьги. Побачивши її на порозі з акуратним кошичком в руках, у який складають зазвичай наїдки для посиденьок на природі, комісар засяяв від щастя і, щойно повісивши її пальто й капелюшок на металевий вішак, заходився розпалювати дрова в п'єцу.

Жінка критично роззирнулася.

— У тебе знову безлад, — сказала вона з докором.

Після цього розпакувала кошик. На столі з'явились кармонадлі з гірчицею і салатою, свіжий хліб, сир і шматок вудженини.

Вістович промовисто ковтнув слину й приніс із кухні посуд. Переклав усе з пакунків на тарілки.

— Отже, я правильно здогадувалася. Ти не вечеряв, — засміялась гостя.

— З'їв штруделя, розмовляючи з міністром поліції.

— Маєш талант добирати товариство.

Обоє засміялися. Після вечері, не запалюючи світла, пили трав'яну гербату. Вістович подумав, що якби не Бейла, то він хляв би зараз який-небудь міцний аквавіт, заїдаючи першими-ліпшими недоїдками зі своїх запасів.

— Я знайшла школу для тієї дівчинки, Ляни, — сказала Бейла. — З осені може навчатися.

Вістович сердечно їй подякував.

— Я попросив постерункових, щоб навідувались у будинок, де вона мешкає, — додав комісар. — І раз на місяць виводили її горе-батька на задвірок, щоб нам'яти боки. Так, аби йому навіть на думку не спадало лупцювати когось у домі.

Бейла відвернулася.

— Не люблю я цю твою методу, Адаме, — промовила жінка, спостерігаючи, як на вулиці один за одним спалахували електричні ліхтарі.

— Іншої не існує, — відповів комісар, — як не існує навіть закону, що дозволить мені заарештувати цього типа й кинути за ґрати.

Вони трохи помовчали, і Вістович не зводив погляду з її тендітної темної постаті, що тримала в руках теплу чашку. Для нього Бейла зараз була уособленням спокою і затишку.

— Можеш курити, якщо хочеш, — озвалася вона.

Він підвівся і відчинив оберлюфт на вікні. Дістав цигарку й підпалив її запальничкою. З насолодою затягнувся димом. Цього йому справді не вистачало для цілковитої гармонії.

— А про що ти говорив із міністром? — почув він запитання Бейли.

— Колись він мав любовний зв'язок з однією тутешньою пані, заміжньою за офіцером, — трохи повагавшись, почав розповідь комісар. З одного боку, він виказував делікатні факти слідства, про які не знали навіть Самковський і Фельнер, а з іншого — Бейла була єдиною, кому він довіряв навіть більше, ніж собі. Невдовзі офіцер помер від отруєння. Підозра впала на його вдову. А міністр, замість підтримати її, втік до Відня. Його коханка відбула термін у в'язниці. Повернувшись, вона помстилася у доволі вишуканий спосіб. Написала еротичний роман під назвою «Розпусний міністр». Про їхній зв'язок.

— Ти говориш про Ельвіру Сапфо? — запитала Бейла.

— Звідки ти знаєш? — від подиву комісар подавився димом і мусив якусь мить відкашлятись.

— У мене є примірник її роману. Встигла купити, перш ніж поліція вилучила весь наклад із книгарень. Доволі непогано написано, мушу зізнатись... Але продовжуй! Це перше твоє розслідування, яке мені до вподоби.

— Сьогодні вранці з'ясував, що майор Сафронський, чоловік цієї Сапфо, насправді живий. Принаймні ніхто його не труїв.

— Який жах! — не стрималася Бейла. — Бідолашна Сапфо! Усі в'язничні жахи пережила абсолютно незаслужено...

— Аби ти ще більше її пошкодувала, додам, що на її плечі звалилися всі його борги... Втім, важливо не це. Убивства поліціянтів, про які ти, безумовно, знаєш з газет, стаються за кілька днів перед приїздом міністра. Так, ніби хтось вирішив покарати всю поліційну структуру: від низів до верхів, від постерункових і унтерофіцерів до...

— До міністра?

— Саме так. Тільки фон Шпрегорф поки що живий.

— І ти думаєш, що вбивця — цей майор, якого вважали мертвим?

— Поки що це головна моя версія.

Комісар загасив недопалок і закурив знову. З вулиці потягнуло холодом, але Вістович, хоча й був у самій сорочці, його не відчував. Бейла щільніше загорнулася в ковдру.

— А міг він повернутися до дружини? — раптом сказала вона.

— Хто? Сафронський? Навряд...

— Чому ж?

— По-перше, тому що Ельвіра не пустила б його навіть на поріг. Адже саме через нього вона втрапила до в'язниці.

— Гадаю, Сапфо звинувачує в цьому не його, а міністра, свого колишнього коханця. З чоловіком її зв'язує інше відчуття.

— Яке ж?

— Відчуття вини. Вона колись його зрадила і тепер, щоб спокутувати свій вчинок, дбає про нього, переховуючи від світу. Адже вона не лише дружина, але й католичка...

Комісар відійшов від вікна й почав міряти кроками темну кімнату.

— Хтозна, може, ти й маєш рацію, — сказав він за якийсь час. — Коли я прийшов у її помешкання, Ельвіра сказала, що відпустила служницю, але ж зрозуміло, що ніякої служниці в неї немає... Вона живе надзвичайно скромно й мусить сама займатися домашніми справами. А втім, біля столика стояло два крісла, а в кредексі кавник з двома філіжанками, мовби вранішню каву вона п'є з кимось, а не сама.

— Якщо хочете знати щось про жіночі таємниці, комісаре Вістовичу, то й запитувати слід жінку! Чоловік у нашому світі, як сліпець серед лісу, — підсумувала Бейла.

Тим часом Вістович увімкнув світильник і дістав з шухляди листок паперу й перову ручку «*Watermann*».

— Пробачиш мені, якщо я відволічуся на кілька хвилин? — запитав він Бейлу.

— Гаразд, але я в цей час роздягатимусь...

Він усміхнувся. Як сильно, виявляється, потребував її присутності й жартів.

— А що ти писатимеш? — запитала вона.

— Панегірик на честь одного видатного слідчого з минулої епохи. Сей достойний муж зветься оберкомісар Франц Кронфельд...

«Достойний муж» наступного дня ще до полудня увірвався в кабінет Вістовича й жбурнув листа йому на стіл.

— Що ви собі дозволяєте, комісаре? — вигукнув він.

Щоки його тремтіли від злості. Очі, вочевидь, палали, проте були сховані за темними окулярами. Одягнений Кронфельд був у довгий плащ і старомодний капелюх. На руках мав шкіряні рукавиці. Самковський схопився з-за свого столу й виструнчився. Вістович же тільки підняв очі.

— Доброго ранку, *Herr Oberkommissar*, — привітався він, — бачу ви отримали моє послання. Схоже, ц.к. Дирекції пошти працює відмінно.

— Що ви хотіли сказати, повідомляючи мені про воскресіння Лазаря, якого я, з ваших слів, замкнув особисто в склепі? — процідив той крізь зуби.

— Що одне з ваших найгучніших розслідувань не варте й мишачого лайна! — Вістович тепер і сам підвівся й сперся кулаками на стіл.

— У мої часи, комісаре, я мав би право викликати вас на поєдинок, — промовив Кронфельд, — пояснюйте, чорт забирай, що ви маєте на увазі.

— Майор Сафронський не помер від отруєння. Найпевніше, він досі живий. Через вас у в'язницю потрапила невинна жінка.

Запала мовчанка. Вістович не міг бачити погляду оберкомісара, але здогадувався, що в його очах, якби не темні окуляри, можна було б прочитати одночасно розгубленість і зранене самолюбство.

— Вимагаю доказів, — прохрипів він.

— Ми з Самковським збиралися якраз навідати пані Сафронську в її помешканні на Личаківській. Можете поїхати з нами, — запропонував комісар.

— Навіщо?

— Перевіримо, чи він не там. У мене є певні підозри щодо нього.

Не кажучи ні слова, Кронфельд вийшов з кабінету, проте коли комісар і ад'юнкт спустилися вниз, то побачили, що він їх чекав.

Дорога зайняла небагато часу, впродовж якого жоден не промовив ані слова.

Перш ніж постукати у знайомі двері, Вістович крадькома глянув на поліційного емерита. Той мав незворушний і навіть байдужий вигляд, мовби збирався зайти не в помешкання особи, якій зруйнував колись життя, а в крамницю з яким-небудь дріб'язком, необхідним для дому.

Чекати, доки пані Сафронська відчинить, довелося довго. Поліціянтам вже почало здаватися, що її немає вдома або ж всередині щось сталося, коли почулося клацання замка й брязкіт дверних защіпок. Господиня відчинила двері, залишивши між собою й нежданими гостями дверний ланцюг.

— Знову ви? — здивувалася пані Сафронська, побачивши перед собою обличчя Вістовича.

— Цього разу не сам, — відповів той, знімаючи капелюха. — Зі мною мій колега і...

— Але я все вам сказала.

— Хай вам грець, відчиняйте! — гримнув Кронфельд і, просунувши руку за двері, зірвав ланцюга з гачка.

Одразу після цього він безцеремонно зайшов до передпокою.

Вістовичу й Самковському не лишалося нічого іншого, як піти слідом. Пані Сафронська перелякано притиснулась до стіни.

— Ось ці добродії, пані Ельвіро, стверджують, що ваш чоловік, якого ви отруїли, живий. Це так? — запитав у неї оберкомісар.

Жінка не відповіла, а тільки схлипнула й притиснула долоні до обличчя.

— Це так?! — підвищив голос Кронфельд.

Вістович уже збирався втрутитись, коли голос за його спиною змусив завмерти всіх.

— Так, скурвий ти сину. Дай їй спокій.

Перш ніж комісар озирнувся, погляд його зачепився за стіл, де стояла відкоркована пляшка вина і два келихи.

У дверях вітальні з'явився згорблений чоловік, що спирався на палицю. Важко переставляючи ноги, він підійшов до крісла і, кривлячись від болю, сів.

— Сьогодні ми маємо свято, — промовив він, вказуючи поглядом на вино, — моя неймовірна Ельвіра сплатила кредиторам останню крону з моїх боргів...

Кронфельд іронічно глянув на Вістовича.

— Ви, здається, в чомусь підозрювали цього пана, якому ледве вдається самостійно ходити, — сказав він. — Думаю, якраз час його допитати.

Скрививши єхидну посмішку, оберкомісар подався до виходу. Тим часом, Ельвіра стримала Вістовича за рукав:

— Мій чоловік дуже хворий, пане комісаре, — сказала вона, — боюся, не витримає, якщо *ту* справу знову відновлять...

— Кого поховали тоді замість нього? — запитав Вістович.

— Якогось молодого волоцюгу. Той помер під нашими вікнами, от у Казимира й виник тоді такий план... Він у всьому розкаявся... Будь ласка, не тривожте минулого.

— Слідство завершено, — сухо відповів комісар. — На все добре, пані Сафронська.

Вийшовши з будинку, троє чоловіків якийсь час мовчки курили, уникаючи погляду один одного. Самковський спостерігав, як з Верхньої Личаківської вниз поволі їхав переповнений трамвай, своїм дзеленчанням розганяючи юрбу дітлахів і роззяв-перехожих, що плентались посеред вулиці. Вістович розглядав квітучу вишню, що визирала з чийогось саду, спираючись на кам'яний мур. Комісар врешті викинув недопалок і вже збирався йти у бік Митної, коли ж до нього озвався Кронфельд:

— Я трохи погарячкував. Не тримайте на мене зла, Вістовичу.

— У жодному разі, пане оберкомісаре. Знаючи, що з вами зробить власне сумління, можу лише поспівчувати, — відповів той.

Не попрощавшись, вони з Самковським залишили його самого посеред хідника й спішним кроком подалися до Дирекції, щоб встигнути на післяобідню нараду в кабінеті Шехтеля.

Директор мав бадьорий вигляд, усміхався й приязно запропонував підлеглим пригоститися кавою з чималого дзбанка посеред столу. Поруч стояло кілька гарних філіжанок і цукорниця з корецької порцеляни. Шехтель полюбляв вишуканий посуд. Порцелянова мануфактура у волинському містечку Корець вже понад 60 років як занепала. Тому директор з особливим завзяттям скуповував їхні вироби всюди, де тільки міг.

— Хочу привітати вас із успішним завершенням слідства, панове, — урочисто звернувся він до підлеглих. — Маніяка вже спіймано, і тепер можна зітхнути з полегшенням.

— Прикро ваш розчаровувати, *Herr Direktor*, але справжнього маніяка не спіймано, — заперечив комісар.

— Як? А Брюкнер? Той самий, що привселюдно обіцяв убивати поліціянтів. Чи не так, пане Самковський?

— Пане директоре... — спробував сказати щось ад'юнкт, втім, Шехтель його не слухав.

— Ви вдвох зв'язали його, мов кабана, і притягнули у в'язницю! — з гордістю промовив директор. — Я вами пишаюся, чорт забирай! А щодо тих двох російських конфідентів, я маю на увазі Орлова і Грумма, то ними заопікується *Evidenzbüro*. А саме — полковник Редль, щойно одужає. Сьогодні мав з ним коротку телефонічну розмову, і він повідомив, що за тиждень-півтора його випишуть зі шпиталю...

Двері кабінету без стуку раптово прочинились, і всередину зайшов міністр фон Шпрегорф. Тепер комісар збагнув, чому Шехтель виставив на стіл свою колекційну порцеляну. Усі присутні підвелися.

— Вітаю вас, панове, — сказав міністр, знаком показуючи, що можна сісти.

Поліціянти привітались у відповідь.

— Бажаєте кави, пане міністре? — запопадливо мовив директор.

— Ні, дякую, — відмовився той. — Перейдімо одразу до справи.

— Як скажете.

Шехтель вирівнявся у кріслі й прибрав поважного вигляду.

— Пане міністре, — почав він, — радий звітувати, що львівська поліція завершила слідство у справі жорстокого маніяка, що досі тримав у страху наше місто...

Фон Шпрегорф здивовано глянув на Вістовича.

— Це правда, пане комісаре? — запитав він.

Вістович завагався з відповіддю, але, зловивши на собі вогненний погляд Шехтеля, відповів ствердно.

— А як же той майор, що виявився живим? — допитувався міністр.

— За стільки років він перетворився на хворого й майже немічного чоловіка, — сказав комісар, — тому, як з'ясувалося, немає жодних підстав його підозрювати.

— Крім того, наші поліціянти затримали двох російських агентів... — директор ніяк не хотів переривати свою доповідь.

Втім, фон Шпрегорф підвівся, і йому довелося замовкнути. Решта також посхоплювались зі своїх місць.

— Якщо справу завершено, то я сьогодні ж повертаюся до Відня, — повідомив він. — Мене тут більше нічого не тримає.

Діставши з кишені візитівку, простягнув її Вістовичу.

— Знайдіть мене коли-небудь у столиці, комісаре. Мої слова про вдячність не були порожнім звуком.

— До побачення, панове! — попрощався він з усіма і вийшов за двері.

На Шехтеля після цього було гірко дивитись. Здавалося, директору хотілося одночасно розридатись і придушити Вістовича. Врешті, нервовим жестом той наказав підлеглим залишити кабінет. Ад'юнкт і комісар, так і не допивши кави з корецької порцеляни, вийшли.

У коридорі вони зупинились і поглянули один на одного.

— І що робимо далі? — трохи розгублено запитав Самковський.

— Маю охоту випити чогось міцного, — відповів комісар. — Складете компанію?

Ад'юнкт стенув плечима.

— Чому б ні...

— Тоді ходімо звідси, доки ніхто не спаскудив нам таких чудових планів.

Поліціянти вийшли на вулицю й небавом рушили вздовж Академічної на Баторія, а відтак, перетнувши Галицьку площу, а далі Валову, опинились на Сербській. Тут Вістович зупинився біля кнайпи «Мінотавр».

— Бували тут раніше, Самковський? — запитав комісар, коли вони зайшли всередину й вмостилися за вільним столиком.

— Уже й не пригадую, але про цю кнайпу згадував хтось із наших слідчих, — відповів той.

— Он як? Чому?

— У Полтві знайшли тіло співачки, котра в ніч смерті мала тут виступ. Свідки вказали на цього Орлова, якого ми арештували на Замарстинові разом із Груммом. Тож розслідування було коротким.

— Ми з вами щасливці, Самковський, — усміхнувся Вістович. — Вдалося відновити справедливість у справі тридцятирічної давнини, допомогти прусській розвідці відправити в Росію золото, за яке там зроблять переворот, замкнути двох російських шпигів, один з яких на додачу ще й убивця, але маніяк, що розгулює в нас під носом і хтозна, може, навіть випиває у цій knайпі, досі на волі.

Комісар важко зітхнув і додав слово, яке найкраще пасувало зараз його настрою:

— Курва...

Підійшов кельнер, і чоловіки замовили по гальбі пива й карафку горілки. Заїдати вирішили печеною гускою, квасною капустою, гуцульською бринзою і хлібом зі шкварками. Було зрозуміло, що ці двоє залишаться тут надовго.

Вістович і Самковський справді не поспішали. Наповнивши чарки оковитою, поліціянти одним духом їх спорожнили, приклалися до пива, а потім з апетитом вгризлися зубами в запашний хліб, на якому спочивали соковиті шкварки. Після цього кожен узяв по кавалку солоної бринзи, що розсипалася в роті на сотні дрібних шматочків, провокуючи рецептори на новий ковток чудової львівської горілки.

— Чому директор так швидко закрив справу? — запитав Самковський, відправляючи виделкою до писка жмут капусти.

— Бо сподівався, що міністр оцінить ефективність поліції під його шефством, — відповів комісар, вдруге наповнюючи їхні чарки.

— Здається, фон Шпрегорф мав його в дупі, — хмикнув Самковський.

— Точне зауваження, пане ад'юнкте, — похвалив Вістович.

— Дякую, шефе! *Antoni Samkowski, melduje się na rozkaz**, — жартівливо відповів його підлеглий.

— Наказую випити чарку. Негайно!

— *Tak jest!***

Шеф і підлеглий перехилили по другій, запивши оковиту пивом. Слідом за ним відправили до шлунків нову порцію хліба, шкварок, бринзи і капусти.

Після п'ятої чарки кельнер приніс їм розкішну печену птицю, яку в цілому Львові подавали тільки в «Мінотаврі». Обоє, мов за сигналом, відламали собі по гусячому стегенцю й, зачерпнувши ножем гірчицю, рівненько покрили нею золотисту шкірку, яка досі шипіла розпеченим тлущем, оскільки заледве п'ять хвилин тому страву дістали з печі. Чоловіки випили знову й вгризлися в м'ясо.

Непомітно наблизилася північ, але обоє й не думали завершувати свого бенкету.

— О дванадцятій кнайпа зачиняється, — промовив комісар, — але ще є клуб унизу. Таємний клуб, не для всіх.

— Знаю, шефе, — кивнув Самковський, — колись ми там заарештували одного збоченця.

— Скоро в Лемберзі не залишиться місць, де ми не арештовували збоченців і маніяків, Самковський, — підводячись, сказав Вістович.

Він підійшов до кельнера й промовив йому кілька слів. Той кивнув і провів їх сходами вниз. У той час як заклад нагорі зачинявся, унизу розваги лише починалися.

---

* Антоні Самковський, чекаю наказів (*пол.*).

** Так точно! (*пол.*).

М'яке червоне світло розливалося між столиками й виплескувалось на кам'яні стіни. Кельнерки в шкіряних комбінаціях походжали між клієнтами, приносячи їм випивку, солодощі, розкурюючи для них опіум і гашиш. За окрему плату вони робили це наголяса, а за достатньо грубі гроші віддавалися замовнику в поближніх ложах, зроблених у стіні й закритих від решти очей ширмами. Декотрі кельнерки мали при собі батоги, призначені для тих, кому подобалися втіхи, перемішані з болем. У ніші навпроти входу було облаштовано естраду, де серед хмари диму готувалися до виступу музиканти й співачка, одягнена в костюм Клеопатри.

— Ви тут часто буваєте, шефе? — запитав Самковський, що вже двічі був змушений протерти окуляри, запотілі чи то від його власних алкогольних випарів, чи то від хвилювання.

— Тільки якщо треба обмізкувати як слід яку-небудь справу, — відповів комісар.

— Отже, часто, — з усміхом підсумував ад'юнкт, і тієї ж миті спокуслива кельнерка спіймала його за краватку й підтягнула до себе. За кілька секунд молодий поліціянт був змушений протирати свої окуляри втретє.

Вістович невдовзі втратив його з виду й сів за столик, спершись спиною на стіну. Дістав з кишені портсигар і витягнув звідти останню цигарку. Закурив, дослухаючись до перших звуків музики. Невдовзі сталося те, чого він чекав: на його колінах вмостилася гарненька чорнявка й, поклавши руки йому на плечі, звабливо вигнулась.

— Роздягнутися? — прошепотіла вона йому на вухо.

Комісар кивнув. Тоді вона зісковзнула з його колін і граційно стягнула з себе шкіряну комбінацію. Вістович окинув поглядом її тіло. Жінка мала прегарне тіло: широкі стегна, плаский живіт і великі важкі груди. Він дістав гаманця, витягнув звідти кілька купюр і простягнув їй.

— Принести тобі чогось? — запитала кельнерка.

— Склянку бурбону й цигарки. І собі візьми чогось.

Вона зникла на якийсь час, а коли з'явилася, то погляд її палав, наче ватра серед темної ночі. Подала йому випивку і вклала до кишені пачку німецьких «*Eckstein*». Собі, схоже, вона взяла порцію морфіну.

— Як ми це зробимо? — запитала кельнерка, знову вмощуючись у нього на колінах.

Замість відповіді він вдихнув запах її шкіри й провів долонями по пругких грудях. Ніщо так його не надихало й ніщо не додавало стільки сил, як гарне жіноче тіло. Вона застогнала й потягнулася до нього поцілунком. В останню мить Вістович її стримав, заглибившись поглядом у її очі, в яких усе ще блискотів червоний морфіновий вогонь. Вони були мовби дзеркало, в якому комісар бачив своє відображення. Можливо, воно залишиться там навіть тоді, коли він звідси піде.

— Що сталося? — запитала кельнерка.

— Завдяки тобі я щойно розв'язав одну складну задачу, — сказав комісар.

— Ти математик? — засміялася вона.

— У певному сенсі, так.

Вістович провів ніжно руками по її гладенькій спині, мандруючи руками від плечей до стану й потім знову вгору.

— Тут є телефонічний апарат? — запитав він несподівано.

Кельнерка розчаровано всміхнулася, підвелася й вказала руками на сходи.

— Біля охоронця.

Клієнт випив бурбон, поцілував її наостанок і рушив сходами нагору.

Доктор Фельнер не відразу взяв слухавку. Комісарові довелося тричі набирати його номер, доки з іншого боку лінії долинув його сонний голос:

— *Am Apparat*...*

— Докторе, це Вістович, — промовив комісар. — Потрібна терміново ваша допомога.

— Курва, Вістовичу! Ви хоч знаєте, котра година? Що, в біса, сталося?..

— За скільки часу ви будете в себе на Пекарській? — перебив комісар.

— Я буду там завтра, сучий ви сину! Завтра! Точніше, вже сьогодні, але о восьмій ранку, а не о першій ночі!..

Вістович видихнув і спробував говорити спокійніше, побоюючись, що той кине слухавку.

— Фельнере, я ні слова не сказав про вашу помилку у справі Сафронського. Я вам допоміг, чи не так? — сказав він. — А зараз мені потрібна ваша поміч.

Доктор, схоже, також вирішив заспокоїтись.

— Що саме потрібно? — запитав він.

— Архів Бюро судової медицини. Його не передають на зберігання поліції. Він залишається на Пекарській. Мені треба перевірити матеріали, скажімо, з 1860 до 1876 року.

— За пів години буду, — відповів доктор і закінчив розмову.

---

* Слухаю... (*нім.*).

Вістович вийшов з «Мінотавра» і роззирнувся по темній Сербській. Жодного фіакра поруч не було, тож до Пекарської доведеться діставатися пішки. Що ж, за пів години він туди й дійде. Одночасно з Фельнером.

Втім, доктор був на місці значно раніше. Коли комісар, захеканий від швидкої ходи й надміру випитого за вечір підійшов до Бюро, то найперше побачив, що двомісний «Браун»* Фельнера вже стояв на хіднику поруч з огорожею, а в кабінеті доктора, вікно якого виходило на вулицю, горіло світло.

Фельнер зустрів комісара насупленим поглядом і сердито процідив щось, схоже на привітання. Обличчя мав спухле зі сну, волосся й борода були скуйовджені. З-під камізельки, втім, виднілася свіжа сорочка, приготована, вочевидь, на ранок. На газовому пальнику в його кабінеті закипала вода. Схоже, доктор мав намір зробити каву.

— Наш архів невеликий, тому папки за потрібний період я швидко знайшов, — промовив Фельнер стомленим голосом і вказав на стіл, де лежав потрібний матеріал. — Там нічого особливого. Штатний розпис, деякі протоколи. Я вже казав, що судова медицина того часу була вкрай недосконалою... Всьому, що вмію зараз, я навчився вже після студій в Академії. І фактично самотужки.

Доктор зняв з пальника киплячий алюмінієвий дзбан і налив з нього воду в дві металеві чашки. Потім всипав у кожну порцію кави й накрив їх старим медичним довідником, що мав тверду, підходящу для такої справи палітурку.

---

* *«Braun»* — австрійський автовиробник, названий за прізвищем засновника Авґуста Брауна. Фірму було створено у Відні 1899 року.

— Пригадуєте, докторе, ви говорили, що наш маніяк виколює жертвам очі, вважаючи, ніби в них може лишитися його відображення? — промовив комісар. — Начебто існує такий забобон серед убивць? Але, чорт забирай, Фельнере, невже в цьому немає бодай примарного наукового обґрунтування? Невже нікому й ніколи не спало на думку справді зазирнути в очі жертви з надією, що в них відобразився портрет убивці?.. Якщо це так, то маніяком керують не забобони, а яка-небудь наукова манія.

Доктор зморщив чоло і на хвилину задумався.

— Здається, існувала колись така теорія, — промовив він невдовзі. — Я був студентом, коли дізнався про її існування. Начебто людське око має в собі фоточутливий білок, на якому відбивається зображення. Відповідно, коли проявити сітківку ока жертви, як це роблять фотографи з фотопластиною, то ми побачимо те, що вона бачила востаннє, тобто обличчя убивці... Це називали... дайте згадати... оптографією, здається...

— Ця теорія себе виправдала? — запитав комісар.

— Ні. То було чистої води шарлатанство. У 80-х роках її спростували, але доти, в 70-х, вона сприймалася цілком поважно...

Не кажучи більше ні слова, Вістович розгорнув папку й узявся вивчати документи всередині. Минув квадранс, потім цілих пів години. Фельнер устиг приготувати нову каву і навіть обійти своє «Царство мертвих», перевіряючи, чи все готово для роботи вранці. О дев'ятій в одній з лабораторій була запланована лекція для студентів та молодших викладачів, що змушувало доктора нервуватися додатково.

Раптом нічним темним коридором почувся радісний вигук Вістовича. Поспіхом замкнувши двері лабораторії, доктор поспішив назад до свого кабінету. Комісар стояв над розгорнутими документами і сяяв від щастя.

— Чи знали ви, докторе, що недовгий час у цьому Бюро існувала посада штатного оптографа? — запитав він.

Фельнер оторопів.

— Ви жартуєте?

— Аніскільки! Ось штатний розпис за 1873 рік! Оптограф, себто той, хто займався «читанням по очах» убитих, отримував щомісячну платню і мав для роботи окрему лабораторію!

— І як... як його звали?..

Вістович не відповів.

— У вас є при собі зброя? — запитав він натомість.

— Так, револьвер.

— От і чудово. Берімо ваш «Браун» і поїхали.

— Куди? — з болем у голосі промовив доктор.

— Побачите, коли приїдемо.

Комісар хутко одягнув плаща, капелюх і рукавиці. Фельнеру залишалося зробити те саме.

Автомобіль доктора виїхав з Пекарської на Панську, перетнув Бернардинську площу, далі Галицьку й по Коперника почав уже повільніше видряпуватись нагору до костелу Марії Маґдалини. Звідки рушив на Потоцького, де Вістович попросив зупинити за кілька десятків кроків від кам'яниці під номером 11.

— Далі ходімо пішки, — коротко промовив комісар.

— Послухайте, Вістовичу, я не поліціянт... — сказав доктор, спостерігаючи, як той перевіряє вміст набоїв у своєму браунінгу.

— Можете залишитися в машині, якщо хочете, — сказав комісар.

Фельнер завагався.

— Чорт із вами, — видихнув він врешті й також ступив на бруківку. — Йду також.

Коли чоловіки підійшли до входу, комісар наполегливо постукав у двері. Глухий звук прокотився темним вогким провулком і відлунив від кам'яних тинькованих стін.

— Думаю, там нікого немає, — з надією в голосі проказав Фельнер.

Комісар постукав удруге, а потім і втретє. Всередині нарешті почулися чиїсь кроки. Двері несподівано відчинив сам господар. Ставши на порозі з ліхтарем у руках, він підняв його до рівня обличчя й промовив:

— Що ж, я вас чекав, панове. Проходьте.

Провівши їх у вітальню, він запалив світло й сів у крісло напроти каміна, в якому ще тліло вугілля.

— А де ваш слуга? — поцікавився комісар.

— Мабуть, у себе. Йому не завжди вдається почути прихід гостей, попри те що спить, притулившись до стіни... Я попрошу, щоб він приготував нам чаю. Адже розмова, як мені здається, буде довгою. Чи не так?

Кронфельд смикнув за оксамитову стрічку, що висіла поруч з каміном. Очевидно, та провадила до кімнати слуги й з'єднувалась із дзвінком.

— Хтозна, — відповів Вістович. — Можливо, все з'ясуємо швидко...

Він прочинив невеликий гардероб, де висіло кілька дорогих чоловічих костюмів. Діставши темно-синю маринарку, поклав її на спинку канапи.

— Надзвичайно гарна річ, пане Кронфельде, — тоном знавця сказав комісар. — І, мабуть, вам до лиця. А ще саме таку мав на собі убивця поліціянтів.

Господар не відповів, тільки вдруге знервовано смикнув за стрічку. Слуга невдовзі вийшов. Був одягнений поспіхом, але тримався рівно й уважно глянув на присутніх.

— Алоїзе, принеси гостям чаю, — наказав йому Кронфельд. — Потім допоможеш мені зібратися. Найпевніше, ці добродії попросять мене поїхати з ними.

— Не треба чаю, — раптом сказав комісар. — Вас заарештовано...

— Це я зрозумів, чорт забирай! — перебив господар. — Але я мушу зібратися.

— Не вас, Кронфельде.

Вістович повернувся обличчям до Алоїза.

— Вашого слугу.

Щойно він це проказав, як у його очах заіскрилося. Комісар відчув такий сильний удар у підборіддя, що не встояв на ногах і важко гепнувся на землю. Встиг помітити тільки цього бісового Алоїза, що якоїсь миті мелькнув перед ним з виставленими попереду себе кулаками. У наступну мить гримнув постріл. Трохи прийшовши до тями, Вістович з подивом збагнув, що стріляв Фельнер. До того ж постріл його виявився точний, як у заправського фельдфебеля. Тіло слуги з простріленою головою лежало на підлозі, закривавлюючи й безнадійно псуючи добрий буковинський килим.

Комісар підвівся й вдячно подивився на доктора. Руки в того тремтіли, мов у лихоманці. Врешті, він мусив сісти й розв'язати краватку. Кронфельд, здавалося, перетворився на статую. Обличчя мав сіро-кам'яне, погляд був спрямований кудись у темне вікно.

— Навіщо ви приховували його злочини, пане оберкомісаре? — запитав Вістович.

— Навряд чи ви зрозумієте, — відповів той могильним голосом.

— Так чи інакше, вам доведеться розповісти.

Кронфельд зморщив чоло, ніби від болю, якого йому завдавали спогади, а тоді почав:

— У 60-х я познайомився з Алоїзом, коли той ще навчався в Академії медицини. Він був товариським і веселим хлопцем. Обожнював спорт, особливо фехтування й сават*. Власне, рівних йому не було ані в дружніх поєдинках, ані у вуличних бійках, котрих у мої часи не бракувало щодня... Я навчався в кадетській школі**, проте після закінчення пішов служити не в армію, а в поліцію. Алоїз по закінченню студій спершу намагався розпочати приватну практику, а коли не вдалося, попросився в поліцію. Там роботи для лікаря було предостатньо. За кілька років на науковій конференції у Відні він уперше почув про оптографію і став гарячим прибічником цієї теорії. Вона видавалася направду прогресивною. Уявіть лише, наскільки б зросла ефективність криміналістики, якби портрет убивці можна було буквально розгледіти в очах жертви. Тодішній поліційний директор усіляко його підтримав і навіть створив спеціально для нього посаду штатного оптографа. Крім того, дозволив проводити наукові дослідження

---

* Сават — вид французького єдиноборства.

** *K. und k. Infanterie Kadettenschule in Lemberg* (*нім.*) — Імператорська і королівська школа кадетів у Львові. Тепер — Національна академія сухопутних військ імені гетьмана Петра Сагайдачного.

в цій галузі... По-моєму, саме тоді Алоїз і почав потроху божеволіти.

— Чому? — запитав комісар.

— Уявіть собі, що це були за дослідження. Сотні трупів людей, тварин і рептилій, з чиїх голів йому доводилося витягати очі й намагатися проявити фотографічним методом їхні сітківки. Звісна річ, експерименти були приречені на провал. Директор поплатився посадою. Алоїза затаврували як шарлатана й вигнали з Бюро... Мені, щоправда, вдалося забрати його до себе у відділ. Людей у кримінальній поліції завжди бракувало, тому керівництво закрило очі на його скандальне минуле. Алоїзові навіть присвоїли чин асистента поліції.

Одного разу ми з ним викрили підпільну лабораторію з виробництва пороху. Хтось із злочинців запалив сірника, й стався вибух. Тоді Алоїз накрив мене собою. Можливо, віддячив за те, що свого часу я не кинув його напризволяще.

Так чи інак, відтоді він майже оглух, але бездоганно навчився відчувати вібрації предметів, стін, підлоги й навіть землі. Це унікальна здатність, яка дозволила йому в подальшому пристосуватися до навколишнього світу.

— І вбивати, непомітно підкрадаючись до жертви, — додав Вістович.

— Новий поліційний директор невдовзі пригадав Алоїзові його ганьбу і, висміявши привселюдно на поліційних зборах, звільнив. За місяць я також подав рапорт на звільнення. На той час мені вже дістався у спадок цей будинок, а доходу від акцій вистачало, щоб утримувати його в належному стані й більш-менш достойно жити.

Тут мені й спало на думку врятувати свого друга знову й узяти до себе камердинером.

— Коли вам стало відомо, що ваш слуга мстить колишнім кривдникам? — після мовчанки запитав Вістович.

— На наступний день після того, як у газетах написали про перше вбивство, я помітив, що зник мій гарнітур. Потім я знайшов його вичищеним у своїй шафі, але на підкладці залишилася кров.

— Чому він узяв ваш одяг?

— Бо в нього давно не було нічого, крім лівреї. Одне з його дивацтв — він не купував собі одягу, хоч я вчасно платив зарплатню.

— Схоже, цей ваш друг до останнього вірив у свою псевдонаукову теорію, — озвався Фельнер. — Адже сам боявся залишитися в очах своїх жертв.

— Навряд чи ви знаєте, що таке одержимість, — відповів Кронфельд. — Вона спочатку живить розум, а потім сама стає розумом...

Епілог

Броди, кордон Австро-Угорщини та Росії
17 червня 1906 року

Ніч була прохолодною. Загін солдатів-прикордонників, загорнувшись у плащі, палив самокрути, додаючи до запаху вологої ночі сморід дешевого курива. За десяток кроків від нього мерехтіло два ліхтарі, які освічували будку вартового і темно-зелений шлагбаум поперек витоптаної ґрунтової дороги. Праворуч від нього чулося кумкання жаб у поближніх болотах, ліворуч — скреготіла залізом станція «Броди».

Від нудного чекання солдатам та їхньому унтерофіцеру потроху вривався терпець. Уже годину вони стовбичили тут невідомо для чого замість того, щоб відіспатися в касарні після важкого дня. Втім, наказано було чекати.

За квадранс на станцію прибув локомотив з кількома вагонами, й солдати пожвавішали. Найпевніше, доведеться його зараз перевірити, а після цього їм нарешті дозволять відбій. З гурту вийшов капрал і подався в бік станції за подальшими інструкціями. Повернувся звідти за десять хвилин понурий і роздратований — наказано чекати далі, а потім перейти під командування полковника, що прибув якраз із Лемберга.

Невдовзі з вагона й справді вийшов офіцер, за ним двоє чоловіків із руками, закладеними за спину, потім двоє конвоїрів і ще один кремезний тип у цивільному. Усі вони рушили в бік загону.

Солдати виструнчилися. Старший відмельдував полковнику про готовність до наказів.

— Як ми знатимемо, коли починати? — стишено запитав полковник у цивільного.

— Починати слід просто зараз, пане Редль, — відповів той. — Нашими полоненими з того боку цікавляться на найвищому рівні. Тож запізнень з їхнього боку не буде.

Він запалив сірника й підніс до годинника.

— Друга тридцять. Чудово... — сказав він.

— Ви робите помилку, Фішере, — озвався раптом один із бранців. — З мене вам було б більше користі тут.

— Хіба ви не хочете повернутися на батьківщину, пане Орлов? — з удаваною турботою в голосі проказав майор. — Збадьоріться. Ще трохи, й ви з паном Груммом будете під надійною опікою вашого царя-батюшки...

Граф з огидою сплюнув у темряву.

— Ну все, пора, — наказав Фішер. — Ведіть їх за шлагбаум, полковнику, і приймайте панство з того боку.

Редль дав короткі інструкції солдатам, і вони, оточивши ув'язнених, рушили до прикордонного переходу. За якусь мить з протилежного боку також з'явився військовий загін. Обмін минув швидко. Уже невдовзі Орлов і Грумм опинилися в руках росіян, а на австрійський бік зайшло двоє чоловіків і жінка. Руки їхні були вільні, а не в кайданках, як у тих, на кого їх обміняли.

Фішер підійшов до них, і якийсь час вони тихо розмовляли. Потім особисто провів їх до станції, де прибулими заопікувався начальник. Їх нагодували й видали куфери з речами. За кілька хвилин усі троє рушили до поїзда.

— Хто ці люди? — запитав Редль, коли вони з Фішером також опинилися у вагоні.

Почувся пронизливий свист локомотива, і потяг здригнувся, відтак потроху почав набирати ходу.

— Отой худий з темною бородою — отець Гапон, — сказав Фішер, — один з очільників народних протестів у Петербурзі.

— Я читав, що його вбили, — здивувався Редль.

— Справді? Як жаль...

Полковнику лишалося тільки вдати, що не зауважив іронію в голосі співрозмовника.

— А інші двоє? — запитав він. — Лисуватий чоловік і жінка?

— Подружжя Вебер. Принаймні так свідчать їхні нові німецькі паспорти.

— А насправді?

Фішер запалив нову цигарку й витримав паузу.

— А насправді, полковнику, вони коли-небудь знищать династію Романових. Недарма ж Яків Бобровський поклав на цю справу ледь не все своє багатство...

Щоправда, сьогодні усіх трьох, як ви бачили, довелося рятувати з лап охранки.

— І що ж тепер? Зміните їм зовнішність?

— Чому ж? Просто перечекаємо якийсь час. За кілька років про них забудуть, і вони знову зможуть повернутися в Росію, щоб завершити все те, що почали.

Поїзд мчав уже з величезною швидкістю, ритмічно вистукуючи сталевими колесами, мовби гігантський телеграф, що передавав кудись у темний простір термінове повідомлення.

— Невдовзі Лемберг, і вам треба виходити, — промовив Фішер, — а ми вирушимо далі, через Краків і Катовіце до Берліна.

— Довгий шлях, — відповів Редль.

— Хочу, аби ви знали, полковнику, я тільки зараз вирішив, що ви не поїдете зі мною.

— Мені нічого робити в Берліні, — криво посміхнувся той.

— Питання в тому, що б з вами там зробили, — незворушно сказав Фішер, — допити в Третьому відділі бувають часами неприємні.

Редль зірвався на ноги.

— Я австрійський офіцер і перебуваю на території Австрії.

— Сядьте, полковнику, — стомлено мовив його співрозмовник.

— Тоді поясніть, що ви маєте на увазі!

— Почнемо з того, що якби не той львівський комісар, золото Бобровського потрапило б у інші руки. Не в наші.

— Ви його переоцінюєте, пане Фішере.

— Навряд. Це радше ви його недооцінили.

— Якщо пам'ятаєте, то на тому складі в Лембергі я лише вдавав, що був за росіян, а в критичний момент став на ваш бік.

— Або ж ви просто побачили, що обставини складаються не на вашу користь... — розвів руками Фішер. — Але гаразд, це ми наразі забудемо.

— Хіба є щось іще?

— Хто такий Ніцетас, полковнику? Никон Ніцетас?

Питання зависло в повітрі, як відлуння пострілу, й змусило Редля зблінути. Не відповідаючи, він знову сів на своє місце.

— На його рахунок зроблено кілька щедрих поштових переказів, які згодом було перенаправлено в банк «*Hottinguer*» у Берні. На ваше ім'я... Можна навіть подумати, що Ніцетас — ваше шпигунське псевдо.

— Під цим псевдо я працював для одного приватного розвідувального бюро в Швейцарії, — відповів Редль таким голосом, ніби в горлі в нього застряг папір.

— І, звісно ж, не знали, що бюро контролює охранка?

— Не знав.

— Що ж, навіть офіцер може помилитися.

Полковник глянув на Фішера й зустрів з його боку погляд, в якому, здавалося, більше не було ворожості. Майор запалив третю цигарку, від чого їхнє купе щільно заповнилось синім тютюновим туманом, крізь який пробивалося світло електричної жарівки.

— Тільки не забувайте, що кожна помилка — це мовби незавершена історія. Ніби повість без епілогу, яку неодмінно треба дописати й цим виправити. Коли прийде час.

Усю подальшу дорогу вони мовчали.

За годину поїзд прибув на станцію «Лемберг».

Зміст

I 7

II 34

III 89

IV 122

V 167

VI 220

VII 272

VIII 307

Епілог 343

Літературно-художнє видання

Богдан Коломійчук

ЕКСПРЕС ДО ҐАЛІЦІЇ

Головна редакторка *Мар'яна Савка*

Відповідальна та літературна редакторка *Ольга Ренн*
Художній редактор *Іван Шкоропад*
Макетування *Таня Омельченко*
Коректорка *Ольга Горба*

Підписано до друку 10.06.2022. Формат 84×108/32
Гарнітури *Diaria Pro*. Друк офсетний.
Умовн. друк. арк. 15,12. Наклад 3000 прим. Зам. № 22-250.

видавництво СТАРОГО ЛЕВА

Свідоцтво про внесення до Державного
реєстру видавців ДК № 4708 від 09.04.2014 р.

Адреса для листування:
а/с 879, м. Львів, 79008

Книжки «Видавництва Старого Лева»
Ви можете замовити на сайті starylev.com.ua
0(800) 501 508 spilnota@starlev.com.ua

Партнер видавництва

!FEST холдинг емоцій

Віддруковано на ПрАТ «Білоцерківська книжкова фабрика»
Свідоцтво серія ДК № 5454 від 14.08.2017 р.
09117, м. Біла Церква, вул. Леся Курбаса, 4.
Тел./Факс (0456) 39-17-40
E-mail: bc-book@ukr.net; сайт: http://www.bc-book.com.ua